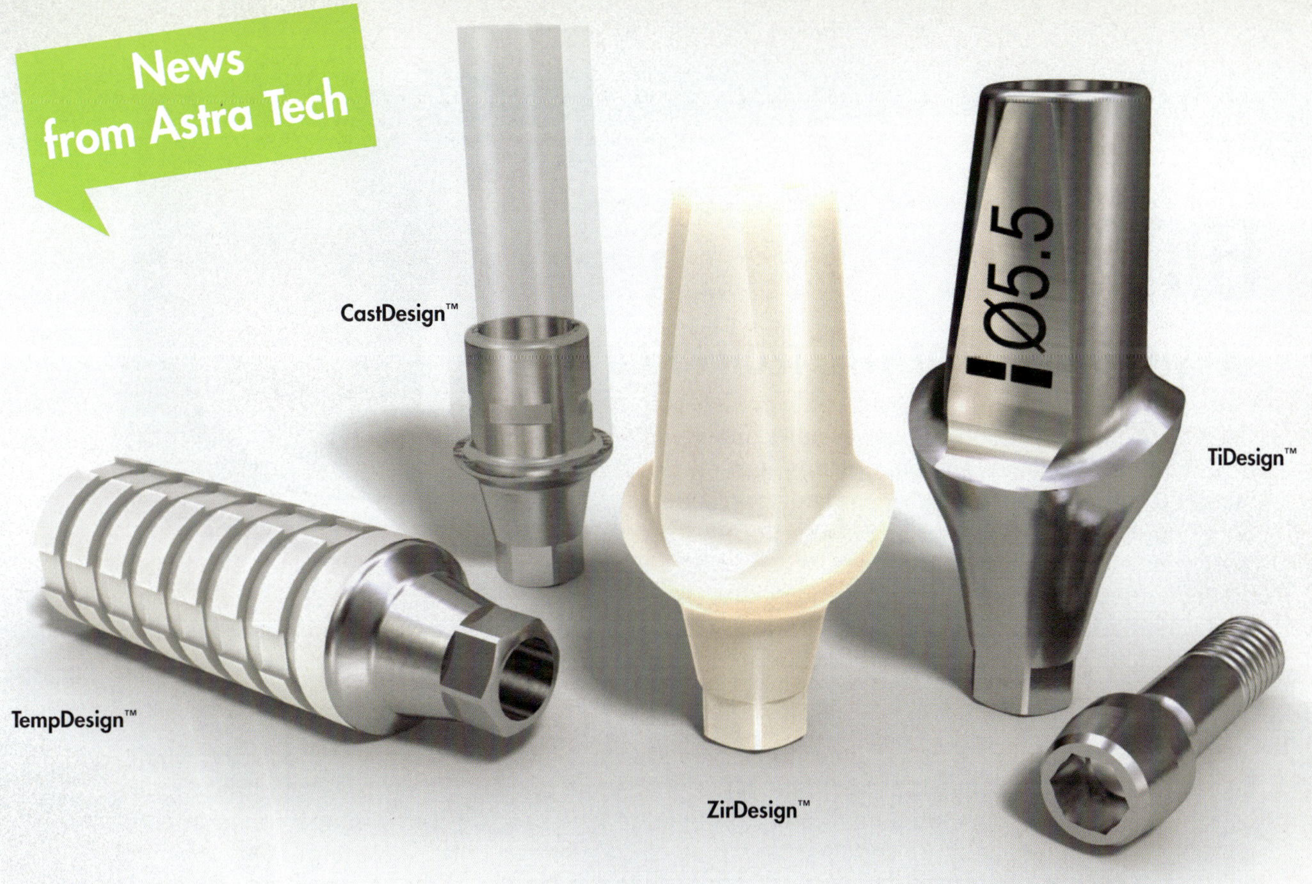

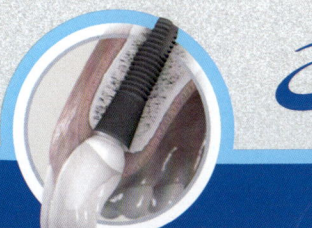
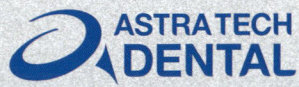
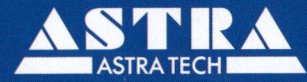
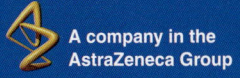

EDITORIAL

OFFSHORING AND DENTAL TECHNOLOGY

Offshoring, the relocation of business processes from one country to another, can involve any area of business—production, manufacturing, or service related. According to Wikipedia, "The economic logic is to reduce costs. If some people can use some of their skills more cheaply than others, those people have the comparative advantage. The idea is that countries should freely trade the items that cost the least for them to produce."

Having had the opportunity to collaborate with dental laboratories overseas on numerous occasions over the years, I can say that none of the cases so shared ever fell under this umbrella. Without exception, I paid a premium to collaborate with colleagues and send work overseas; cost reduction was not the objective.

Nonetheless, offshoring is a charged topic on almost any level. Even some of those who wholeheartedy support the concept of free trade argue that some primary beneficiaries of offshoring are countries whose government is manipulating the currency—keeping it at a subpar value in comparison to the origin country's currency, thus providing it with an unfair advantage. Others would argue that even if such practices exist, offshoring has not increased the unemployment rate, at least not in the case of the United States.

In the absence of solid data, the extent of offshoring in dental technology remains unknown; however, there is little doubt that it has become common practice in recent years. In some instances, an allegedly local business is no more than a receiving desk to a complete offshore operation. But my intention here is not to provide a personal opinion of this practice; rather, I would like to highlight some of the dilemmas surrounding the issue.

First, it is clear that the practice of offshoring is done to reduce cost. This being the case, is there any proof that the reduced cost associated with offshoring has ever reached the patient, or has it just benefited lab owners and/or practitioners? After all, even prior to offshoring, the cost of laboratory work in the US in terms of the overall charge to the patient was reasonable compared to Western Europe.

Second, organized dentistry in the US has been voicing a looming concern over the future availability of highly skilled dental technicians. Task forces addressing this issue have been in place, but it appears that in some instances the focus was mainly on providing proper and affordable training opportunities for prospective candidates. The bigger picture, in my opinion, is somewhat different. Dentistry has seen a constant increase in quality candidates. This is not only because of the deep desire young people have to maintain and restore the dentition of their fellow human beings; it is also the knowledge that a good, and well-deserved, compensation is part of the deal. Why would a young person who shows preliminary interest in dental technology apply to a school, good and affordable as it may be, if the financial prospect is uncertain?

Offshoring is not about right or wrong, but there is a clear dichotomy that dentists must recognize. Even with best intentions in mind, devoting time and energy to preservation of the dental technology profession is no more than an empty gesture if while doing so you are wrapping your next laboratory case to be shipped offshore.

Avishai Sadan, DMD
Editor-in-Chief
Avishai.Sadan@Case.edu

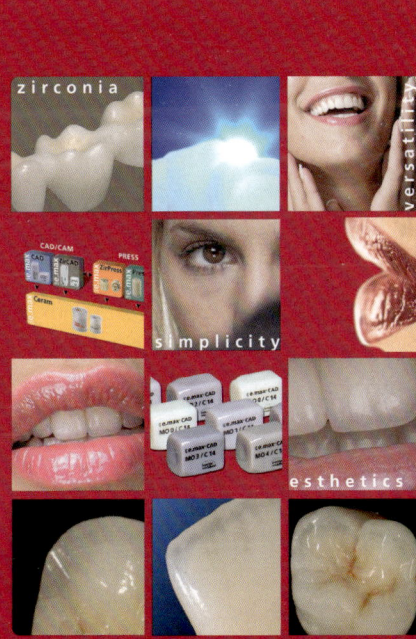
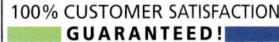
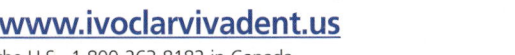
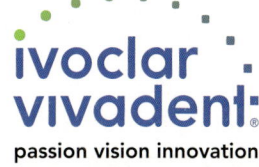

QDT 2008

QUINTESSENCE OF DENTAL TECHNOLOGY

EDITOR-IN-CHIEF

Avishai Sadan, DMD
Professor and Chairman
Department of Comprehensive Care
School of Dental Medicine
Case Western Reserve University

ASSOCIATE EDITORS

Thomas J. Salinas, DDS
Associate Professor
Department of Dental Specialties
Mayo Clinic

Markus B. Blatz, DMD, PhD
Professor and Chairman, Department
of Preventive and Restorative Sciences
School of Dental Medicine
University of Pennsylvania

SECTION EDITORS

Yoav Grossman, DMD, MPH
Ramat Gan, Israel

Paul Castellon, DDS
Department of Prosthodontics
LSU School of Dentistry

EDITORIAL REVIEW BOARD

Pinhas Adar, CDT, MDT
  Atlanta, Georgia
Naoki Aiba, CDT
  Monterey, CA
Mike Bellerino, CDT
  Metairie, Louisiana
Karen Bruggers, DDS, MS
  Cary, North Carolina
Gerard J. Chiche, DDS
  New Orleans, Louisiana
Sillas Duarte Jr, DDS, MS, PhD
  Cleveland, Ohio
Shiro Kamachi, DMD
  Boston, Massachusetts
Edward A. McLaren, DDS
  Los Angeles, California
Tom Peterson, MDT
  Lynn, Massachusetts
Servando Ramos, DDS
  US Army
Achim Renner, MDT
  West Palm Beach, Florida
Aki Yoshida, CDT
  Weston, Massachusetts

Cover photograph by Sillas Duarte.

PUBLISHER
H.W. Haase

ASSOCIATE PUBLISHER
Tomoko Tsuchiya

JOURNAL DIRECTOR
Lori A. Bateman

MANUSCRIPT EDITOR
Jake Wolff

PRODUCTION EDITOR
Patrick Penney

EDITORIAL ASSISTANT
Sally Curran

ADVERTISING SALES
William G. Hartman

**ADVERTISING/EDITORIAL/
SUBSCRIPTION OFFICE**
Quintessence Publishing Co, Inc
4350 Chandler Drive
Hanover Park, Illinois 60133
Phone: (630) 736-3600
Toll-free: (800) 621-0387
Fax: (630) 736-3633
E-mail: service@quintbook.com
Website: http://www.quintpub.com

QDT is published once a year by
Quintessence Publishing Co, Inc,
4350 Chandler Drive, Hanover Park,
Illinois, 60133. Price per copy: $80.

MANUSCRIPT SUBMISSION
QDT publishes original articles covering
dental laboratory techniques and methods.
See Guidelines for Authors at
www.quintpub.com for submission information.

Printed in Canada
ISSN 0896-6532 / ISBN 978-0-86715-486-3

IN MEMORIAM

LLOYD L. MILLER Jr, DMD
1930–2007

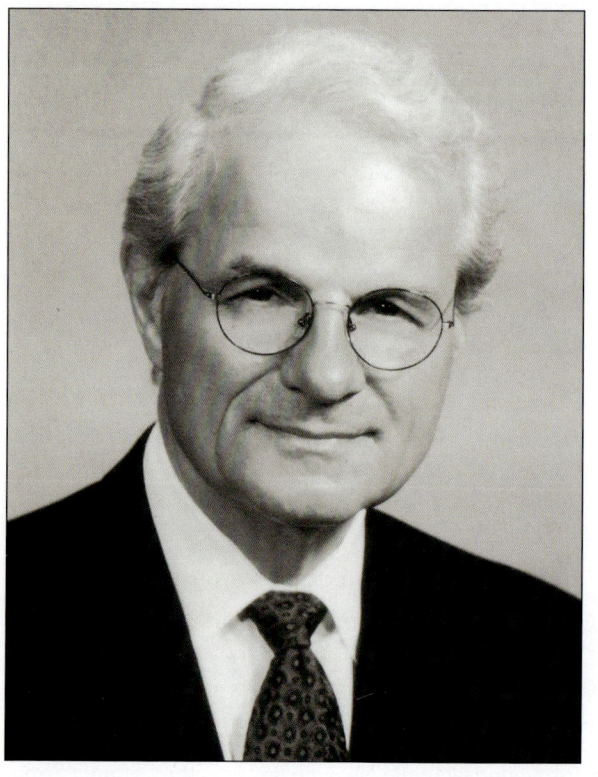

Lloyd Miller died peacefully at his home in Union, Maine, on November 11, 2007. He fought a courageous battle against an overwhelming cancer and received wonderful support from this wife, Ann, throughout his illness.

Lloyd was a man for all seasons. An outstanding clinician, dynamic lecturer, and perhaps more importantly, kind and generous to all his friends. He managed to combine an academic career with his natural talents in restorative dentistry. No mean achievement. He was a clinical professor of graduate and postgraduate prosthodontics at Tufts University School of Dental Medicine and maintained a private practice in restorative dentistry in Weston, Massachusetts.

Lloyd was particularly involved in dental technology and developed his own private laboratory and research facility that many dentists visited to see the outstanding work that was done. Lloyd's technicians had a high regard for him and he valued this trust more than the higher honors bestowed on him during his career.

His research, both clinical and scientific, was recognized at the 20th International Symposium on Ceramics in San Diego in 2002, where he was awarded the first Lifetime Achievement Award by Quintessence Publishing Company. He served as president of the American Academy of Crown and Bridge Prosthodontics, the Academy of Dental Science, and the American Academy of Esthetic Dentistry. In 1996 Tufts honored Lloyd by dedicating the new postgraduate prosthodontics clinic in his name. He was proud to receive distinguished lecturer awards from the Greater New York Academy of Prosthodontics and the American Academy of Prosthodontists. In 1999 he received the Distinguished Service Award from Tufts University and in September 2007 received the Deans Medal from Tufts University School of Dental Medicine in recognition of his outstanding leadership and dedication to the dental school and profession of dentistry.

Lloyd was one of America's great international ambassadors; he was known throughout the world and much in demand on the dental circuit. It was my privilege to meet him when Quintessence Publishing Company held its first International Symposium on Ceramics in New Orleans in 1983. His paper on tooth preparation and the design of metal substructures still remains a classic and is an example of his meticulous attention to detail and academic rigor. He expressed himself in a way for all to understand, a quality that made him a brilliant teacher of graduate and postgraduate studies.

Lloyd enjoyed collecting western art and skiing in the Rockies. On his farm in Union, he raised bees, heirloom apples, and nut trees. A big game hunter his whole life, he had a handsome trophy collection in his old dairy barn. The barn also houses his gallery of wildlife and American Western paintings, prints, sculptures, and saddlery.

Personal memories of Lloyd Miller enable me to pay tribute to the man; his Stetson and cowboy boots were a treat to see and one could distinguish him even in a crowded air terminal. He delighted my twin girls, Jennifer and Susan, who took to him instantly. And as was typical of Lloyd, he let Jennifer use his precious and almost vintage two-seater Mercedes to race around Union when we stayed at Cool Waters farm in Union. My own memories of the time I spent with Lloyd will remain with me forever. Dry martinis on his deck as the sun went down, listening to the wild turkey coming down from the woods to feed and the cries of coyotes looming for them. Then a visit to his wonderful wine cellar before dinner. Ann was a perfect host and a great cook. If I was to select one moment in time that I still cherish, it was to walk down from the farm through the meadow and sit on a rock by the St George River in total peace and quiet. Lloyd would often pick me up in his tractor, the autumn colors shone brightly and it was great to be alive. The hills truly seemed to be alive with music. Lloyd was an inspiration to us all.

John McLean

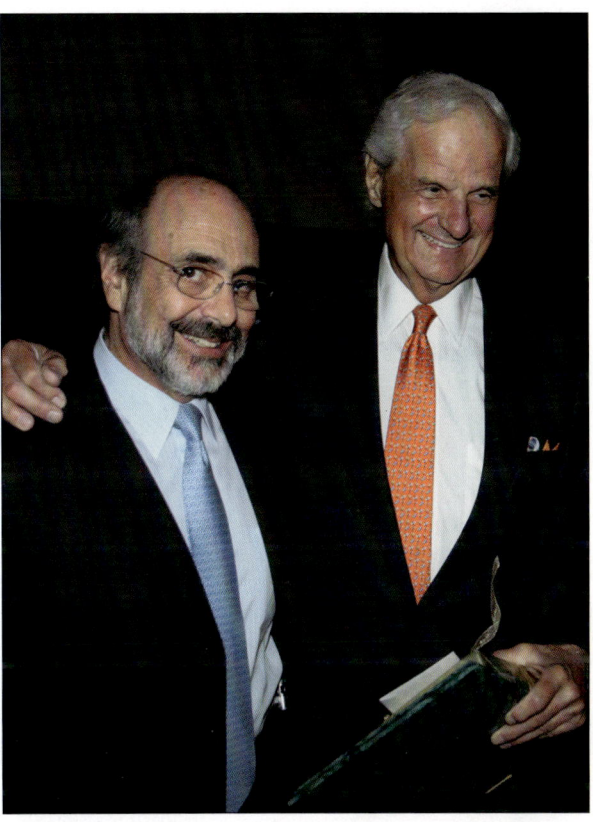

In 2007 Lloyd Miller received the Distinguished Clinician Award at the 9th International Symposium on Periodontics & Restorative Dentistry in Boston. Dr David Garber presented the award, which recognizes outstanding contributions to the advancement of dentistry.

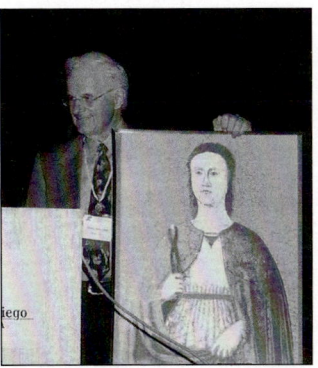

Lloyd Miller received the first Lifetime Achievement Award at the 20th ISC in 2002.

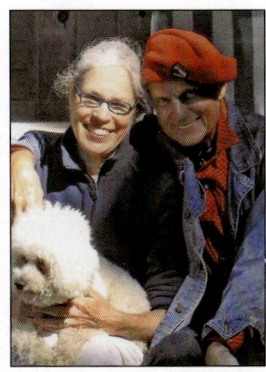

Lloyd and Ann Miller, October 2007.

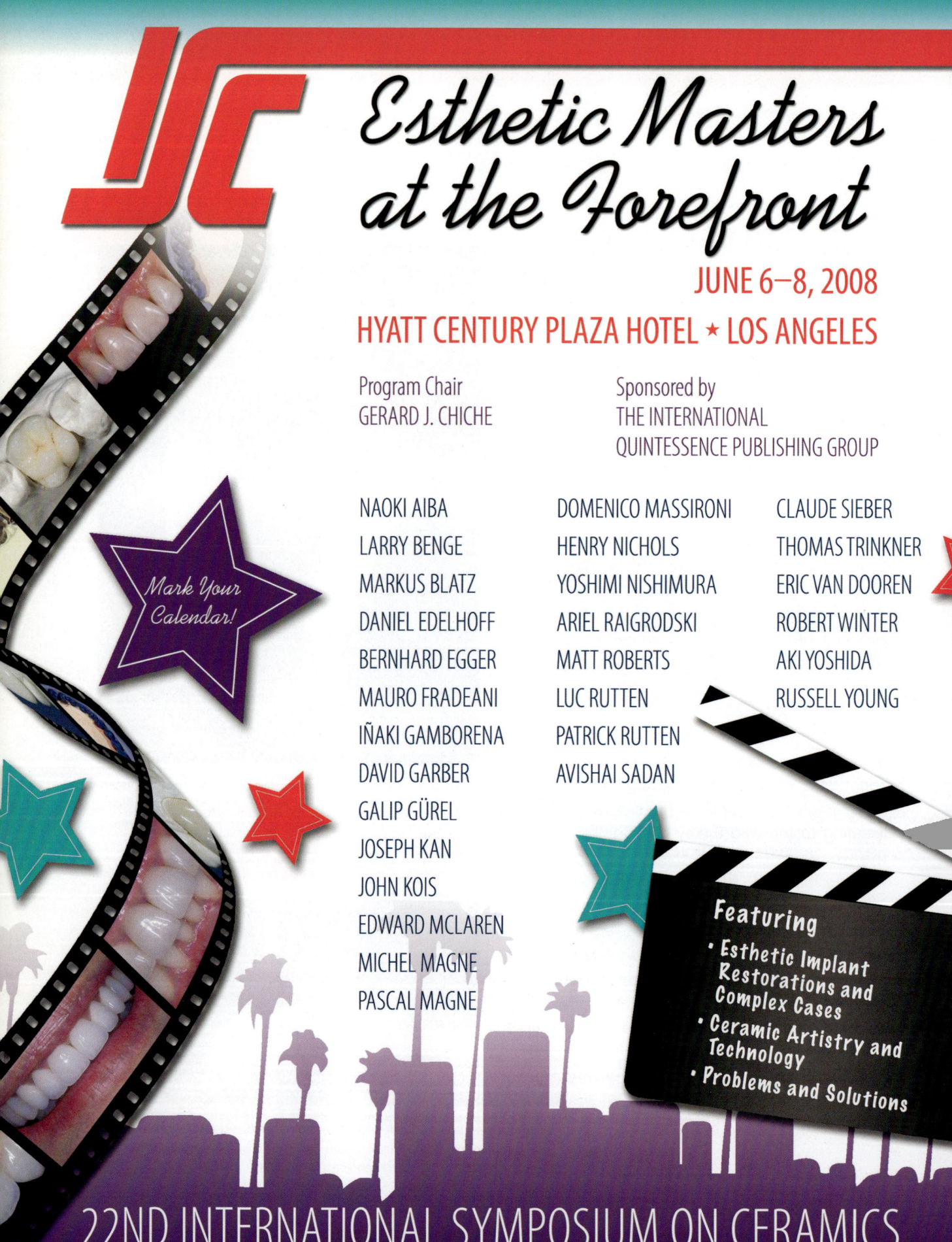

IMPLANT-SUPPORTED FIXED RESTORATION BASED ON ELECTROFORMING FOR THE ESTHETIC REHABILITATION OF EDENTULOUS PATIENTS

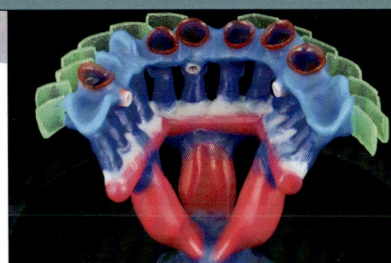

Juergen Mehrhof, MDT[1]
Katja Nelson, DDS[2]

Rehabilitating edentulous patients includes the restoration of soft and hard tissues. Inadequate bone volume can be restored using various augmentative procedures in combination with heterologous or autologous materials. In cases of severe atrophy, the use of iliac bone grafts may be the treatment of choice.[1] However, in spite of these surgical procedures, predictably restoring the ideal gingival contour in completely edentulous patients is still a challenge and will presumably remain so. Thus, implant-retained fixed prostheses must compensate for these insufficiencies by allowing the restoration of the white and red esthetics while satisfying other patient demands. Numerous implant restorative concepts have been documented based on either screw retention or cementation of the prosthesis. Screw-retained restorations are known to be predictably removable and are seen as the gold standard by many clinicians.[2,3]

The fabrication of a one-piece metal framework with a high degree of passive fit is a challenging task for the dental technician. To date, there are no

[1]Master Dental Technician, Berlin, Germany.

[2]Assistant Professor and Head, Department of Implantology and Special Prosthodontics, Clinic for Oral and Maxillofacial Surgery/Clinical Navigation and Robotics, Charité Campus Virchow Clinic, Berlin, Germany.

Correspondence to: Mr Juergen Mehrhof, Reuchlinstr. 10-11, 10553 Berlin, Germany. E-mail: zahntechnik.mehrhof@web.de

published data demonstrating a passive fit of screw-retained prostheses.[4] Cement-retained prostheses have been increasingly used, since they are thought to compensate for any inaccuracies leading to misfit and tension of the superstructure. Studies have shown that the retention mechanism does not influence the strain development of the implant-supported restoration, thus questioning the importance of passive fit on the long-term success of osseointegrated implants.[4] Whether strain development within an implant-supported restoration has any impact on the longevity of the prosthesis and implant components has not been clarified.

Cement-retained prostheses have become the restoration of choice for implant rehabilitation of edentulous patients due to their easier fabrication and enhanced esthetics.[3,5,6] However, one disadvantage is the potential inability to remove the cemented restoration in case of abutment screw loosening or if repair is needed. No validated data are available on the long-term retrievability of a multiunit structure with more than two metal components (abutments) using a luting agent.[7–10] If retention is achieved using provisional cement, there is a risk of premature loosening, whereas definitive cementation makes it difficult to remove the restoration when needed. Studies have demonstrated that composite-resin, zinc-phosphate, and glass-ionomer luting agents are suboptimal compared to provisional cement for retaining prostheses on titanium abutments.[9,10,11] Obviously, the choice of luting agent plays a decisive role in the retention of cement-retained prostheses.[9] In addition to the issues discussed above, residual cement retained within the sulcus can have a deleterious effect in cases of deep crown margins.[11]

Although retrieval of the structure is required less often today due to the increased longevity of implants and their components and improvements in the implant-abutment connection, this issue should not be disregarded. The advantages of each type of restoration should be considered and used in a modified superstructure; by using conventional prosthetic techniques, it is possible to combine the retrievability of screw-retained prostheses with the easy fabrication and high degree of passive fit of cement-retained prostheses in one predictably removable and esthetic restoration.[12]

Electroforming technology has been used to form substructures for porcelain inlays and crowns.[13,14] Composed of pure 24-karat gold deposited directly onto a duplicate die or abutment, electroformed copings are fairly thin (± 0.2 mm) with a marginal accuracy of 4.9 to 20 μm.[15,16] This technology has been used in implant dentistry for removable dentures retained by a cone-shaped telescopic crown or single tooth replacements.[15] The retention mechanism of conical double crowns based on electroformed copings can provide excellent retentive force over a long period of time.[16,17]

This article describes the clinical and technical procedures for a retrievable implant-supported fixed superstructure based on the electroforming technique that combines the advantages of cement- and screw-retained prostheses.[18,19] For a comprehensive esthetic and functional rehabilitation of the edentulous patient, several factors must be considered (Figs 1 and 2).

The superstructure consists of primary units—individually fabricated abutments—vertically fastened to the implant. A 24-karat gold-coping is galvanized onto these primary units. The coping is glued to a tertiary structure carrying the ceramic (Fig 3). The structure is additionally secured using three horizontal bolts.

In edentulous patients with severe hard tissue deficiencies, iliac bone grafting based on the natural lip dynamics is essential (Fig 4). Lost tissue should be restored in the direction in which it was lost, accounting for the space necessary for the superstructure (Fig 5). In many cases, treatment planning cannot be performed on the basis of the existing restoration (Fig 6). Therefore, patients can be asked to bring in a photograph that shows their original dentition. This allows the clinician and technician to judge the tooth form, position, and angulation, as well as the original lip support (Fig 7), making it easier to approximate the original appearance with ceramic (Fig 8).

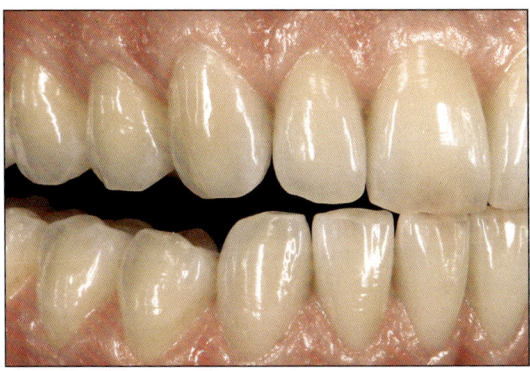 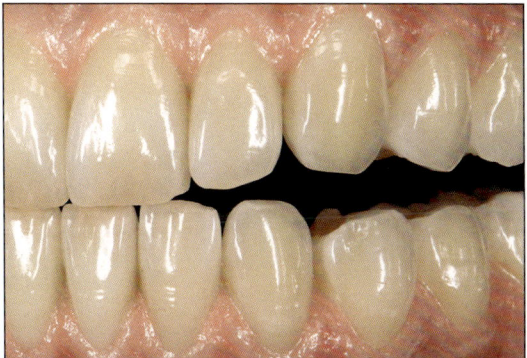

Figs 1 and 2 The natural appearance of ceramic allows for predictable positioning of the gingival contours.

Fig 3 The superstructure is based on a primary unit *(a)* (vertically screwed abutment) onto which a 24-karat gold-coping *(b)* is galvanized. The coping is glued to a tertiary structure *(c)* carrying the ceramic. A horizontal bolt additionally secures the seat.

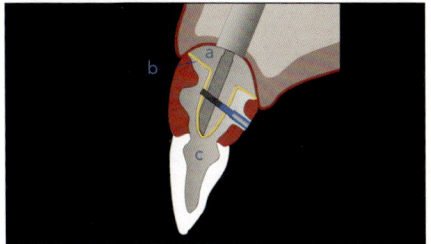

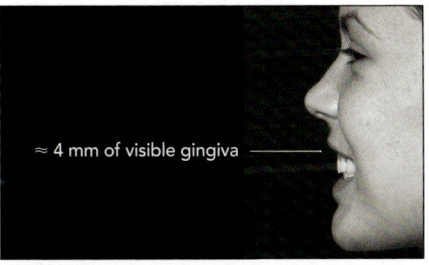

Fig 4 The dynamic of the lips determines the amount of gingival display.

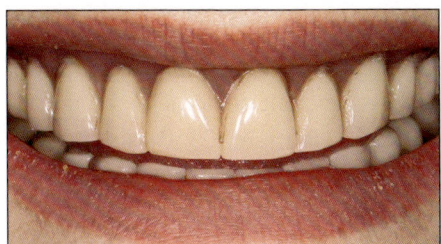

Fig 5 Bone deficiency should be corrected in the direction in which the bone was lost, while allowing sufficient space for the implants and framework.

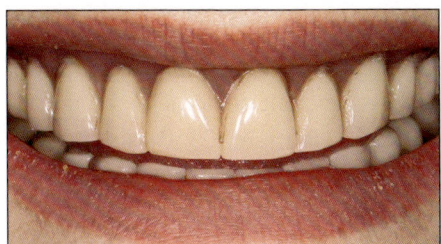

Fig 6 A 50-year-old patient with insufficient complete dentures in the maxilla and mandible.

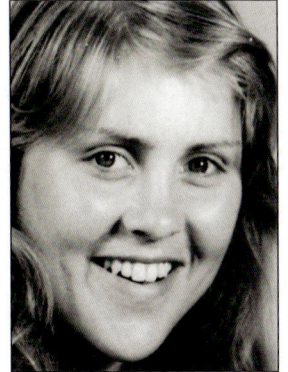

Fig 7 Patients should be asked for photographs showing their original dentition, which provide a plethora of valuable information.

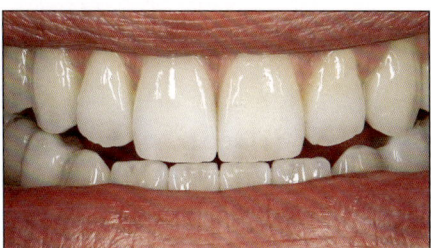

Fig 8 Compared to the initial situation (see Fig 6), the definitive implant-retained fixed restoration provides excellent esthetics.

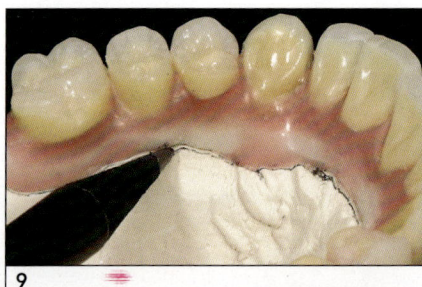

Fig 9 The wax try-in is vertically screwed to ensure a secure seat for the bite registration.

Fig 10 The outline of the wax try-in guides the soft tissue contouring on the cast (gray line).

Fig 11 A perfect emergence profile is essential for a successful fixed restoration in the edentulous patient.

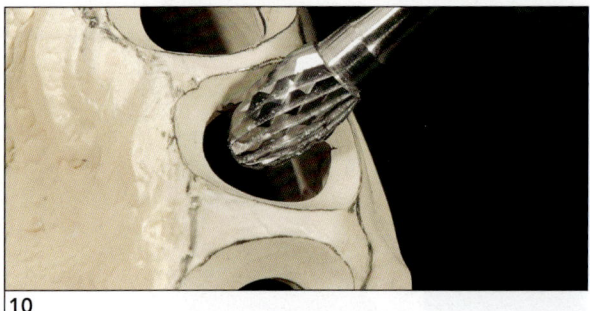

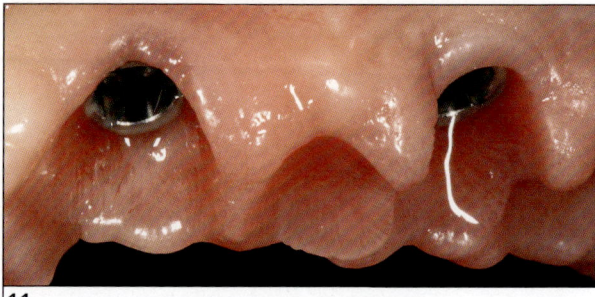

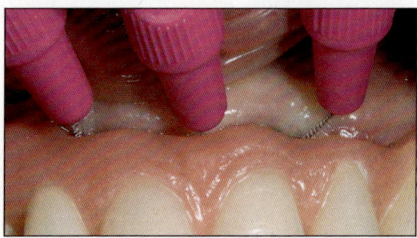

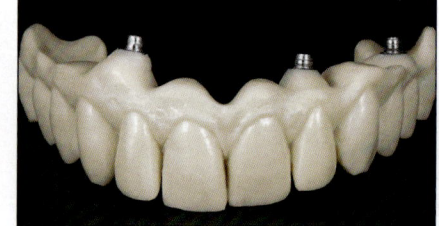

Fig 12 One prerequisite of an implant-retained prosthesis is the ability to perform proper oral hygiene. This can be evaluated during the provisional phase.

Fig 13 Polyurethane is used to fabricate a duplicate of the provisional restoration since it shows a high dimensional stability over time.

CLINICAL AND TECHNICAL PROCEDURES

Many patients present with esthetically and functionally insufficient restorations. After the surgical phase is carried out, an open-tray impression and interocclusal record should be taken, and a wax try-in should be used to fabricate a provisional implant-retained restoration. The wax try-in is also used to define the soft tissue architecture around the implant (Fig 9), allowing soft tissue formation during the provisional phase (Figs 10 and 11). During this phase, any corrections necessary should be carried out to obtain perfect esthetics and function while ensuring adequate oral hygiene (Fig 12). The provisional is then used as a template to fabricate the definitive restoration.

A duplicate of the provisional restoration is made using polyurethane resin (Alpa-Pur, Alpina, Munich, Germany). The duplicate is accurately repositioned on the implant analogs of the master cast (type IV gypsum, Unibase 300, Dentona, Dortmund, Germany) (Fig 13), and then used to fabricate silicone matrices (Sil-Tech, Ivoclar Vivadent, Schaan, Lichtenstein), which ensure correct dimensioning of the definitive restoration.

Individually fabricated primary units cast in high-gold casting alloy (Orplid CF, Hafner, Pforzheim, Germany) are milled parallel in the lower third and with a 2-degree angle in the upper two thirds to ensure easy incorporation (Fig 14). These primary units are then prepared for electroforming (Fig 15). The abutments are spray-coated with a thin layer

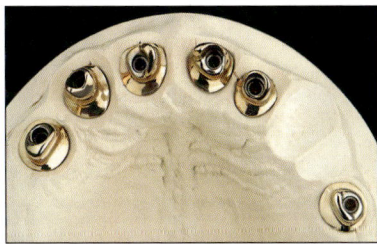

Fig 14 For optimal tissue contouring, individually fabricated abutments were used.

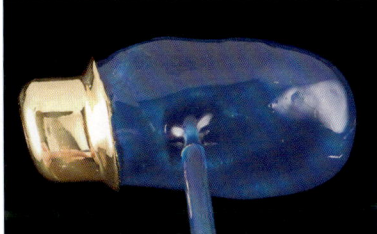

Fig 15 By galvanizing gold directly onto the abutment, a high level of precision is achieved.

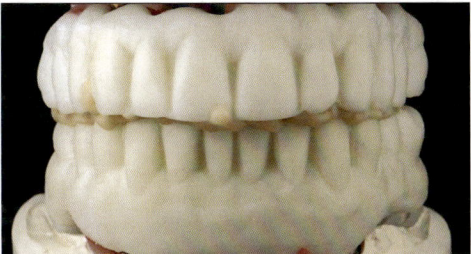

Fig 16 The electroformed copings with a duplicate of the provisional restoration allow reexamination of the vertical dimension of occlusion and tooth position.

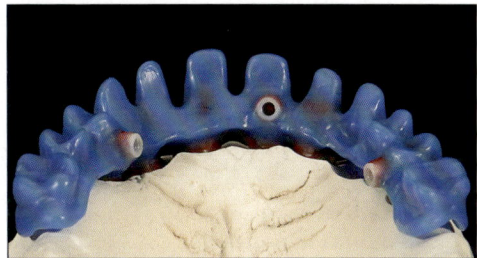

Fig 17 The tertiary structure is waxed on a second cast.

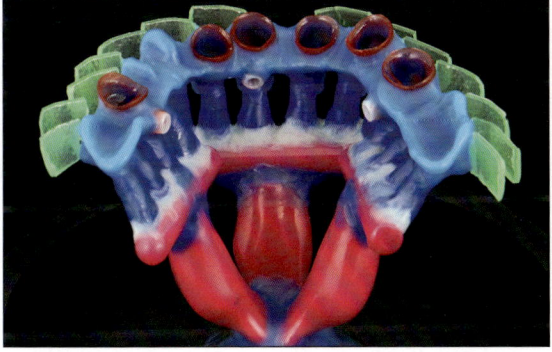

Fig 18 Cooling fins are added to control the solidification process.

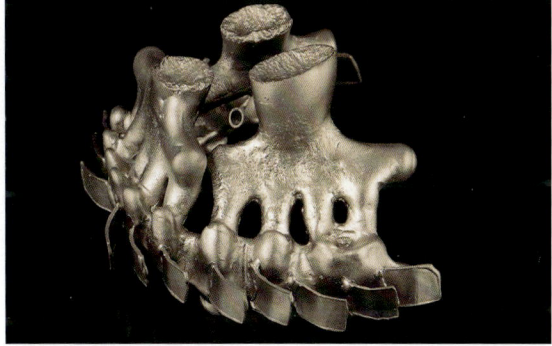

Fig 19 The separated and half-filled sprues indicate sufficient additional metal inflow and minimal distortional forces during cooling.

of silver lacquer and placed in a fully automated electroplater (HF Vario Plus, Hafner).

Correct seating of the electroformed copings on the primary units must be verified intraorally. With the use of autopolymerizing composite resin (Pattern Resin, GC, Tokyo, Japan), the copings are collected with a prefabricated pick-up tray made from light-curing composite resin (Individulux, Voco, Cuxhaven, Germany) (Fig 16). This step is necessary to ensure the precision of fit of the superstructure, since it defines the position in which the coping is glued to the tertiary structure in the dental laboratory.

Next, the primary units are connected to implant analogs and accurately positioned into the splinted electroformed copings to fabricate a new gypsum cast (Unibase 300, Dentona). This cast is used for the waxing of the tertiary structure (Fig 17).

Investing (GC Investment, GC) and casting are then carried out. The framework was cast in one piece from high-gold alloy (V-Classic, Metalor, Stuttgart, Germany) (Figs 18 and 19). The space between the copings and framework that results from casting-related deformation accommodates the self-curing luting agent.

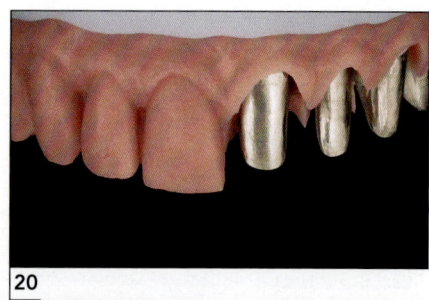

Fig 20 Silicone matrices define the idealized proportions of the red and white porcelain.

Fig 21 The gingival mask is removed after layering the white ceramic.

Fig 22 Only one color of the red powder is used as the basis of the artificial gingiva.

Fig 23 Ideal moisturizing of the paste is important throughout the layering process.

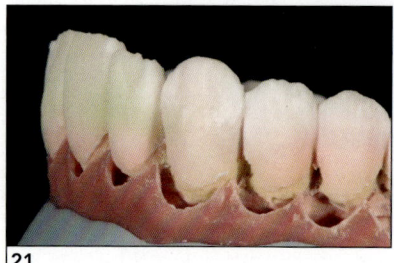

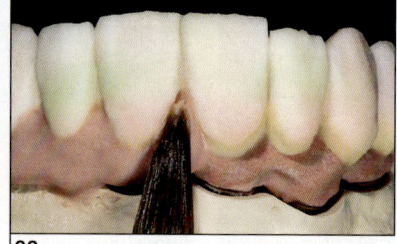

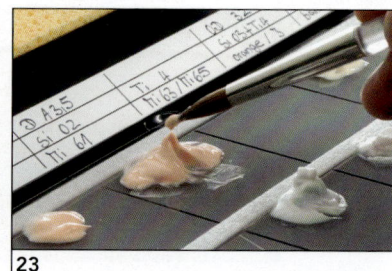

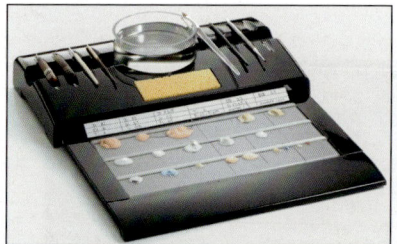

Fig 24 Various powders and stains will be used throughout the ceramic work.

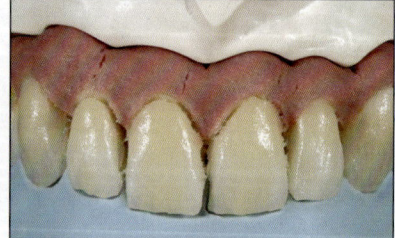

Fig 25 White and red ceramic is applied prior to the first firing.

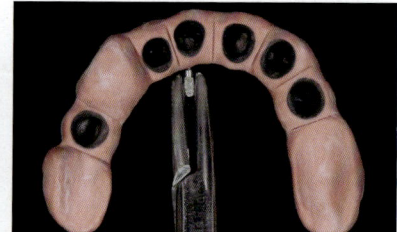

Fig 26 At this stage, the shape is almost finished.

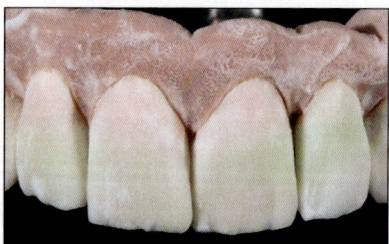
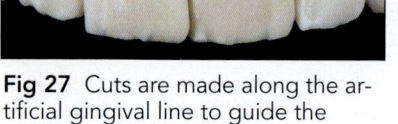

Fig 27 Cuts are made along the artificial gingival line to guide the crack formation during firing

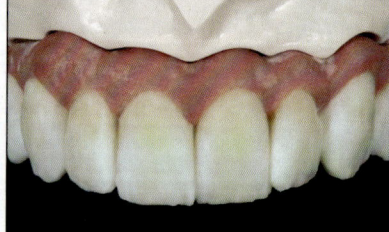

Fig 28 Cracks are initiated at the predetermined sites.

Fig 29 Prior to the second firing, corrections are performed only on the white ceramic.

During the provisional phase, the proportion of red and white esthetics is optimized to satisfy the patient and clinician's demands, and this information is transferred to the definitive restoration using matrices (Gi-mask, Coltené/Whaledent, Langenau, Germany) (Fig 20). The use of matrices simplifies the technician's work process and allows for easy three-dimensional contouring. Porcelain is layered on the tertiary structure with red and white powder (Creation CC, GC) using a new moisturizing system (Aqualine, Mehrhof Dental Technologies, Berlin, Germany) (Figs 21 to 34). Pink and white porcelain are then fired together.

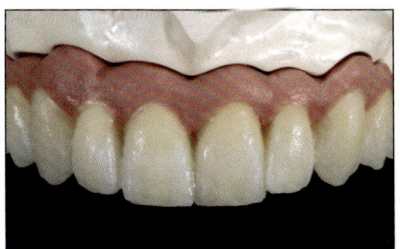

Fig 30 No crack formation is visible after the second firing. The layering of the white ceramic is almost complete.

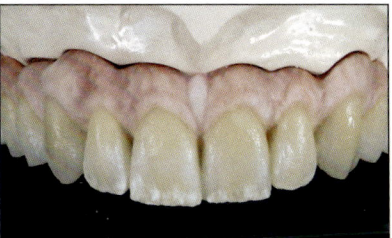

Fig 31 Minor corrections on the red and white porcelain are carried out.

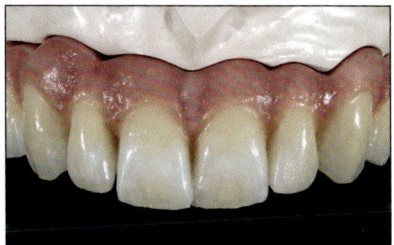

Fig 32 Appearance of the surface after the third firing. No grinding has been performed on the pink ceramic.

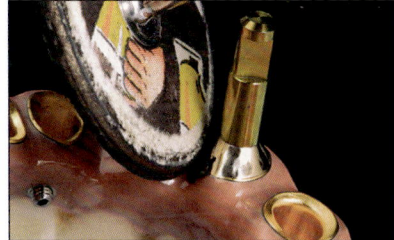

Fig 33 In the glazing process, a mixture of low- and high-fusing pink porcelain is used.

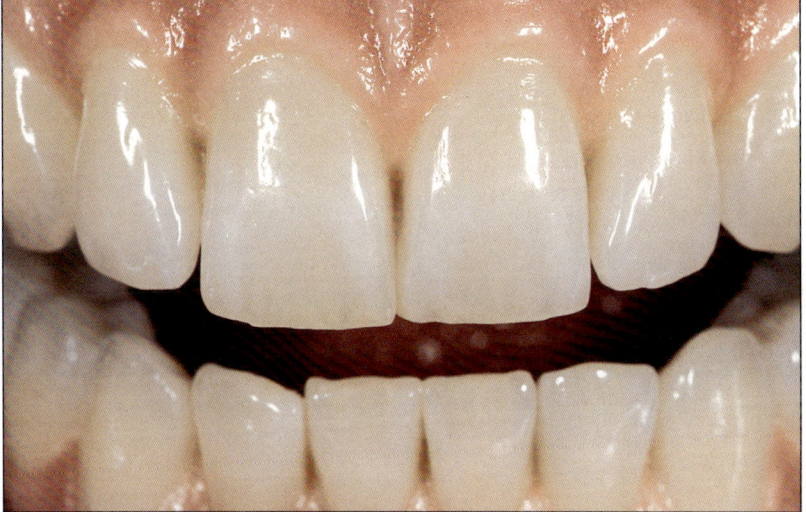

Fig 34 The final restoration displays a natural surface texture and proper proportions.

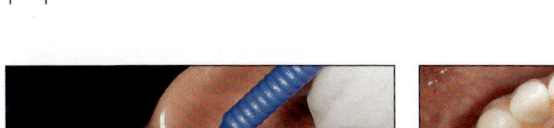

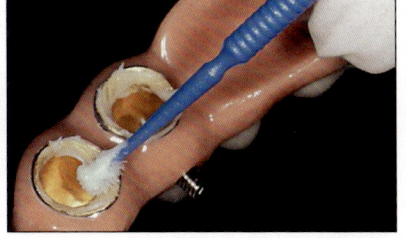

Fig 35 Final finishing is performed using a large-diameter paper disk.

Fig 36 Provisional cement is administered at the margin of the coping as a sealant.

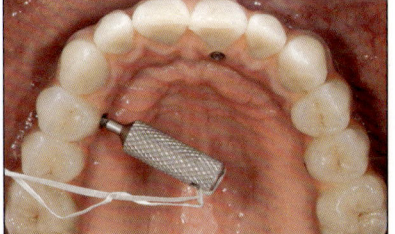

Fig 37 The restoration is placed on the abutments/primary units and the horizontal bolts are tightened.

Next, the electroformed copings are glued (AGC-Cem, Wieland, Pforzheim, Germany) to the tertiary structure in the laboratory. After gluing, perforation of the copings for the horizontal bolts (Security Lock 1.4 mm, Bredent, Germany) is accomplished using a 1.4-mm multidrill (Bredent). Final finishing is then performed to prepare the restoration for delivery (Fig 35).

When the primary units are placed intraorally, the abutment screws should be tightened according to the manufacturer's instructions. Only a very thin layer of provisional polyurethane cement (Im-Prov, Dentegris, Germany) needs to be administered at the margin of the restoration to seal it from bacterial leakage (Fig 36). This cement is not needed for retention (Fig 37).

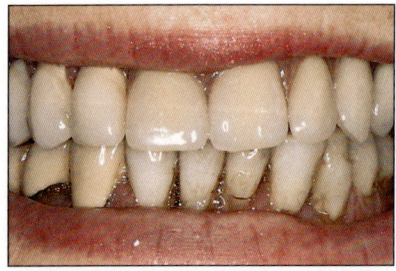

Fig 38 Initial situation with existing restorations.

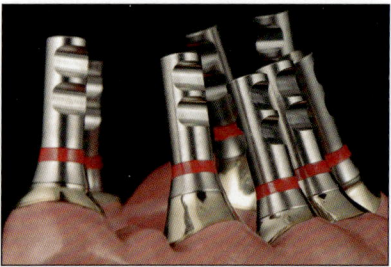

Fig 39 Eight implants were placed for a fixed restoration.

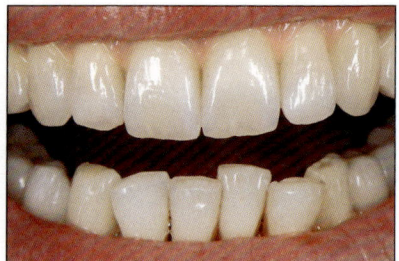

Fig 40 Implant-retained fixed prosthesis in the maxilla using red and white ceramic.

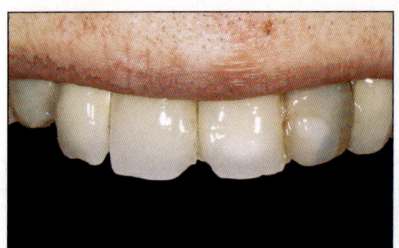

Fig 41 Initial situation in the anterior maxilla.

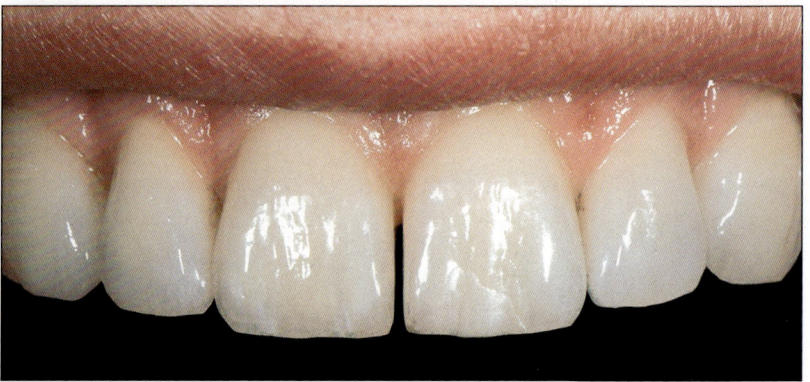

Fig 42 Ceramic restoration used to simulate the original appearance, including a diastema.

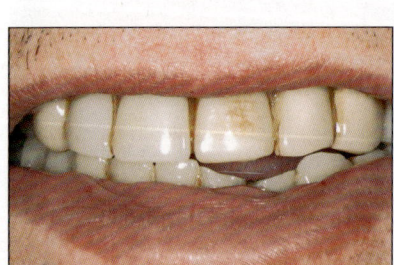

Fig 43 Initial situation with insufficient complete dentures.

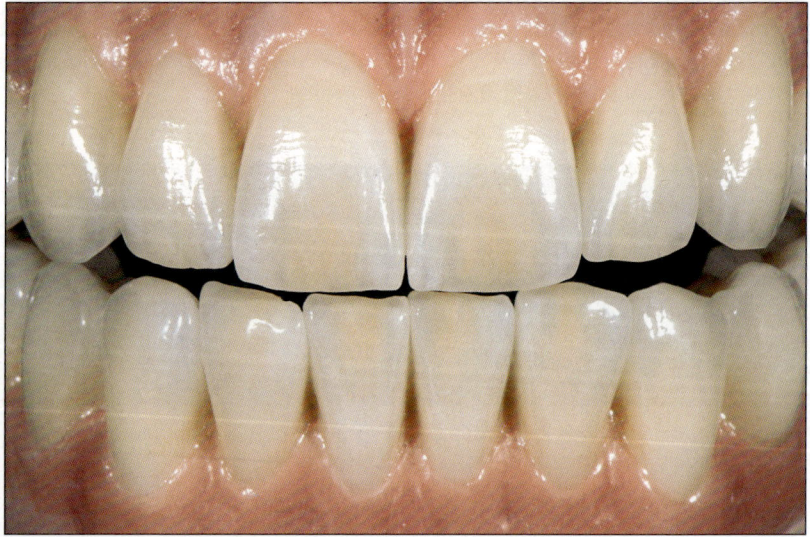

Fig 44 Fixed implant-supported rehabilitation in the maxilla and mandible. Hard and soft tissue deficiencies are restored.

Figures 38 to 48 show the initial clinical situation and definitive implant-retained fixed restoration of several patients. All patients, except the one in Figs 43 and 44, underwent major iliac bone augmentation in the maxilla as described.[1] The patients were asked to wear a nightguard (Erkodur 1.5 mm, Erkodent, Pfalzgrafenweiler, Germany).

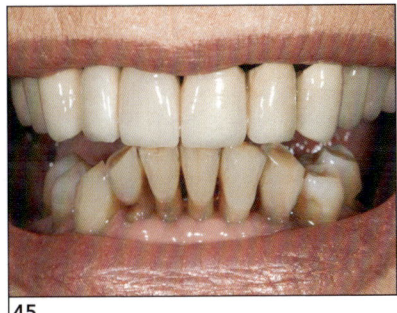

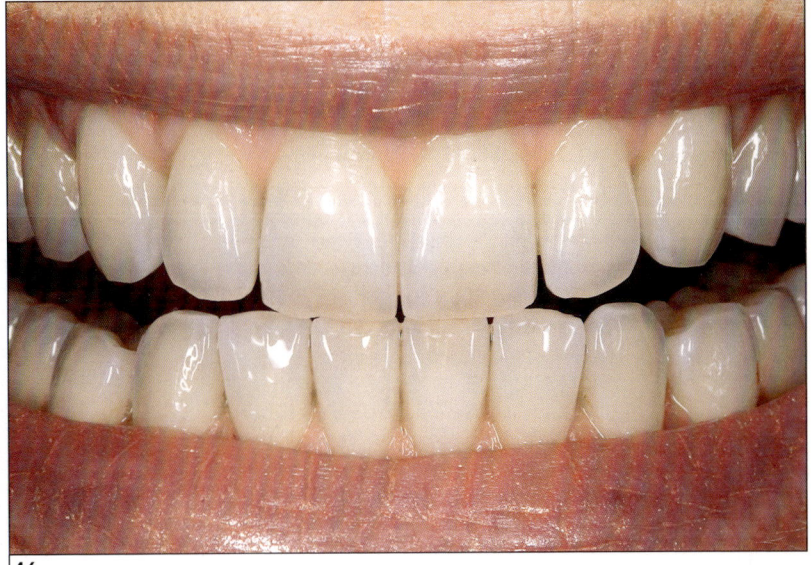

45

46

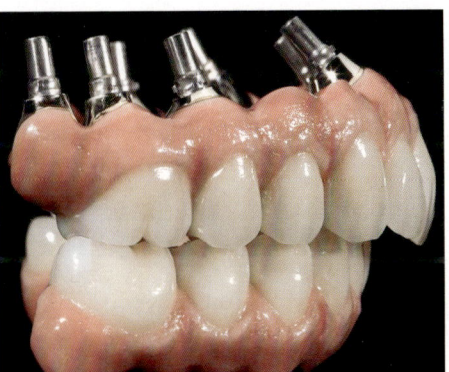

47

Fig 45 Initial situation. All teeth must be removed due to periodontal disease.

Fig 46 Not only are the esthetics improved with retrievable implant-retained fixed restorations, but the patient's quality of life is enhanced, as well.

Figs 47 and 48 Implant fixed restoration used to restore the natural appearance.

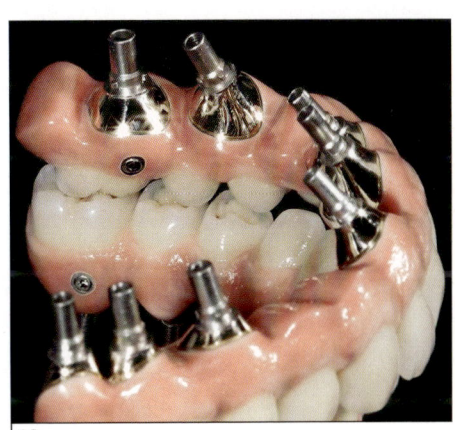

48

CONCLUSION

The procedure described in this article makes it possible to fabricate an esthetic and retrievable implant-retained fixed prosthesis. The technique combines the advantages of screw retention—easy and predictable removal—with those of cement retention, including easier fabrication, enhanced esthetics, and superior occlusal design with no vertical screw access holes.

The retention of the structure is based on the precise fit of the electroformed copings and not on the retentive capacity of a luting agent. No replicas are involved during the fabrication of the gold copings since they are electroformed directly onto the surface of the primary units, thus ensuring optimal retentive properties.

ACKNOWLEDGMENT

Special thanks to Dr Detlef Hildebrand for his work on the patient in Figs 43 and 44.

REFERENCES

1. Nelson K, Ozyuvaci H, Bilgic B, Klein M, Hildebrand D. Histomorphometric evaluation and clinical assessment of endosseous implants in iliac bone grafts with shortened healing periods. Int J Oral Maxillofacial Implants 2006; 21:392–398.

2. Chee W, Felton DA, Johnson PF, Sullivan DY. Cemented versus screw-retained implant prostheses: Which is better? Int J Oral Maxillofac Implants 1999;14:137–141.

3. Michalakis KX, Hirayama H, Garefis PD. Cement-retained versus screw-retained implant restorations: A critical review. Int J Oral Maxillofac Implants 2003;18:719–728.

4. Karl M, Wichmann MG, Winter W, Graef F, Taylor TD, Heckmann SM. Influence of fixation mode and superstructure span upon strain development of implant fixed partial dentures. J Prosthodont (in press).

5. Misch CE. Screw-retained versus cement-retained implant-supported prostheses. Implant Rep 1995;7:15-18.

6. Hebel KS, Gajjar RC. Cement-retained versus screw-retained implant restorations: Achieving optimal occlusion and esthetics in implant dentistry. J Prosthet Dent 1997; 77:28–35.

7. Michalakis KX, Pissiotis AL, Hirayama H. Cement failure loads of 4 provisional luting agents used for the cementation of implant-supported fixed partial dentures. Int J Oral Maxillofac Implants 2000;15:545–549.

8. Breeding LC, Dixon DL, Bogacki MT, Tietge JD. Use of luting agents with an implant system: Part I. J Prosthet Dent 1992;68:737–741.

9. Covey DA, Kent DK, St. Germain HAJ, Koka S. Effects of abutment size and luting cement type on the uniaxial retention force of implant-supported crowns. J Prosthet Dent 2000;83:344–348.

10. Squier RS, Agar JR, Duncan JP, Taylor TD. Retentives of dental cements used with metallic implant components. Int J Oral Maxillofac Implants 2001;16:793–798.

11. Agar JR, Cameron SM, Hughbanks JC, Parker MH. Cement removal from restorations luted to titanium abutments with simulated subgingival margins. J Prosthet Dent 1997;78:43–47.

12. Lindström H, Preiskel H. The implant-supported telescopic prosthesis: A biomechanical analysis. Int J Oral Maxillofac Implants 2001;16:34–42.

13. Raidgrodski AJ, Malcamp C, Rogers WA. Electroforming technique. J Dent Technol 1998;15:13–16.

14. Vence BS. Electroforming technology for galvanoceramic restorations. J Prosthet Dent 1997;77:444–449.

15. Weigl P, Hahn L, Lauer HC. Advanced biomaterials used for a new telescopic retainer for removable dentures: Ceramic vs. electroplated gold copings: Part I. In vitro tribology effects. J Biomed Mater Res 1999;53:337–347.

16. Weigl P, Lauer HC. Advanced biomaterials used for a new telescopic retainer for removable dentures: Ceramic vs electroplated gold copings: Part II. Clinical effects. J Biomed Mater Res 1999;53:337–347.

17. Heckmann S, Schrott A, Graef F, Wichmann M, Weber H. Mandibular two-implant telescopic overdentures. Clin Oral Implants Res 2004;15:560–569.

18. Nelson K, Mehrhof J, Hildebrand D. Fabrication of a fixed retrievable implant-supported prosthesis based on electroforming: A technical report. J Prosthodont; in press

19. Lixin X, Heberer S, Mehrhof J, Nelson K. Clinical evaluation of fixed (retrievable) implant-supported prostheses in the edentulous jaw: A 5-year report [in Chinese]. Chinese J Dent Res (in press).

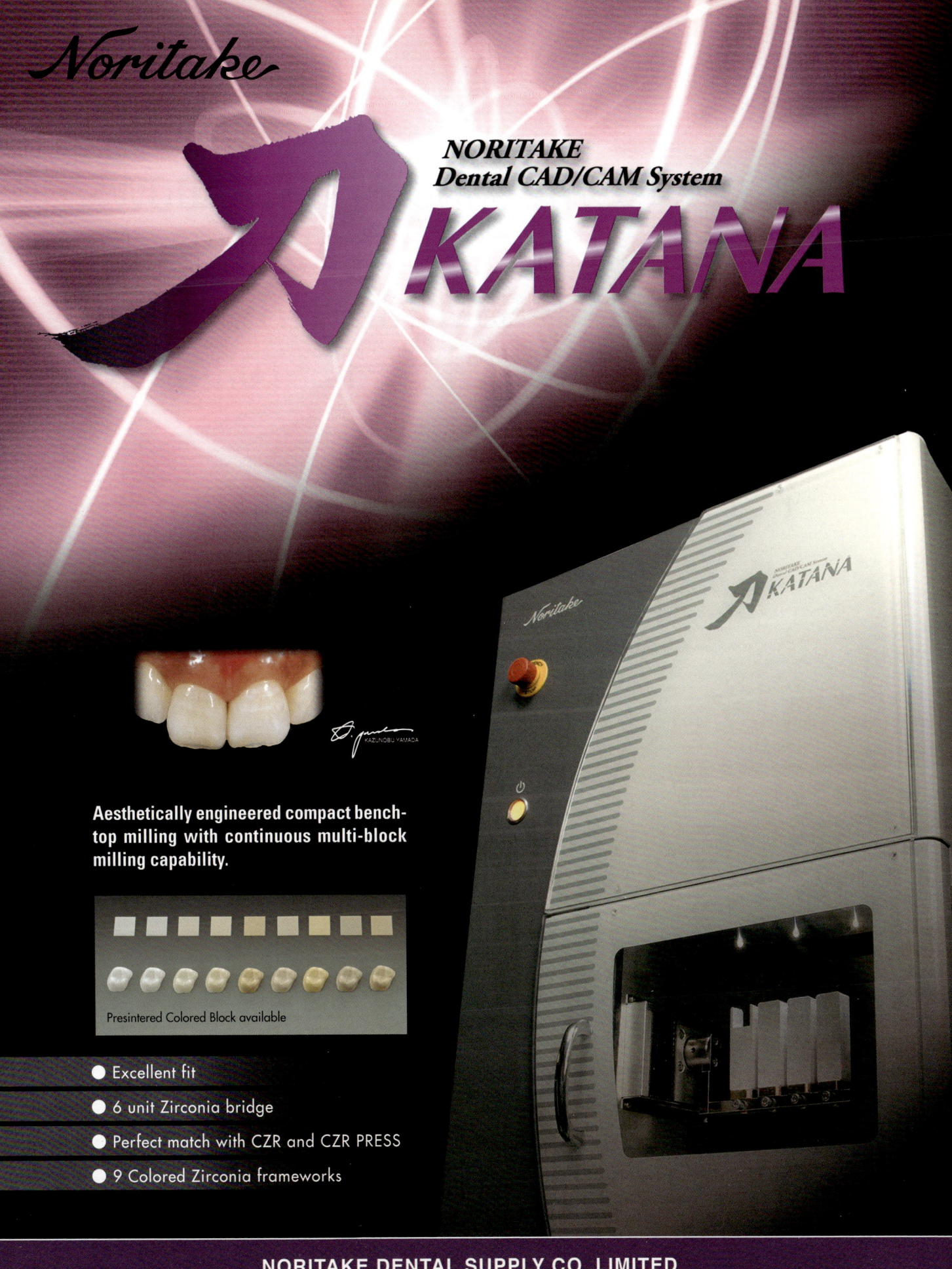

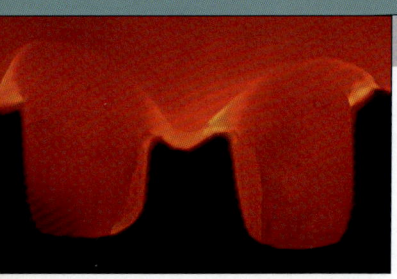

THE CONCEPT OF SHADOWS: VISUALIZING LIGHT TRANSMISSION IN ESTHETIC RESTORATIONS

Sillas Duarte Jr, DDS, MS, PhD[1]
Tomikazu Tada, RDT[2]
Avishai Sadan, DMD[3]

Light transmission is essential for the esthetic integration of restorative materials and natural teeth. Good optical properties are responsible for a restored tooth's natural appearance. The management of light transmission is especially imperative in certain challenging clinical situations; however, restoration of misaligned or discolored teeth presents esthetic challenges in our daily practice that require the incorporation of illusions for an esthetic result. This article demonstrates how shadows can improve or impair the quality of anterior restorations.

[1]Associate Professor, Department of Comprehensive Care, Case Western Reserve University, Cleveland, Ohio, USA.

[2]Master Dental Ceramist, Laboratory Manager, Department of Comprehensive Care, Case Western Reserve University, Cleveland, Ohio, USA.

[3]Chair, Professor and Chair, Department of Comprehensive Care, Case Western Reserve University, Cleveland, Ohio, USA.

Correspondence to: Dr Sillas Duarte Jr, Department of Comprehensive Care, Case School of Dental Medicine, Case Western Reserve University, 10900 Euclid Avenue, Cleveland, OH 44106-4905, USA. E-mail: sillas.duarte@case.edu

PRINCIPLES OF LIGHT TRANSMISSION

A complete definition of the nature of light is quite complex. The scientific explanation certifies that light is a type of electromagnetic radiation.[1] Einstein explained that light exists in a particle-like state as packets of energy called photons.[2] The photon produces an electromagnetic field around itself. This electromagnetic field is not constant in strength; in fact, it fluctuates as the photon travels. All photons travel through space at the same speed; however, the electromagnetic fields of some photons fluctuate faster than those of others.[3] The human eye can perceive the effects of differences in the photon energy levels and the electromagnetic field. This electromagnetic fluctuation is called frequency.[3] The human eye can perceive only frequencies between 4.0×10^{14} Hz (hertz) and 7.9×10^{14} Hz as visible light.[4] For the most part, visible light is discussed in terms of wavelengths, with the unit being nanometers (nm; 1 nm = 10^{-9} m), rather than in frequencies.[4] The

CASE 1 (Figs 1 to 3)

Fig 1 Preoperative view. Observe the reduced space to obtain appropriate width/length ratio of the central incisors.

Fig 2 Postoperative view, final restorations. Soft shadow concepts were used to produce a proper outcome.

Fig 3 The patient's smile reveals suitable light incorporation of ceramic and soft tissues.

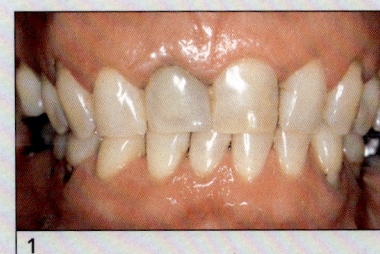

1

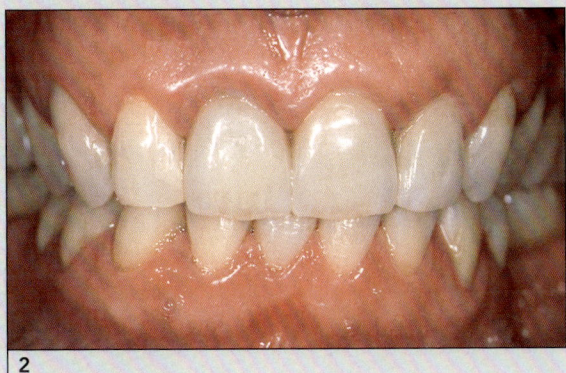

2

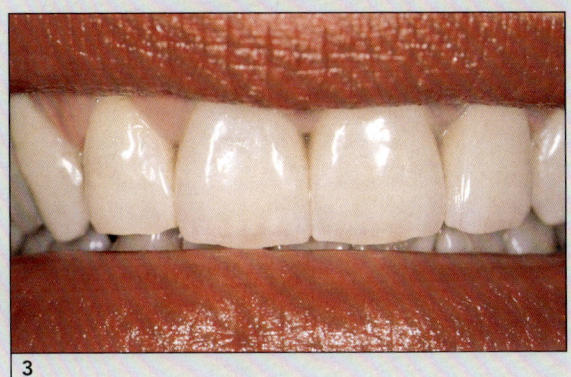

3

human brain recognizes these wavelengths as different colors: 750 nm is about the longest wavelength of red light at one end of the color spectrum, and 380 nm is approximately the shortest wavelength of violet light at the other.[5] All other visible colors fall between these two wavelengths.[6]

The wavelike nature of light explains many of its properties, including reflection/refraction and diffraction/interference.[3] When it reaches an object, the light can be reflected, transmitted, or absorbed.[7] These phenomena create an important characteristic, referred to as contrast, which is related to the natural appearance of a restoration. A light source can produce high- or low-contrast light.[1] Depending on the interaction of the light with a given restoration, a shadow may be produced. A resultant shadow has the potential to improve or spoil the final outcome of an esthetic treatment. Therefore, to better understand the effect of light transmission on a restoration, clinicians must concern themselves with the presence of shadows.

THE CONCEPT OF SHADOWS

Soft Shadow

The shadows in esthetic restorative dentistry might be hard or soft. Low-contrast light produces a shadow that is no longer clearly defined.[1] Thus, the shadows created by low-contrast light are soft shadows: The viewer cannot determine where the limits of the shadow are, which creates a diffused appearance. A soft shadow can improve the esthetic characteristics of restorations. For example, it is possible to mask the size of a tooth by moving line angles or cervical crests of convexity closer or farther apart.[8] Thus, by increasing or reducing the flat surface, one can widen or narrow, respectively, the appearance of the tooth (Fig 1).[8] As the area of reflected light is enlarged or decreased, the resulting shadows create an optical illusion (Fig 2). When the shadows and light distribution are properly assigned in a restoration, the esthetic appearance is clearly improved because of the distribution of light (Fig 3).[9]

CASE 2 (Figs 4 to 6)

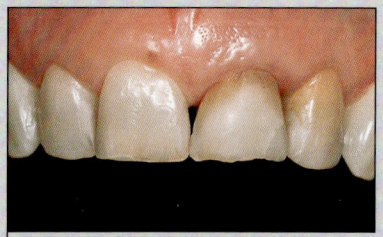

Fig 4 Preoperative view. The maxillary left central and lateral incisors were resistant to bleaching, especially at the gingival third.

Figs 5a and 5b Final outcome of the restored teeth.

Figs 6a and 6b Observe appropriate light incorporation of the restorations with soft tissue and lips on right side of patient's smile. The papillae corresponding to the dark abutment teeth on the left side reveal a grayish appearance and thus hard shadow.

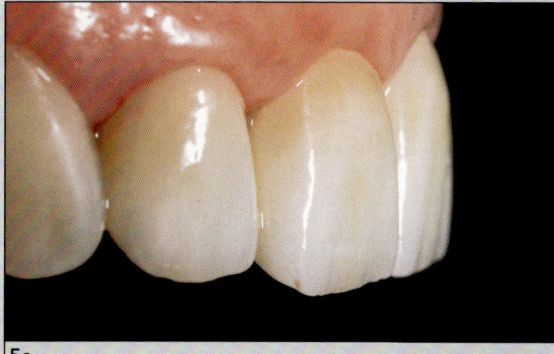

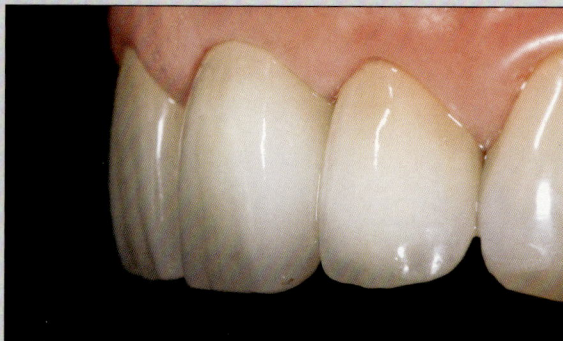

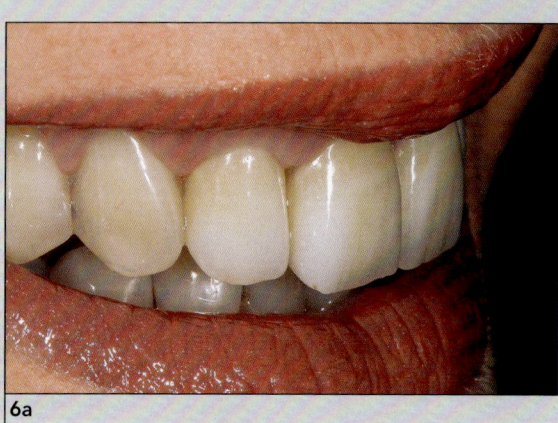

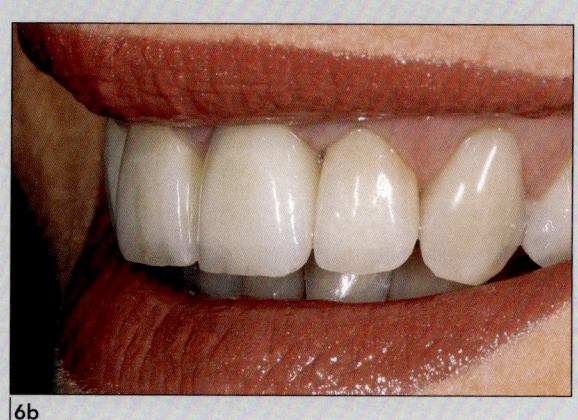

Hard Shadow

A hard shadow is created by a high-contrast light source, which produces a shadow with sharply defined edges.[1] Because a natural tooth has subtle differences in light transmission,[10] the effects of a high-contrast light source become evident. The amount of light transmitted through the tooth structure indicates the quality of the substrate and thus the presence (or absence) of a hard shadow.

A hard shadow appears on the soft tissues, thereby producing a grayish papilla when the lip is in its normal position.[11] As a consequence, hard shadows create an unesthetic effect on dental restorations. Therefore, the presence of shadows highlights the importance of interaction of light with the teeth and their supporting tissues.

Hard shadows are produced by (*a*) discolored or dark abutments or (*b*) nontranslucent/fluorescent or opaque restorations.

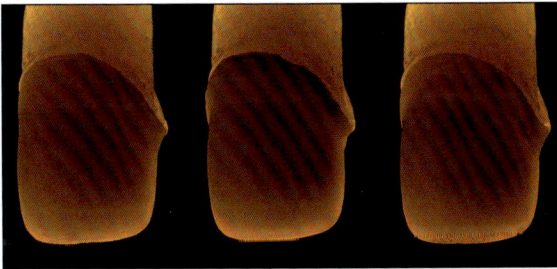 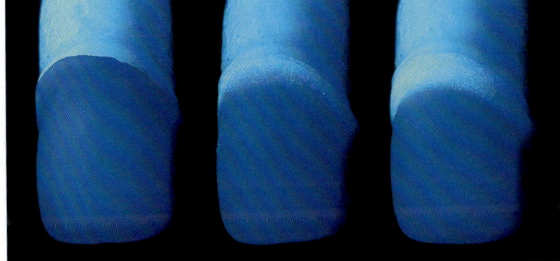

Fig 7 *(a)* Alumina copings under transillumination. *(b)* Fluorescence of alumina copings. *From left:* no ceramic shoulder, 1.0-mm ceramic shoulder, and 2.0-mm ceramic shoulder. Observe the improvement of light transmission with ceramic shoulder in both transmitted and fluorescent light.

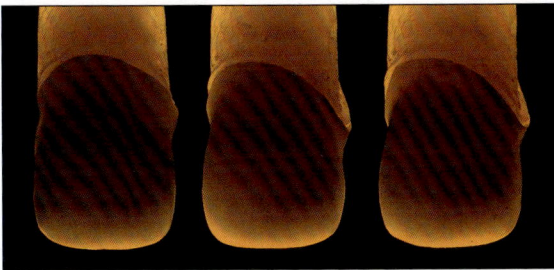 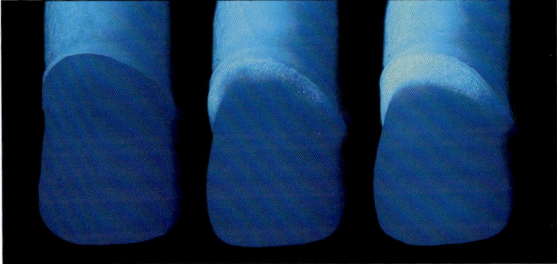

Fig 8 *(a)* Zirconia copings under transillumination. *(b)* Fluorescence of zirconia copings. *From left:* no ceramic shoulder, 1.0-mm ceramic shoulder, and 2.0-mm ceramic shoulder. Observe the improvement of fluorescence only for 2.0-mm ceramic shoulder. The ceramic shoulder does not affect light transmission on transmitted light.

Discolored teeth

The darker the substrate, the more contrast one should expect. When teeth become discolored, it can be a challenge to restore a natural appearance.[12] Dental discolorations can be generalized or isolated. Fluorosis,[13] tetracycline staining,[14] and enamel-dentin dysplasia[15] are examples of generalized discoloration. An isolated discoloration affects only a given tooth, and it might occur because of pulp trauma,[16] dystrophic calcification of the pulp,[17] remaining necrotic tissue in the pulp chamber after root canal therapy,[18] blood pigmentation due to hemorrhage,[18] endodontic sealers,[19–21] or metal post corrosion.[22,23] Dark abutments also complicate the reproduction of a natural target shade (Figs 4 and 5).[24] Moreover, the discoloration of a tooth results in a lack of translucency, as well as a decrease in fluorescence. As the light cannot be correctly transmitted within the discolored tooth's complex optical system, the resulting hard shadow will produce an unnatural appearance (Figs 6a and 6b).

Nontranslucent opaque restorations

Nontranslucent/nonfluorescent restorations, overextended opaque frameworks (either metallic or ceramic), and metallic posts and cores may prevent light penetration and distribution into the surrounding tissues (Figs 7 and 8). The gingival color around restored teeth with artificial crowns has been shown to reveal a change toward red-purple[25] or red-green,[26] depending on the restorative material. Zirconia can produce a color shift ranging from yellow to blue, despite it being the material with the least noticeable color change against the mucosa.[26]

Consequently, a hard shadow appears at the soft tissues, which produces a papilla when the lip is in its normal position (see Fig 6b).[11] This is referred to as the "umbrella effect" and emphasizes the interaction of light with the teeth and their supporting tissues.[11]

CASE 3 (Figs 9 to 16)

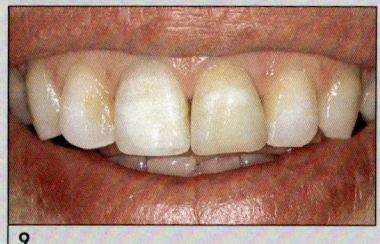

Fig 9 Preoperative view.

Fig 10 Transillumination exposes the lack of light transmission through the ceramic restoration.

Fig 11 Defective metallic cast post and core.

Fig 12 After removal of old metallic post, the root exhibits dark pigmentation as a result of nonprecious metal corrosion.

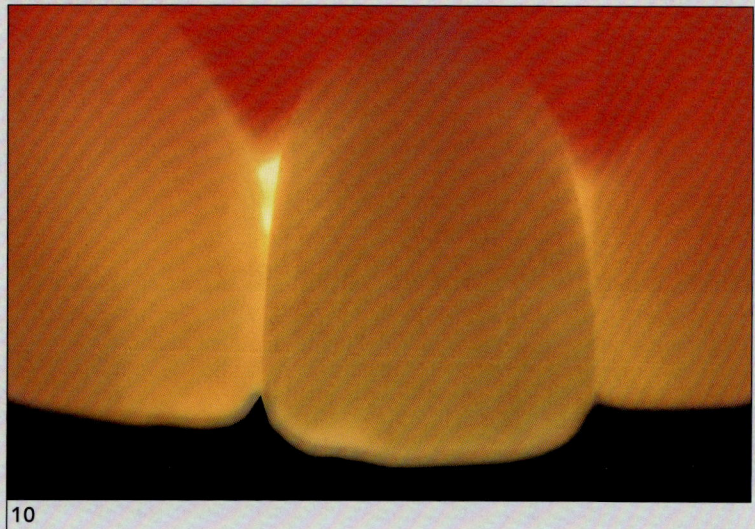

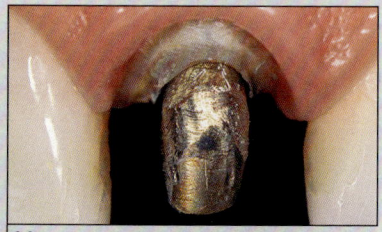

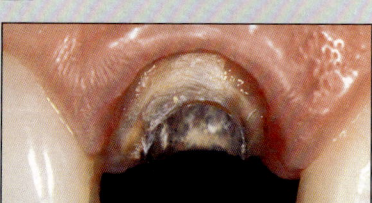

OPTIMIZING LIGHT TRANSMISSION

Discolored teeth

Before restoring a compromised tooth, the clinician should observe the quality of the existing abutment's light transmission (Fig 9). The degree of discoloration and how the final restoration might be affected must be assessed in order to improve the esthetic results (Fig 10). Transillumination and fluorescence tests should be performed to indicate the potential of hard shadows, especially before final impressions are taken. Ideally, the goal is to eliminate the dark color of the abutment prior to restoration.[12]

Staining can be removed by chemical or mechanical procedures. Chemical removal consists of bleaching the coronal part of the tooth with peroxides.[27] This technique is limited to the coronal third because of the potential for root resorption.[28–30]

After the removal of a cast post and core, a dark root canal resulting from corrosion of nonprecious metal is common (Figs 11 and 12). Corrosion products from iron, chromium, nickel, zinc, stannous, as well other elements, penetrate into the dentin tubules (Fig 12).[31] The presence of corrosion products in dentin tubules may contribute to root fracture[31] and darkening and/or discoloration of the gingival tissue.[32] Due to the light transmission characteristics of the metal ions trapped in the root structure, the dentin's fluorescence may be significantly reduced. To rehabilitate the dentin's light transmission, careful mechanical removal of the root discoloration with low-speed burs can be performed. Obviously, this procedure will weaken the

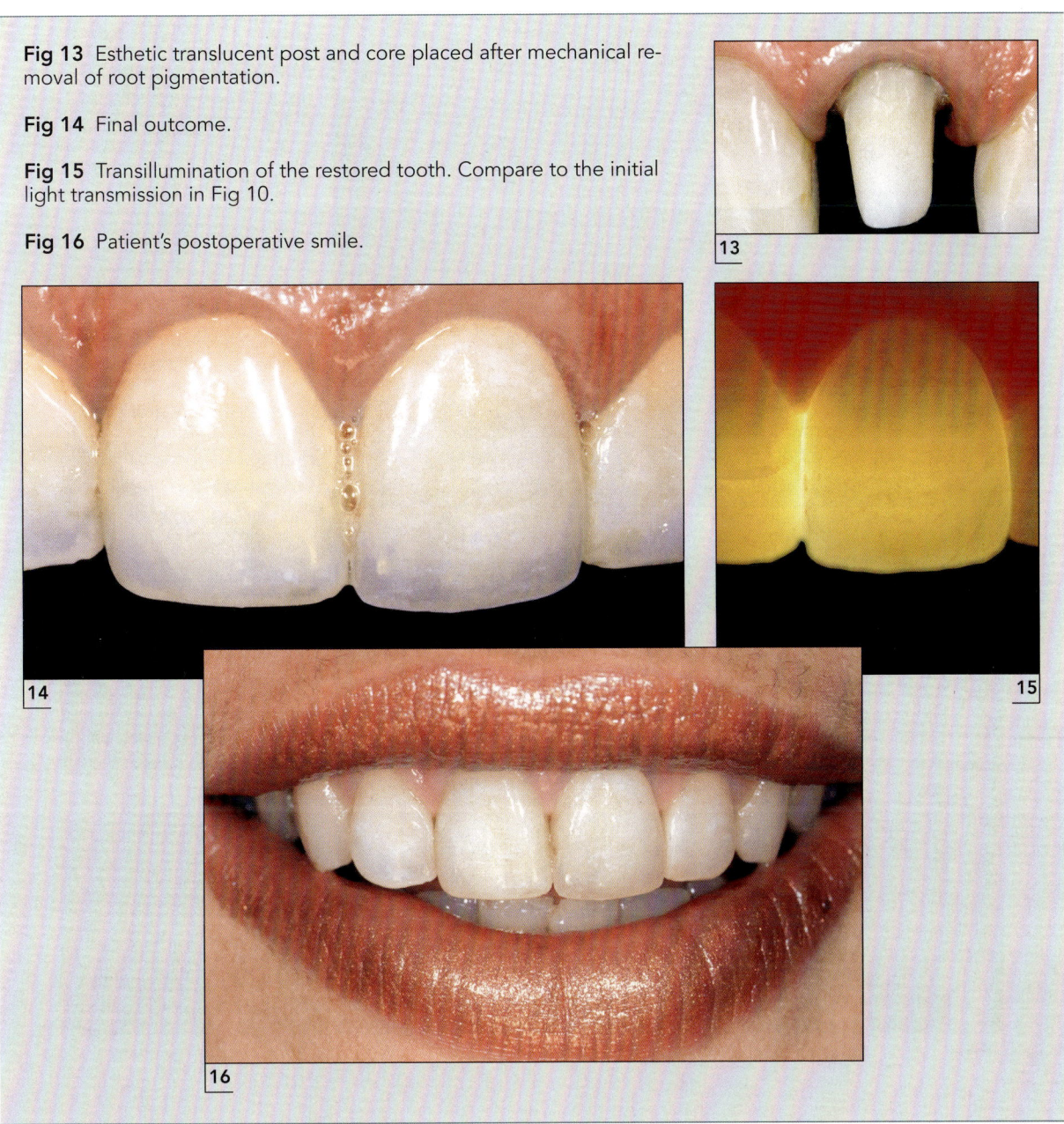

Fig 13 Esthetic translucent post and core placed after mechanical removal of root pigmentation.

Fig 14 Final outcome.

Fig 15 Transillumination of the restored tooth. Compare to the initial light transmission in Fig 10.

Fig 16 Patient's postoperative smile.

remaining tooth structure.[12] Wherever possible, bleaching is preferable to mechanical stain removal. Depending on the level of discoloration, it may be necessary to combine the techniques. The thickness of the remaining dentin also plays an important role in the light transmission (see Fig 17).

Translucent fiber posts must also be considered to improve light distribution in compromised teeth (see Figs 18a to 18d). For core buildup, highly fluorescent fiber posts (ie, Postec, Ivoclar Vi-

vadent; Light-Post DT, Bisco) and composite resin (ie, Four Seasons, Ivoclar Vivadent; Vit-l-escence, Ultradent Products; Miris, Coltène Whaledent; Esthet-X, Dentsply Caulk) can be used to provide light distribution similar to that of natural tooth structure (Figs 13 to 16).

Nonfluorescent frameworks

The optical properties of ceramic cores are influenced by their thickness.[33] Densely sintered ce-

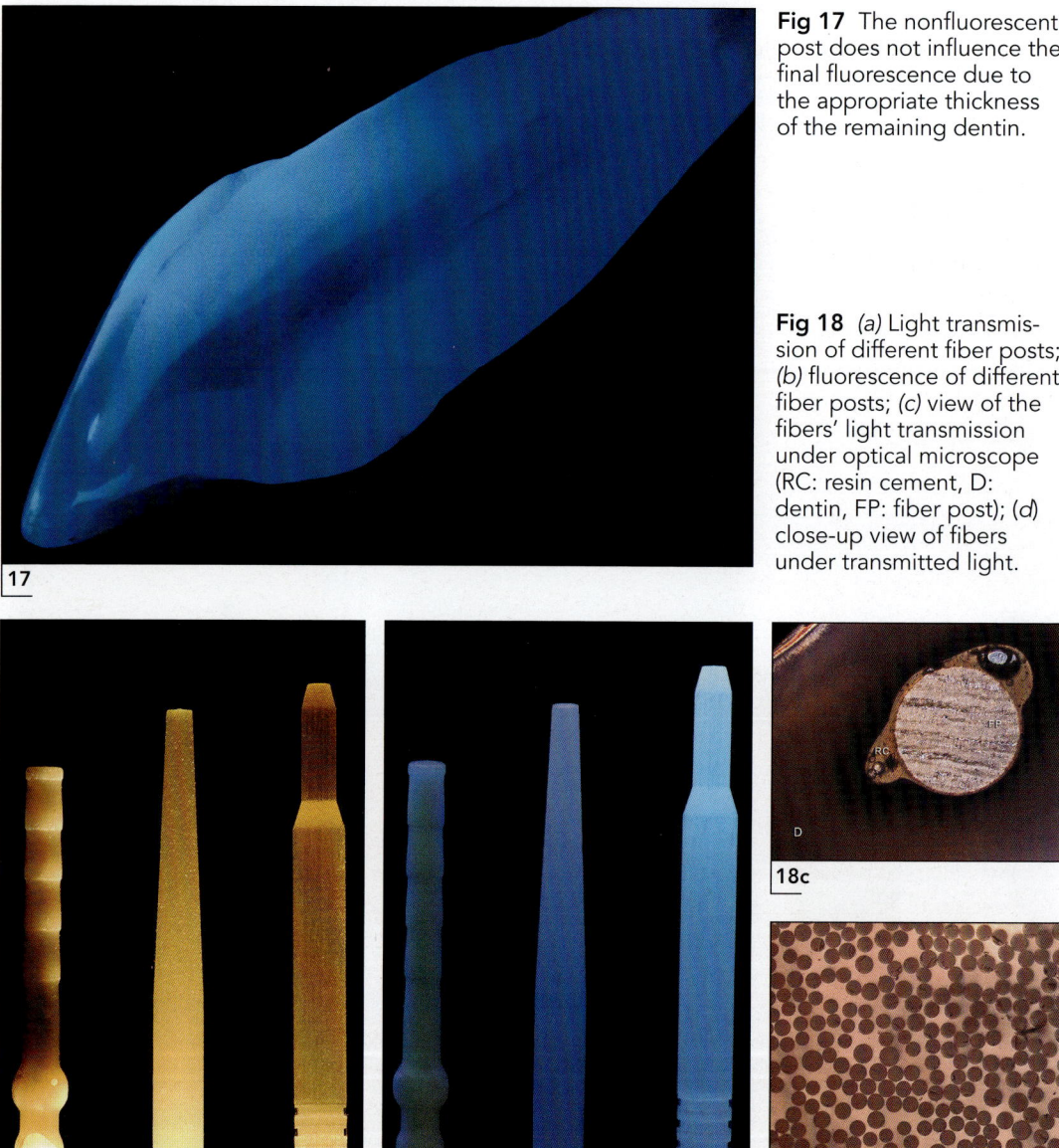

Fig 17 The nonfluorescent post does not influence the final fluorescence due to the appropriate thickness of the remaining dentin.

Fig 18 *(a)* Light transmission of different fiber posts; *(b)* fluorescence of different fiber posts; *(c)* view of the fibers' light transmission under optical microscope (RC: resin cement, D: dentin, FP: fiber post); *(d)* close-up view of fibers under transmitted light.

ramics are less translucent than their silica-based counterparts.[34] To improve light transmission of opaque metallic frameworks, Geller suggested a 2-mm reduction at the gingival margins and subsequent buildup of a highly fluorescent ceramic shoulder. The aforementioned technique has been used with metal, alumina, and zirconia copings with acceptable results (see Figs 7 and 8).[35] Densely sintered ceramics lack fluorescence; as such, it is imperative to fabricate a highly fluores-

cent ceramic shoulder for anterior rehabilitations, especially in patients whose mucosa is less than 1.5-mm thick. Ceramic margins 2-mm thick result in better esthetic compliance with natural tissues (see Figs 7 and 8). Conversely, under transmitted light, when the abutment has no discoloration, the thickness of the shoulder does not influence the translucence.

The association of a discolored abutment and nonfluorescent framework results in lack of translu-

Fig 19 *(a and b)* Alumina coping with 2.0-mm ceramic shoulder. Observe the reduced light transmission and tendency toward gray due to the pigmentation of a dark abutment. *(c and d)* Extended zirconia copings showing the deficient light transmission at the gingival third under transmitted light and fluorescence.

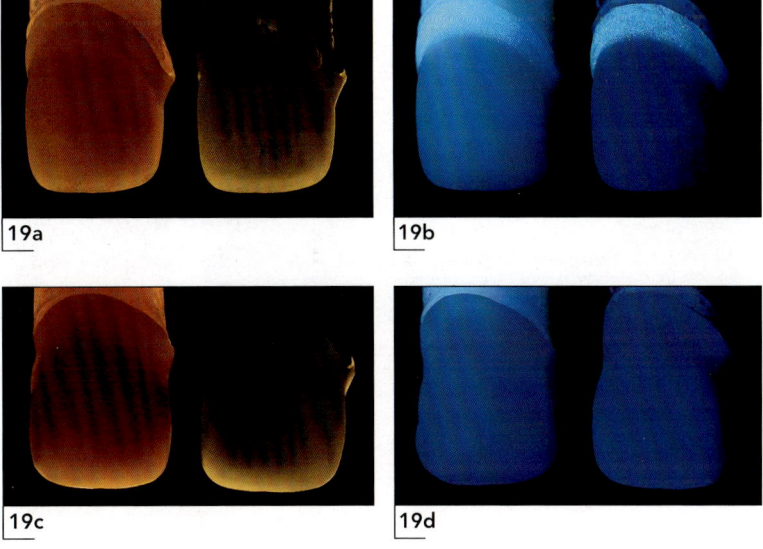

19a
19b
19c
19d

CASE 4 (Figs 20 to 25)

Fig 20 Preoperative view of patient's smile.

Fig 21 Preoperative view showing defective crowns and discolored teeth.

Fig 22 *(a)* Final preparation before impression, *(b)* transillumination of the preparations; *(c)* fluorescence of the preparations. Observe the reduced fluorescence on the gingival third of the right central incisor. Transillumination and fluorescence tests should be performed to preview the potential of hard shadows.

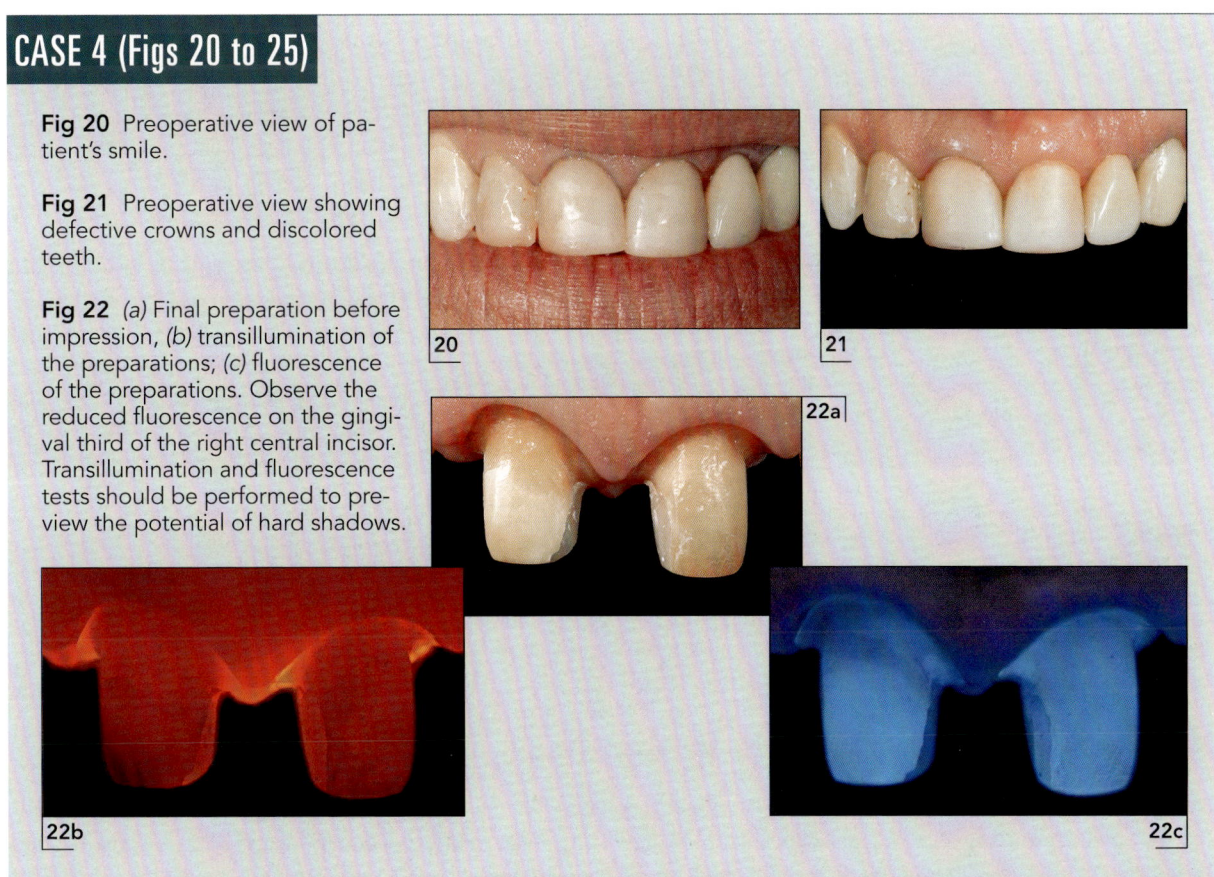

20
21
22a
22b
22c

cence and fluorescence (Figs 19a to 19d), thus generating a hard shadow at the gingival third. A combined approach to improve the optical properties of both abutment and restoration must be attempted to enhance final esthetics as much as possible (Figs 20 to 22). However, the patient should

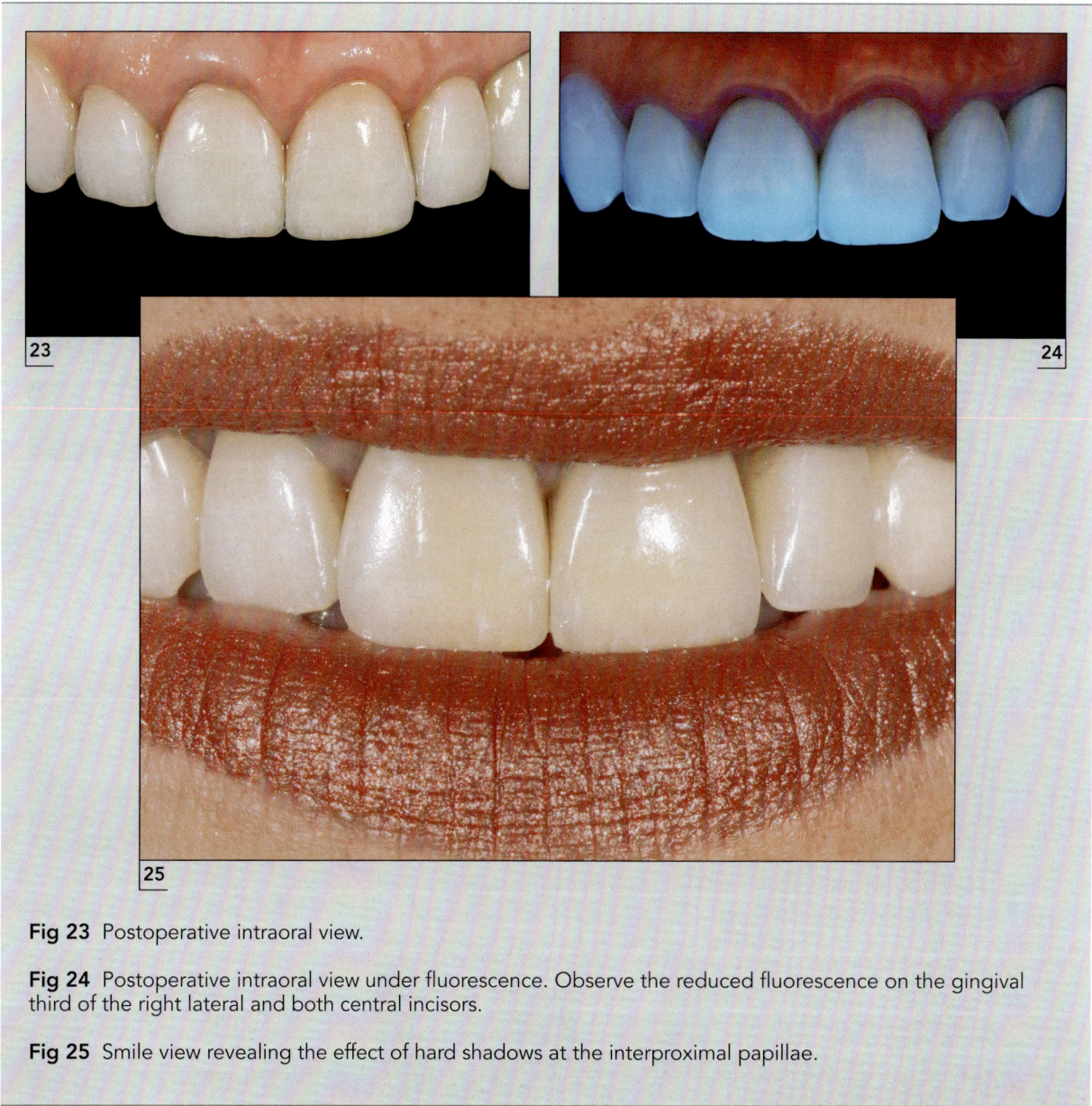

Fig 23 Postoperative intraoral view.

Fig 24 Postoperative intraoral view under fluorescence. Observe the reduced fluorescence on the gingival third of the right lateral and both central incisors.

Fig 25 Smile view revealing the effect of hard shadows at the interproximal papillae.

be informed of the limitations in such situations and the prognosis of the outcome (Figs 23 to 25).

ter esthetic outcomes, while hard shadows must be overcome to produce appropriate results.

CONCLUSION

The light-transmission characteristics of teeth and restorative materials must be examined to allow a fully esthetic integration. Soft shadows allow bet-

ACKNOWLEDGMENTS

The authors thank Mr Patrick Schnider, Oral Design Moutreux, for fabricating the crowns for cases 1, 2, and 4. The authors also thank Jose Carlos Romanini for fabricating the crowns for case 3 and Fabiana Varjão for help with photography.

REFERENCES

1. Hunter F, Fuqua P. Light: Science & Magic: An introduction to photographic lighting. 2nd ed. Newton, MA: Focal Press; 1997.

2. Kiess TE, Shih YH, Sergienko AV, Alley CO. Einstein-Podolsky-Rosen-Bohm experiment using pairs of light quanta produced by type-II parametric down-conversion. Phys Rev Lett 1993;71:3893–3897.

3. Walker B. Behavior of light rays. In: Optical Engineering Fundamentals. Bellingham, WA: SPIE Optical Engineering Press, 1998: 35–42.

4. Rossing TD, Chiavernia CJ. Light Science: Physics and the Visual Arts. New York: Springer, 1999.

5. Ronchi V. The foundations of the science of vision. In: Optics: The Science of Vision. Mineola, NY: Dover, 1991: 67–123.

6. Longair M. Light and colour. In: Lamb TL, Bourriau JB (eds). Colour: Art and Science. Cambridge: Cambridge University Press, 1995: 65–102.

7. Grajower R, Wozniak WT, Lindsay JM. Optical properties of composite resins. J Oral Rehabil 1982;9:389–399.

8. Heymann HO. The artistry of conservative esthetic dentistry. J Am Dent Assoc 1987;Spec No:14E–23E.

9. Lombardi RE. The principles of visual perception and their clinical application to denture esthetics. J Prosthet Dent 1973;29:358–382.

10. Duarte S, Jr., Perdigao J, Lopes M. Composite resin restorations-Natural aesthetic and dynamics of light. Pract Proced Aesthet Dent 2003;15:657–664.

11. Magne P, Magne M, Belser U. The esthetic width in fixed prosthodontics. J Prosthodont 1999;8:106–118.

12. Sadan A. Restoring discolored teeth and missing adjacent teeth. An interview with Konrad H. Meyenberg. Quintessence Dent Technol 2002;25:110–116.

13. Damm DD, Fantasia JE. Diffuse discoloration of teeth. Fluorosis. Gen Dent 2001;49:356, 428.

14. Abou-Rass M. The elimination of tetracycline discoloration by intentional endodontics and internal bleaching. J Endod 1982;8:101–116.

15. Ansari G, Reid JS. Dentinal dysplasia type I: Review of the literature and report of a family. ASDC J Dent Child 1997;64:429–434.

16. Andreasen FM, Zhijie Y, Thomsen BL, Andersen PK. Occurrence of pulp canal obliteration after luxation injuries in the permanent dentition. Endod Dent Traumatol 1987; 3:103–115.

17. Stroner WF, Van Cura JE. Pulpal dystrophic calcification. J Endod 1984;10:202–204.

18. Miara P. Aesthetic treatment of discoloration of nonvital teeth. Pract Periodontics Aesthet Dent 1995;7:79–84.

19. van der Burgt TP, Mullaney TP, Plasschaert AJ. Tooth discoloration induced by endodontic sealers. Oral Surg Oral Med Oral Pathol 1986;61:84–89.

20. Parsons JR, Walton RE, Ricks-Williamson L. In vitro longitudinal assessment of coronal discoloration from endodontic sealers. J Endod 2001;27:699–702.

21. Plasschaert AJ, van der Burgt TP. Teeth discoloration by endodontic materials [in German]. Stomatol DDR 1988;38:161–166.

22. Wirz J. Corrosion, caused by root screws or posts [in German]. Zahnarztl Mitt 1983;73:1346–1349.

23. Wirz J, Johner M, Pohler O. Corrosion behavior of different screws and posts in the root canal [in German]. SSO Schweiz Monatsschr Zahnheilkd 1980;90:217–242.

24. Nakamura T, Saito O, Mizuno M, Kinuta S, Ishigaki S. Influence of abutment substrates on the colour of metal-free polymer crowns. J Oral Rehabil 2003;30:184–188.

25. Takeda T, Ishigami K, Shimada A, Ohki K. A study of discoloration of the gingiva by artificial crowns. Int J Prosthodont 1996;9:197–202.

26. Jung RE, Sailer I, Hämmerle CH, Attin T, Schmidlin P. In vitro color changes of soft tissues caused by restorative materials. Int J Periodontics Restorative Dent 2007; 27:251–257.

27. Dahl JE, Pallesen U. Tooth bleaching: A critical review of the biological aspects. Crit Rev Oral Biol Med 2003;14: 292–304.

28. Dezotti MS, Souza MH, Jr., Nishiyama CK. Evaluation of pH variation and cervical dentin permeability in teeth submitted to bleaching treatment [in Portuguese]. Pesqui Odontol Bras 2002;16:263–268.

29. Friedman S. Internal bleaching: long-term outcomes and complications. J Am Dent Assoc 1997;128:51S–55S.

30. Esberard R, Esberard RR, Esberard RM, Consolaro A, Pameijer CH. Effect of bleaching on the cemento-enamel junction. Am J Dent 2007;20:245–249.

31. Silness J, Gustavsen F, Hunsbeth J. Distribution of corrosion products in teeth restored with metal crowns retained by stainless steel posts. Acta Odontol Scand 1979;37:317–321.

32. Arvidson K, Wróblewski R. Migration of metallic ions from screwposts into dentin and surrounding tissues. Scand J Dent Res 1978;86:200–205.

33. Holloway JA, Miller RB. The effect of core translucency on the aesthetics of all-ceramic restorations. Pract Periodontics Aesthet Dent 1997;9:567–574.

34. Heffernan MJ, Aquilino SA, Diaz-Arnold AM, Haselton DR, Stanford CM, Vargas MA. Relative translucency of six all-ceramic systems. Part I: Core materials. J Prosthet Dent 2002;88:4–9.

35. Yoshida A. All-ceramic restorations: Material selection and opacity control for esthetically superior results. Quintessence Dent Technol 2007;30:87–100.

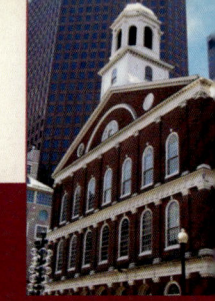
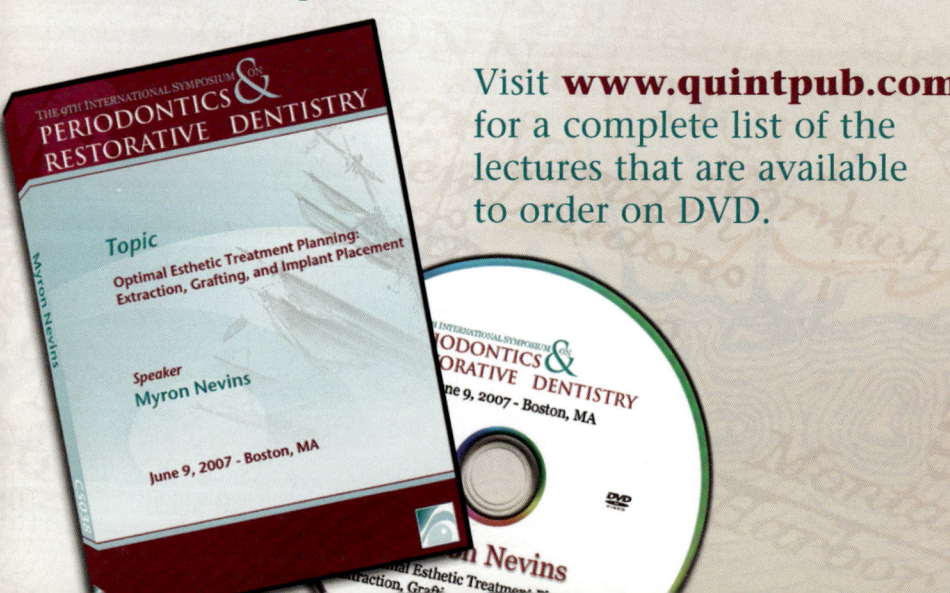

CONTEMPORARY MAXILLARY IMPLANT-SUPPORTED FULL-ARCH RESTORATIONS COMBINING ESTHETICS AND PASSIVE FIT

Peter S. Wöhrle, DMD, MMedSc, CDT (CH)[1]
Donald F. Cornell, CDT[1]

Since the introduction of osseointegrated implants by Branemark,[1,2] the focus of implant-supported restorations has been implant survival and proper function. Initially, the esthetic result was not of primary importance. Recently, however, increasing patient demands and technological advances have led to the development of new techniques to fabricate implant-supported full-arch restorations, especially in the maxilla. These techniques offer more esthetically pleasing prostheses that achieve passive fit and can be repaired within the veneering porcelain if needed.

[1]Private practice, Wöhrle Dental Implant Clinic, Newport Beach, California, USA.

Correspondence to: Dr Peter Wöhrle, Wöhrle Dental Implant Clinic, 360 San Miguel Dr, Suite 601, Newport Beach, CA 92660, USA. E-mail: pswohrle@ix.netcom.com

IMPLANT-SUPPORTED FULL-ARCH RESTORATIONS: PROBLEMS

Passive Fit

A passively fitting framework has been described in the literature as both necessary[3] and difficult to achieve.[4–6] Implant prostheses do not exhibit the same degree of movement compared to the periodontal ligament found around natural teeth[7]; therefore, the techniques employed in conventional dentistry do not work as predictably in implant dentistry. Inaccuracies in implant restorations are the result of a number of factors, including inherent machining tolerances of components,[8] distortion of impression material,[9–12] setting expansion of dental stone,[13,14] expansion and contraction of alloy and wax,[15] expansion of investment material,[16] and distortion of the framework during heat treatment and porcelain application.[17] In addition, misfit is magnified by assembling the restoration on a copy of the patient's mouth (the master cast) rather than on the patient's mouth itself.

Traditionally, these deficiencies have been overcome by using repeated intraoral try-ins and by cutting and soldering the framework prior to veneer application, but studies have shown that soldering does not necessarily improve the fit of implant-supported restorations.[18,19] Further, postsoldering is often technically impossible due to excessive frame dimensions in moderately to severely resorbed cases. Cemented restorations have thus become very popular with clinicians, who use the cement space to increase passive fit compared to screw-retained restorations.[20–22]

Esthetics

Fabricating esthetically pleasing implant-supported full-arch restorations is a difficult task, especially in the maxilla. The loss of hard and soft tissues compromises the esthetic result. Teeth become long and narrow due to the resorption of the residual ridge. In the gingival area, teeth are often curved palatally due to bone loss patterns that reduce bone height and circumference.[23–25] Technically, the sheer magnitude of building a fullarch restoration makes it impossible to achieve the attention to detail that is typically necessary to fabricate a single-tooth restoration. Managing internal and external characterization becomes impossible. Building the crowns in succession will lead to more firings than usual, resulting in large porcelain restorations with a nonvital appearance. Thus, fullarch porcelain restorations are often doomed esthetically before they even begin.

Long-term service and the potential benefits of retrievability are additional factors unique to implant-supported restorations. If any veneering of the restorations fails, the entire restoration is at risk. Once the restoration has been inserted for even a short period of time, it is impossible to repair porcelain fractures by adding porcelain in the oven. The other option is to try to repair the frac-

ture intraorally or in the laboratory with a composite material. Although this option has fewer risks, it is at best a compromise to the overall quality, integrity, longevity, and esthetics of the restoration.

IMPLANT-SUPPORTED FULL-ARCH RESTORATIONS: SOLUTIONS

Altered Framework Design

An altered framework design was developed to address the implant-specific concerns mentioned above: passive fit, artistic freedom, form, function, retrievability, and ability to repair potential porcelain fractures.[26] The concept is based on luting copings intraorally into the framework, thus predictably achieving a passive fit of the cast restoration. In addition, the design principles of building single crowns for improved esthetic results as well as an option for predictable repair were incorporated.

Treatment planning for an implant-supported restoration requires the determination of the ideal vertical dimension, arch form, and occlusal plane of the final prosthesis prior to implant placement.[27] These prosthetic parameters are verified clinically through the evaluation of fixed provisional restorations supported by teeth that will be extracted after the healing phase of the implants or by a complete denture setup in totally edentulous patients. In addition to the established requirements prior to surgical implant placement,[28] the number and location of implants necessary to support the planned restoration are determined. A surgical template incorporating these prosthetic parameters is used to optimize implant placement. While the original protocol used surgical templates derived from common prosthetic principles, today's patient can benefit from computer-aided design/computer-assisted manufacture (CAD/CAM)-generated surgical templates that allow a minimally invasive procedure[29–31] (NobelGuide, Nobel Biocare, Göteborg, Sweden) and immediate function.[29,32,33] Upon soft tissue maturation, a master cast is fabricated. Provisional restorations that have been carefully adjusted to

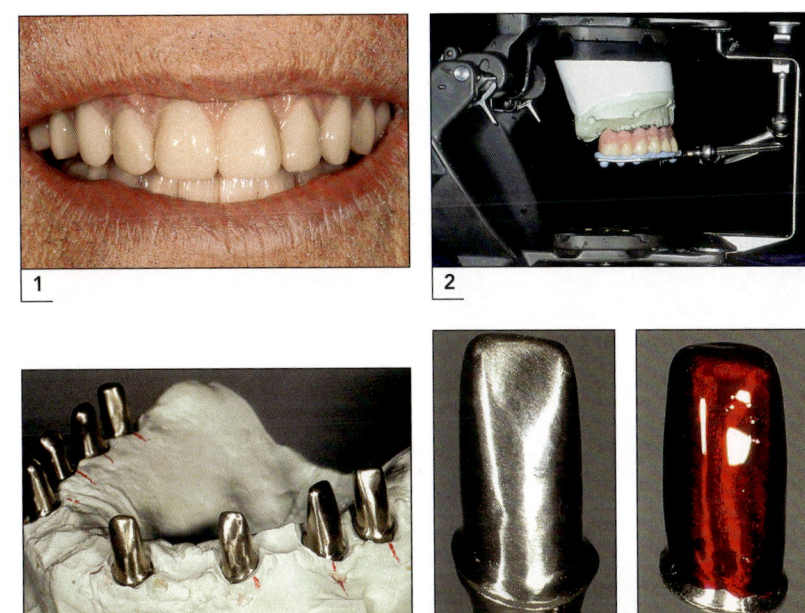

Fig 1 Implant-supported provisional prosthesis used to assess esthetic and phonetic parameters.

Fig 2 The master cast is mounted with a facebow and cross mounted with the maxillary and mandibular arches. While the provisional prosthesis is on the master cast, a silicone index covering the entire restoration is fabricated.

Fig 3 Titanium abutments are milled to a common 2-degree taper. A coping is waxed and cast onto each of these abutments.

Figs 4a and 4b The coping exhibits an intimate fit to the underlying abutment. Prior to fabrication of the suprastructure, die spacer is applied to the axial wall of the copings. The thickness of the die spacer increases with more distal locations of the abutment.

fulfill the prosthetic, phonetic, and esthetic needs of the patient (Fig 1) are necessary because of the complexity and expense associated with a full-arch ceramic restoration. The provisional restoration is used to mount the master cast with standard prosthetic techniques (Fig 2).

Modifiable prefabricated titanium abutments are selected according to the implant angulation and size of the restoration. The location for the finish line is determined based on the esthetic needs and implant location. In the esthetic zone, the abutments are prepared for a 1-mm subgingival finishing line. In the nonesthetic zone, an equi- or supragingival finishing line can be selected. All abutments are prepared to rest within a vacuform template of the diagnostic waxup, milled with a 2-degree taper on a milling machine, and then polished. In addition, grooves or flat areas are incorporated into the abutments to facilitate their transfer to the oral cavity and ensure the exact repositioning of the abutments after transfer.

A coping is fabricated for each milled abutment from wax or from composite material. The copings are finished to a maximum thickness of 0.3 mm.

Special care should be taken to ensure a proper marginal seal. The copings are then invested, cast in gold, and fitted to their respective abutments (Fig 3). A second coping is fabricated from light-cured resin over the cast gold coping. These copings act as spacer copings and are finished to a thickness of 0.2 mm in the anterior region and 0.55 mm in the posterior region (Fig 4). Each spacer coping extends toward the gold coping margin but terminates at the internal line angle of the gold coping's axial wall/shoulder junction. This light-cured spacer is polished but not cast in gold. The spacers are then placed onto their respective cast gold copings, each of which is seated on its milled implant abutment.

Subsequently, a full-arch waxup is fabricated over the gold copings and resin spacers. For frameworks that are to be fabricated with CAD/CAM technology, acrylic resins or composite resins are the materials of choice. Prior to waxing, a separating medium is applied to the acrylic spacers. The waxup re-establishes the ideal tooth length and position and tissue height. Ideally, a silicone index of the provisional restoration on the

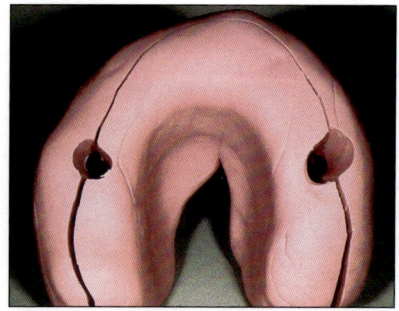

Fig 5 The silicone index of the provisional restoration, seated on the master cast, is split and fitted with vent holes, allowing wax or acrylic pattern resin to be injected.

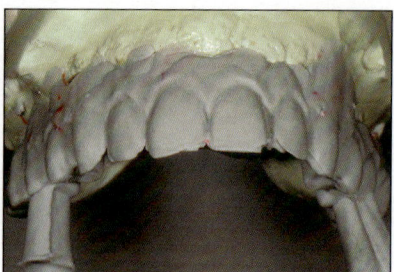

Fig 6 The provisional restoration, which was evaluated intraorally by the patient, is duplicated in either wax or acrylic resin on the master cast to ensure the success of the definitive restoration.

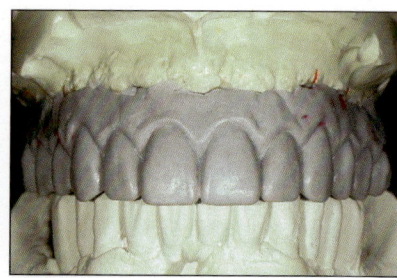

Fig 7 Deficiencies in the contours and details are corrected, and vent holes are eliminated. The prosthetic parameters that were established intraorally with the provisional restoration have been transferred successfully to the master cast.

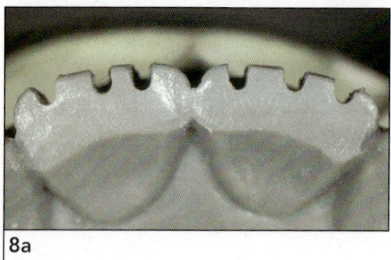

8a

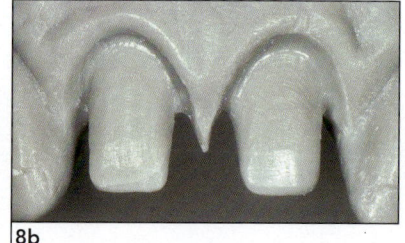

8b

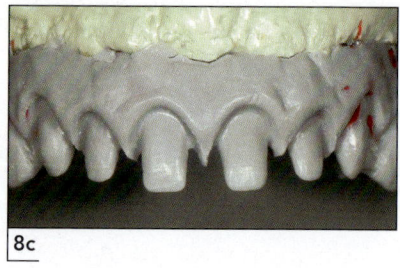

8c

Figs 8a to 8c The full contour waxup is prepared. The tooth portion of the restoration is effectively a preparation of the individual tooth, providing adequate reduction, resistance, and retention. Care should be taken to mimic the desired gingival height and contour. Once all teeth have been prepared to receive a crown, the tissue portion of the framework is reduced. The amount and form of preparation depends on the veneering material.

master cast was obtained during the mounting appointment (Figs 5 to 7). Alternatively, a vacuform or other index of the verified provisional prosthesis can be secured to the cast and filled with wax. This waxup should be executed precisely since it determines the final size, shape, and position of the prosthesis and is verified by cross mounting of the opposing dentition with the provisional restoration and waxup.

Each tooth is prepared in wax as if it were a real tooth to establish the ideal preparation for each individual crown. All preparations extend slightly into the tissue waxup (Fig 8). After preparation of all teeth, the tissue waxup is also cut back. The tissue is reduced until only a minimal framework is left. The framework is recontoured around the implant abutments and measures approximately 0.3 mm in thickness around the abutments. The wax framework is adapted to the margin of each cast

gold coping. Subsequently, the individual tooth preparations are redefined.

The framework can be cast as a single piece (Fig 9) or in multiple segments. Once the waxup is removed from the cast, a pair of tweezers is used to remove each cast gold coping and acrylic spacer from the inside of the frame (Fig 10).

The framework is cast in alloy, onto which porcelain can be baked. After casting, the framework is checked on the master cast (Fig 11). If the full arch was cast in one piece, the acrylic spacers should be removed from the gold copings before seating them on the master cast. The gold copings are placed on the proper abutments, and the full-arch casting is placed over the assembly on the master cast. The casting should fit loosely over each abutment and coping. If an adequate fit is not achieved, the inside of the framework should be adjusted until a passive fit is evident.

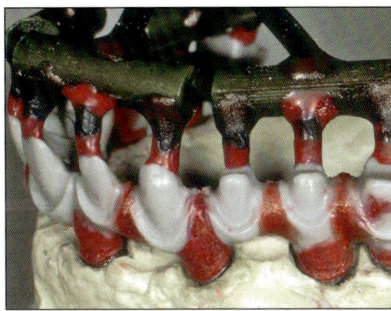

Fig 9 The framework is sprued on the master cast. This can be done in a single piece or in sections. Alternatively, a screw-retained framework can be scanned for CAD/CAM production.

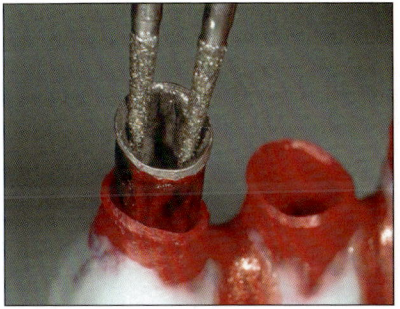

Fig 10 Prior to investing the framework, the individual copings are removed.

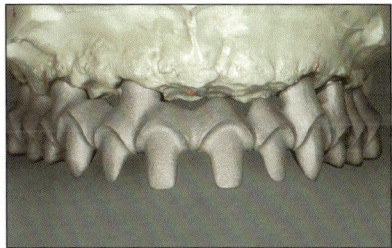

Fig 11 When seated on the master cast, the framework should exhibit passive, loose fit when the copings are seated on the appropriate abutments, with the die spacer removed.

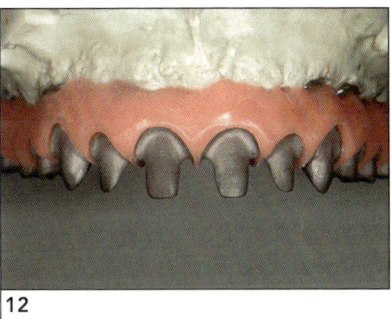

12

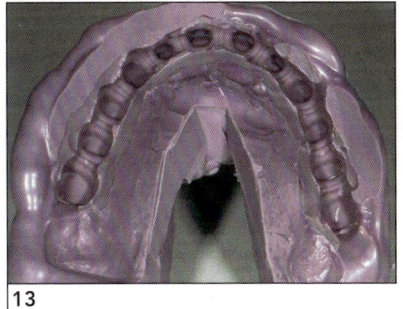

13

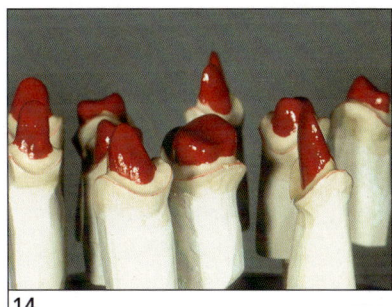

14

Fig 12 The tissue-receiving portion of the framework is waxed up to block out the undercuts and develop the emergence profile around the crowns.

Fig 13 Full-arch impression of the framework seated on the master cast.

Fig 14 Individual dies for all crowns are fabricated using the traditional methods. Copings can be fabricated using traditional or CAD/CAM techniques.

Fig 15 Individual copings seated on the master cast.

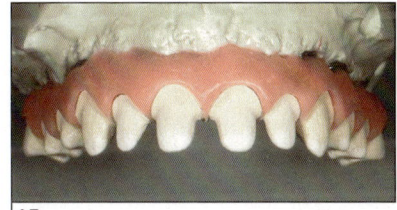

15

Once the fit has been evaluated, the framework is finished and prepared to receive porcelain in the tissue areas apical to the crown margins. The tissue portion is waxed back onto the framework to achieve the ideal contours. The waxed tissue will serve two purposes: (1) it will aid in the proper contouring of the crown buildups, and (2) it will block out potential undercuts in the metal framework when an impression of the framework seated on the master cast is made (Fig 12). The impression, made with standard impression material for fixed partial dentures (Fig 13), is poured in improved die stone. Individual dies of each preparation are then prepared (Fig 14).

From this point on, the fabrication of the definitive restoration is comparable to traditional restorations. A full arch of individual copings is fabricated to fit the stone dies. Each coping is opaqued in its appropriate shade. Porcelain margin material is applied circumferentially to each coping (360 degrees), even though the metal copings have not been prepared to receive a conventional porcelain margin. It is a decisive advantage to use these materials in the marginal area to optimize the esthetic result. The opaqued copings with the porcelain margins are then returned to the original metal framework (Fig 15).

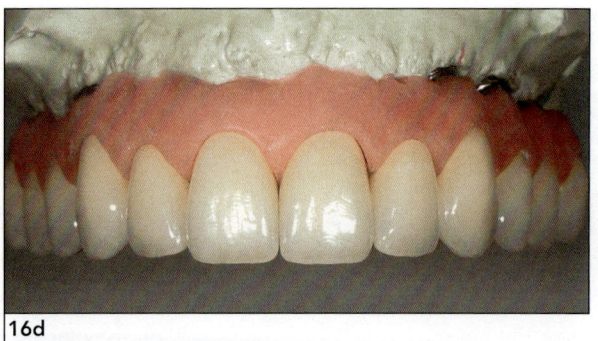

16d

Fig 16 Individual crowns are fabricated for the entire arch. Note the artistic detail and vibrancy of the porcelain.

Figs 17a to 17c Various pink porcelain shades are applied to the buildup to mimic the natural tissue color and overall gingival appearance.

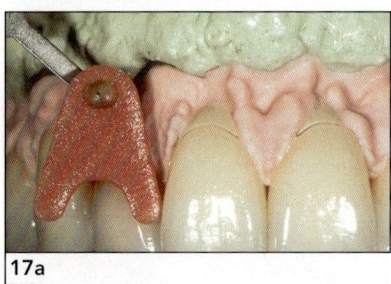

17a

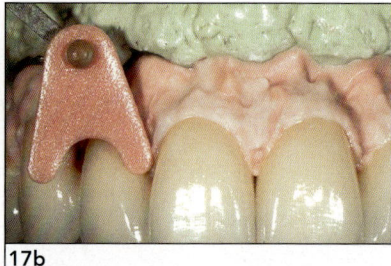

17b

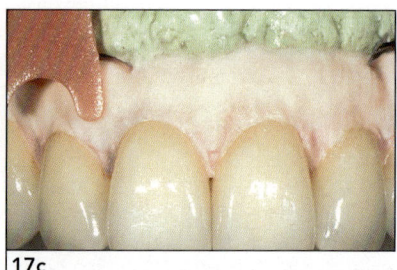

17c

At this stage, each coping receives its porcelain buildup. This allows the crowns to be fabricated individually, thus maintaining maximum artistic freedom (Fig 16). Once all crowns are fired and contoured, they are ready to be glazed. Prior to glazing, it is recommended to proceed with at least one tissue-porcelain firing. For this purpose, the crowns are removed from the framework and the wax simulating the tissue is boiled off. The tissue portion of the frame is then opaqued. A ceramic separating pen is used to insulate the gingival areas of the crowns so that the gingival porcelain will not stick to the crowns upon removal. The tissue porcelains are then applied from the margins of the framework approximately 0.5 mm above the height of each crown margin (Fig 17). Once all tissue porcelain is applied and contours are evaluated, each crown is lifted off the framework without disturbing the surrounding tissue buildup. The frame is then placed on a tray and fired in the porcelain oven.

After firing, the crowns are placed back on the framework, and the process of applying tissue porcelain is repeated a second time to finalize the tissue contours. In some cases, a third firing may

be necessary depending on the amount of porcelain shrinkage. The preglazed crowns are placed onto the tissue frame. All crown and tissue contours are then evaluated for proper shape and emergence profile, recontoured if necessary, glazed, and polished with pumice. Each crown is returned to the tissue frame to evaluate the contours and the size of the gap between the gingival crown contour and the adjacent tissue porcelain. If this space is too large, corrections can be carried out using low-fusing porcelain to minimize the gap. If an anatomic buildup of the tissue porcelain was executed, little or no grinding will be necessary. A low-temperature glaze firing of the tissue porcelain is carried out. Polishing is then carried out with a rubber wheel and pumice. Now, the tissue framework is ready to receive the individual ceramic restorations (Fig 18).

Each tooth preparation is in metal, as is the inside of each crown. The remaining exposed metal preparations and the inside of the crowns are silicoated to facilitate bonding between the framework and the crowns. The individual crowns are luted to the framework using an appropriate resin-based luting agent (Panavia TC, Panavia, Japan).

Figs 18a and 18b Prior to crown cementation, the application of porcelain to simulate the gingival tissues is completed. For screw-retained restorations, a decision must be made by the restorative dentist whether the screw access holes will be extended through the crowns in the laboratory or if the framework will first be seated intraorally.

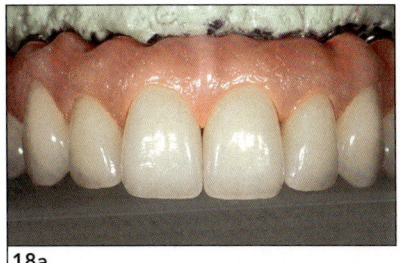

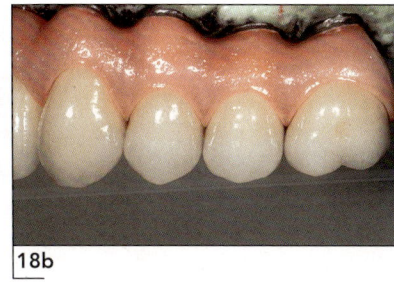

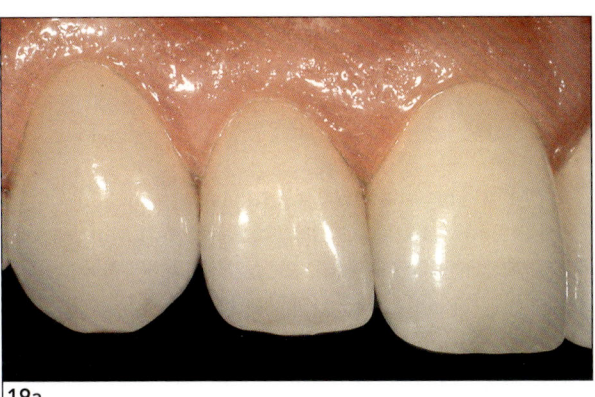

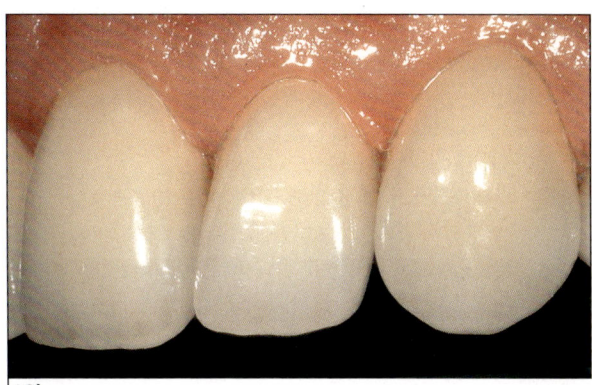

Figs 19a to 19c Full-arch porcelain restoration after cementation of individual crowns to the framework. This approach allows complete control of the most important esthetic and functional parameters.

The luting agent will flow into the gap between the tissue, porcelain, and crowns, and any excess should be removed before the curing is completed.

Once the luting agent is set, the inhibitor is removed and excess material is trimmed away. This process is repeated until all crowns are luted to the framework. The composite margin at the crown-tissue interface should be so small that it is clinically irrelevant. Using appropriate luting agents will enhance the illusion that the crowns are growing naturally from the ceramic tissue. All composite margins around the individual crowns are then polished (Fig 19).

Passive fit of the completed restoration is achieved by assembling it directly in the patient's mouth as opposed to on the master cast. The milled abutments are seated on their respective implants, oriented to coincide with the master cast, and tightened to the manufacturer's recom-

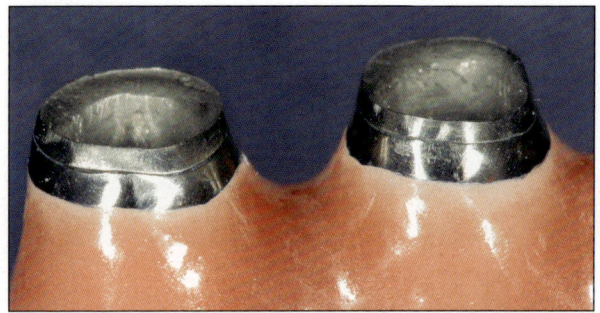

Fig 20 After cementation of the copings into the framework intraorally, the prosthesis is removed to facilitate cement removal. This close-up photograph reveals the minimal cementation line, representing the total distortion from impression making to delivery of the prosthesis.

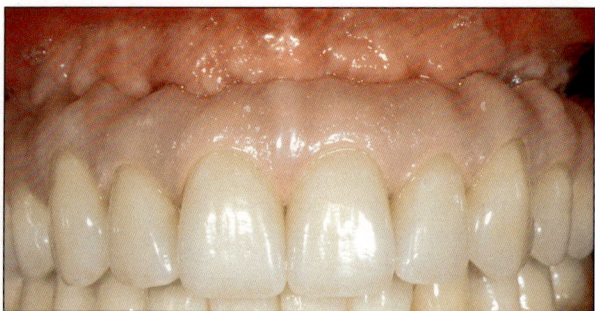

Fig 21 Full-arch porcelain restoration seated in the mouth.

mended torque. The gold copings are transferred to the mouth. The framework is seated over the abutment-coping assembly, and complete and passive fit is verified. If the framework does not seat completely, the interfering area is identified and adjusted accordingly. Subsequently, the internal aspects of the tissue framework containing the implant abutments and external aspect of the gold copings are silicoated and silanated. Three copings—one anterior coping and the two distal copings—that form a broad-based triangle are identified for the first luting cycle. The corresponding internal housings within the framework are filled with the luting agent (Twin Lock, Hereaus Kulzer, Irvine, California) and placed intraorally. The prosthesis is completely seated using finger pressure, and excess luting agent is removed with a brush and an explorer. Adequate fit of the framework over the gold copings and implant abutments is verified before a curing light is used to achieve initial setting. After 10 minutes, the dual-cure resin cement should be completely cured, and the framework is removed from the patient's mouth, including the three gold copings that now are an integral part of the framework. Excess cement is removed in the laboratory, and the luting process is repeated multiple times, incorporating two to four copings at any one time until all copings have been luted into the framework (Fig 20).

The result is a prosthesis with a totally passive fit because the components were assembled in-

traorally. The internal adaptation of each cast coping fits intimately with its implant abutment, assuring excellent marginal adaptation and coping retention. The acrylic spacers, which were placed between each coping and the framework during the initial waxup and soldering procedures, compensate for any discrepancies in the accuracy of the master cast and subsequent casting and porcelain applications. Luting these copings intraorally results in a totally passive framework with maximum retention. The prosthesis is cemented with temporary cement after the abutment screw access has been sealed. It can be retrieved at any time if necessary (Fig 21).

The resulting prosthesis satisfies the original criteria: an implant-supported full-arch restoration with a completely passive fit that allows maximum artistic freedom while re-establishing the harmony and proportions between the teeth and supporting structures (Figs 22 and 23).

If fracture of a porcelain crown is observed (Fig 24), it can be handled as if it were a single-tooth restoration. The crown is cut off the framework intraorally, the site is reprepared, and an impression is made. Then, a new coping and crown can be fabricated, tried in, and luted to the framework (Figs 25 and 26). A conventional provisional restoration can be fabricated for the prepared abutment during the fabrication of the new ceramic crown.

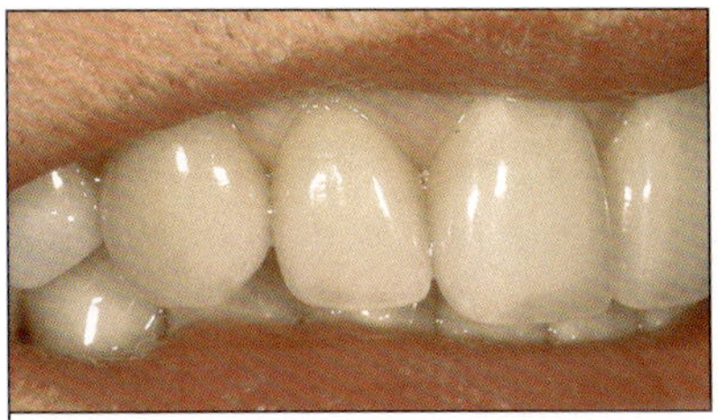

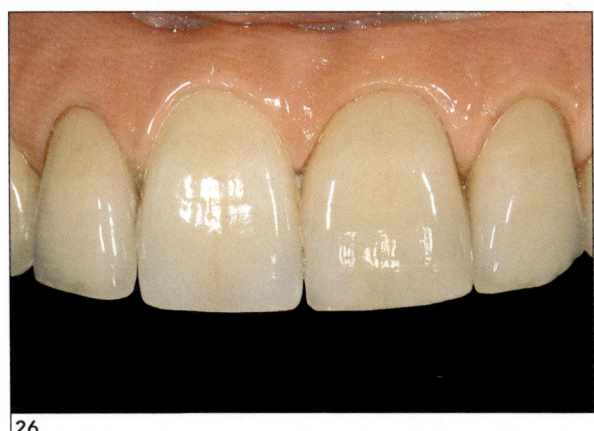

22a

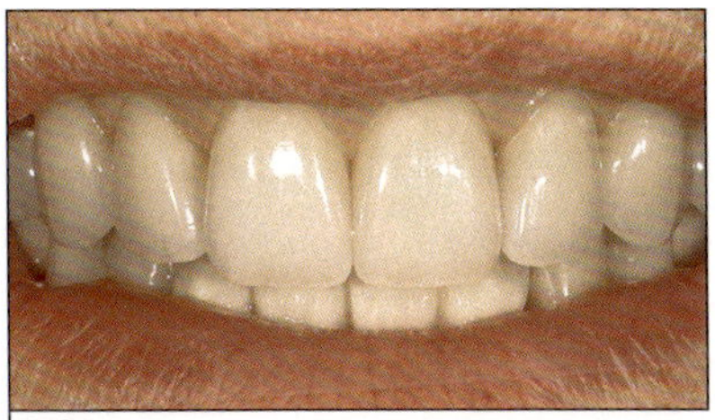

22b

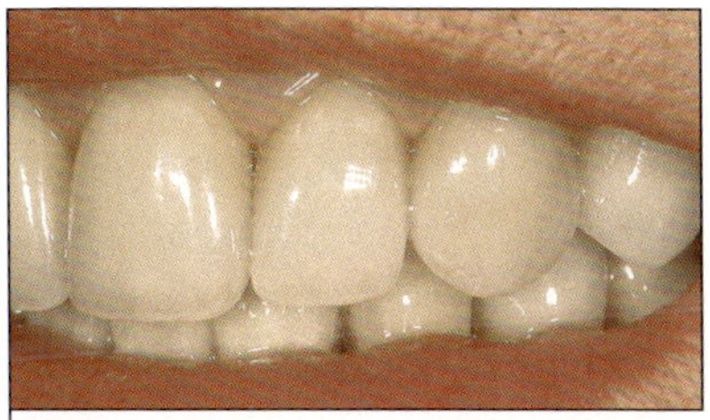

22c

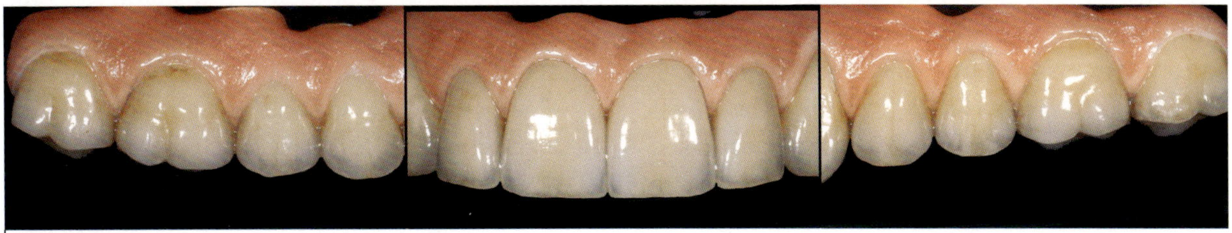

23

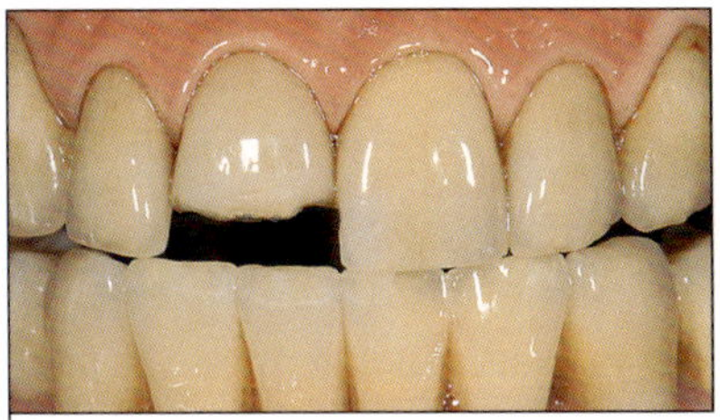

24

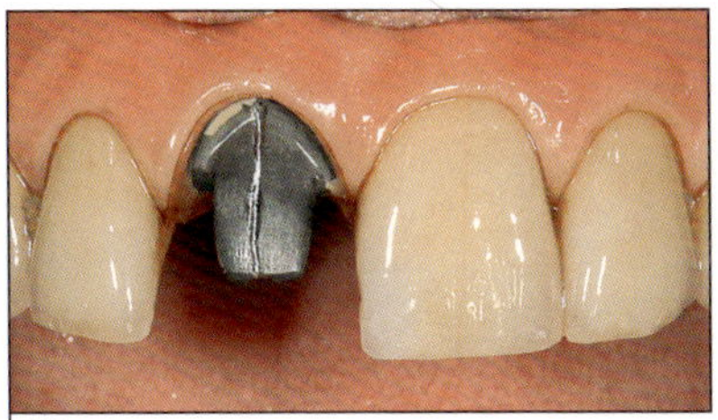

25a

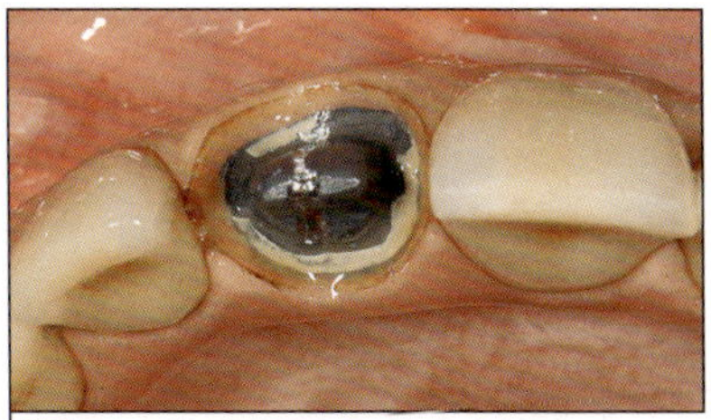

25b

26

Figs 22a to 22c Final result. Note the duplication of the tooth position, height and form of the gingival contours, and lip support compared to the provisional restoration (see Fig 1).

Fig 23 The fully assembled framework prior to insertion. Note the artistic coloration and attention to detail of the teeth and soft tissues.

Fig 24 Thirteen years after insertion, the patient presented with a fractured right central incisor.

Figs 25a and 25b Without removing the prosthesis, the crown is cut off and impressions are made for a new crown.

Fig 26 A new crown is cemented intraorally, thus repairing an otherwise catastrophic porcelain fracture quickly and predictably.

Computerized Treatment Planning and Implant Placement

The outcome of the prosthetic reconstruction is greatly improved by the use of computerized treatment planning[30,34,35] (three-dimensional computerized tomography scan) and implant placement[32,36] (NobelGuide). The implants can be placed in the most favorable positions, and the surgical procedure can be carried out faster, less invasively, and more precisely.[34] Adequate transmucosal exit points, coronal-apical depth, mesiodistal spacing, and implant angulations can be predetermined and transferred exactly to the surgical field. This ensures that the definitive prosthetic reconstruction will be executed to the highest standards, with minimal interferences from screw holes, adequate embrasures, and avoidance of implants when they would interfere with the esthetic emergence profiles and adequate anteroposterior spread.[32] Prefabricated fixed prostheses, produced from the surgical template, can be inserted immediately after implant placement.[36–38] During the past decade, the ideal number of implants used to restore a full arch has decreased steadily. Today, four to six implants seem adequate to predictably support an entire arch.[37] This reduced number not only allows for a decreased treatment time and cost,[39,40] but also allows patients to receive a fixed implant-supported dentition that is comparable in cost to a bar-retained overdenture on four implants, with less long-term maintenance.

CAD/CAM Framework Design

CAD/CAM technology has revolutionized dentistry. One of the most beneficial improvements was the development of techniques allowing for the fabrication of a passively fitting, screw-retained framework on a master cast.[41–43] As discussed above, large metal frameworks that needed to be cast often did not fit adequately.[17] For frameworks receiving porcelain veneering materials, additional firings induced more distortion of the framework, often resulting in a clinically unacceptable prosthesis.

Thus, techniques were developed to circumvent most of the issues associated with elaborate laboratory and clinical procedures.[39] With the introduction of CAD/CAM technology, it is now possible to have a precise, perfectly fitting framework milled from one piece of titanium or zirconium oxide.[44–46] It is important to realize that this passive fit is dependent upon an accurate master cast, and that any inaccuracies during master cast fabrication are incorporated into the framework.

Today, the practitioner has two choices when it comes to framework substrate: titanium or zirconium oxide. A titanium framework is used most often as a supporting structure for prefabricated teeth that are processed onto the framework or as a substructure to receive individual, cemented ceramic crowns.[47] A zirconium oxide framework is the framework of choice for an all-ceramic restoration, when the porcelain is either applied directly to the zirconium framework for a direct buildup or when individual crowns are fabricated over the framework and either pressed or cemented onto it.

The choice of framework material is based on esthetic needs of the patient, financial considerations, and technical specifications of the materials, such as length of cantilevers and framework-connector dimensions.

Basic Implant-Supported Full-Arch Restorations

A CAD/CAM-generated titanium framework (Procera Implant Bridge Titanium, Nobel Biocare) supporting prefabricated composite or acrylic resin teeth and veneered with acrylic resin is the most proven and cost-effective way to restore full-arch implant cases.[40] The commercially pure titanium grade 2 framework is milled from a single block of titanium, duplicating a resin framework that is essentially fabricated according to the principles discussed above. The framework needs to be designed in such a way that it maintains adequate height and width of the titanium for strength and shows adequate retention and resistance to support the veneering materials. Such frameworks exhibit excellent fit[44] and provide long-term satisfactory service.[40] With adequate planning and execution, the orofacial width can be maintained at an acceptable minimum even when the resorption of the residual ridge has progressed.

Advanced Implant-Supported Full-Arch Restorations

Some patients desire a more esthetic restoration using customized, hand-made porcelain crowns

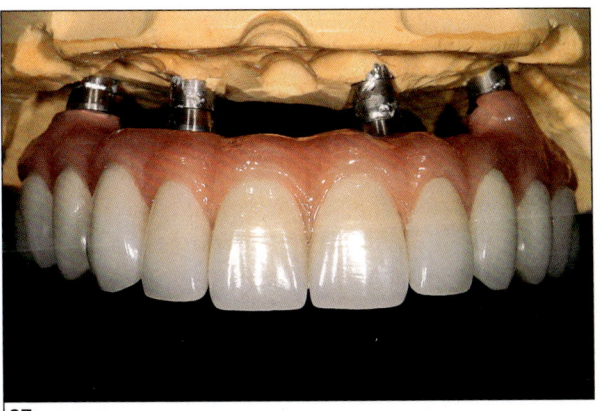

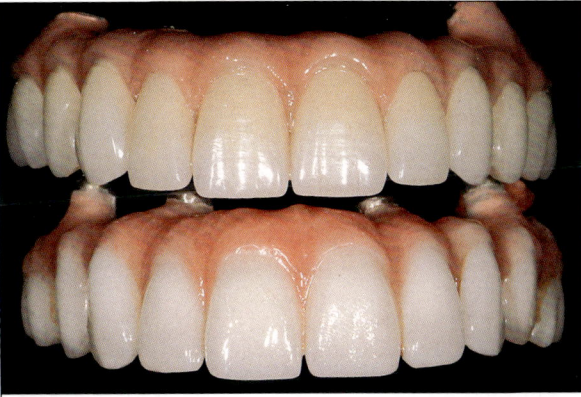

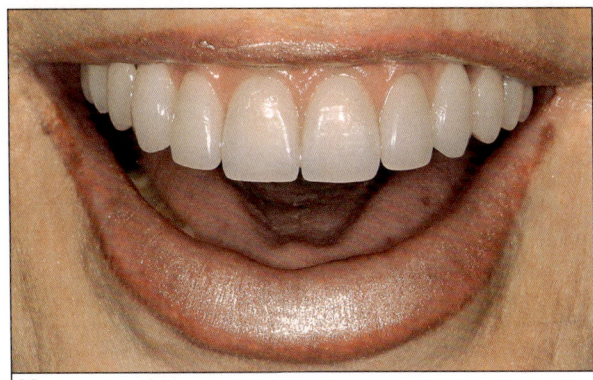

Fig 27 "All-on-Four" implant-supported restoration with individual all-ceramic restorations. (Ceramist: Dr Dario Adolfi).

Fig 28 The final restoration is an exact copy of the provisional restoration.

Fig 29 Final smile view.

Fig 30 Acrylic resin framework prior to scanning and CAD/CAM production. The preparations for individual crowns are inspected for sufficient facial clearance with a silicone key. (Ceramist: Dr Dario Adolfi.)

Fig 31 The acrylic resin framework is checked for sufficient interarch clearance on the articulator.

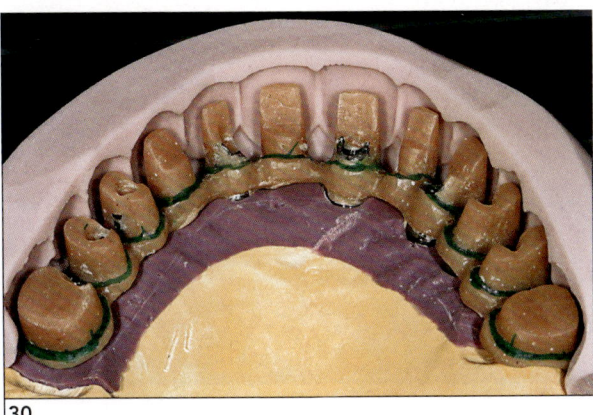

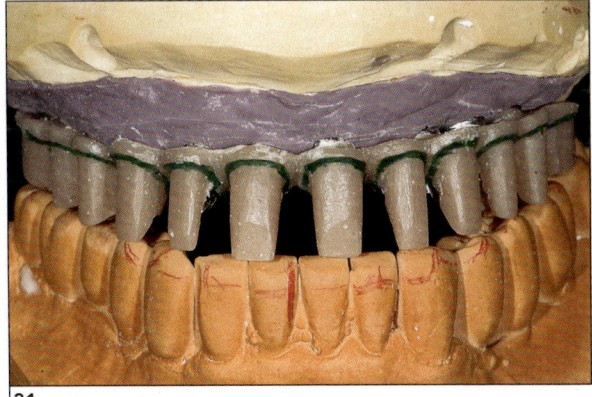

rather than prefabricated teeth. To satisfy this demand, the altered framework design,[26] incorporating individual single crowns onto a framework, has been modified to provide both passive fit and superior esthetics (Figs 27 to 29).[47] A screw-retained, milled titanium framework (Procera Implant Bridge Titanium) is used to support the crowns and tissue portion. The choice of veneering material for the tissue portion consists of either acrylic resin or composite materials. Should any changes in residual ridge morphology occur during the lifetime of the restoration, it can be easily adjusted by adapting the pontic area to the new clinical situation.

The technical aspects are similar to the altered framework design. After impression, facebow, and cross-mounting procedures, a provisional restoration is used as the guide to fabricate an acrylic or composite resin framework (Figs 30 and 31) with

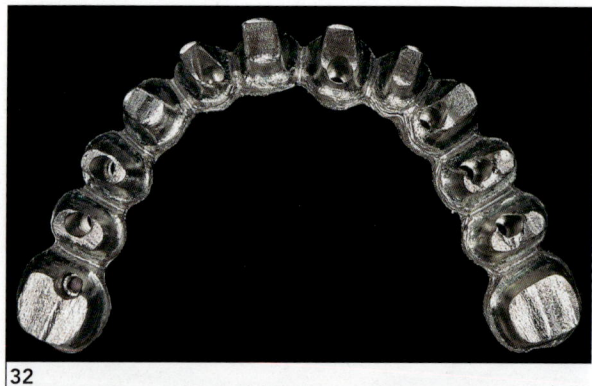

Fig 32 The milled titanium prosthesis is returned to the laboratory after production.

Figs 33 and 34 The crown preparations are opaqued, the gingival contours are re-established, and undercuts are eliminated.

Figs 35 and 36 Individually fabricated crowns on the framework prior to cementation and tissue application.

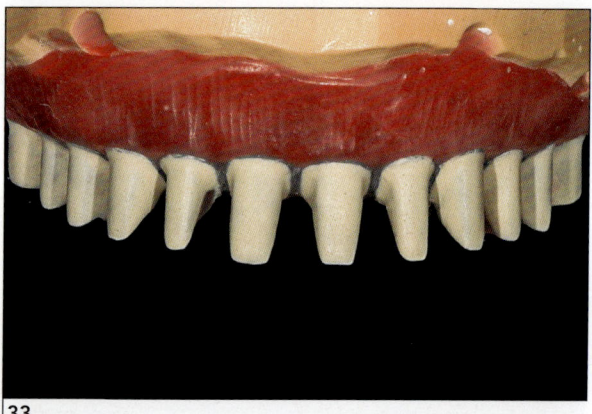

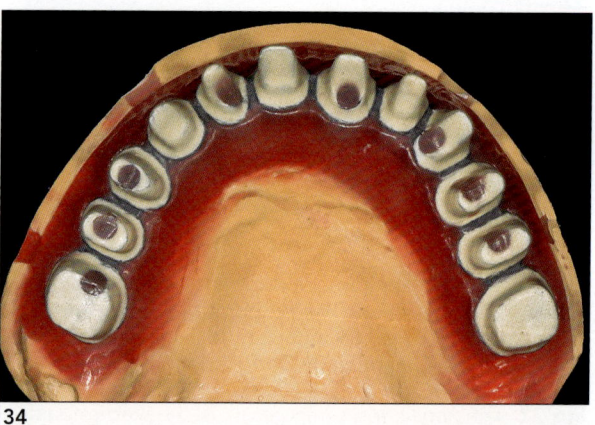

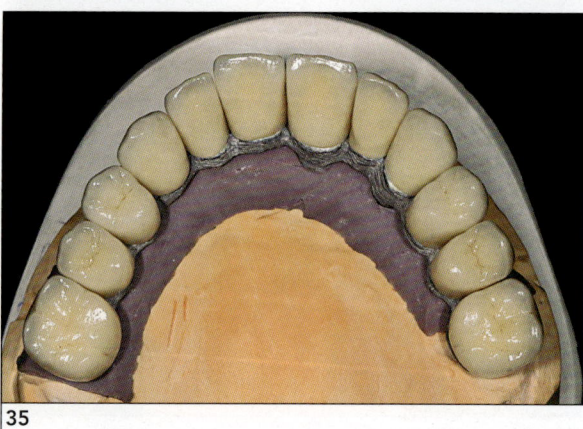

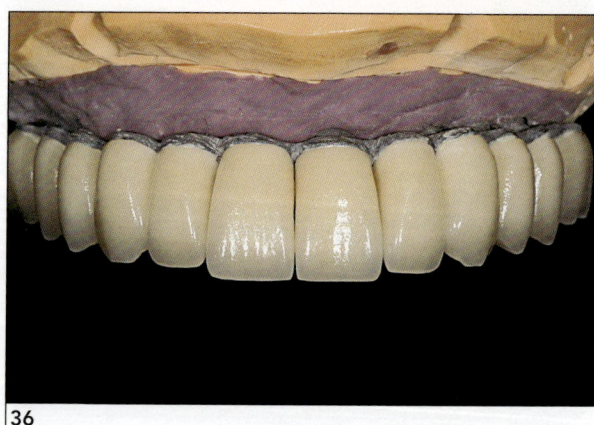

individual tooth preparations for each single crown. The framework is prepared for CAD/CAM procedures and returned to the laboratory (Fig 32). Individual all-ceramic copings (Procera, Nobel Biocare) are fabricated using zirconium oxide (Figs 33 to 36) and veneered with the appropriate porcelain system (NobelRondo, Nobel Biocare). If the restoration is designed as a fully retrievable prosthesis, access holes to the underlying screw channel are incorporated into the crowns after cemen-

tation (Fig 37). Once all tooth portions of the prosthesis are finished, attention should be directed toward the tissue-simulating areas. These can either be processed with acylic resin materials or built up in composite resin. The usual guidelines for designing the ridge-prosthesis contact areas apply: ovate pontic design in edentulous areas, interproximal access for proximal brushes (Fig 38), and high polishing or glazing. Upon completion, the prosthesis is ready for delivery (Fig 39).

Fig 37 Screw access holes are incorporated into all crowns for full retrievability.

Figs 38a to 38c For ideal implant placement in maxillary full-arch restorations, no implants should be placed in the incisor region. Ovate pontic design should be used in edentulous areas to provide adequate space for interproximal brushes.

Fig 39 Intraoral view of the definitive prosthesis.

Fig 40 Maxillary and mandibular provisional restorations. Note that no implants are placed in the maxillary incisor region.

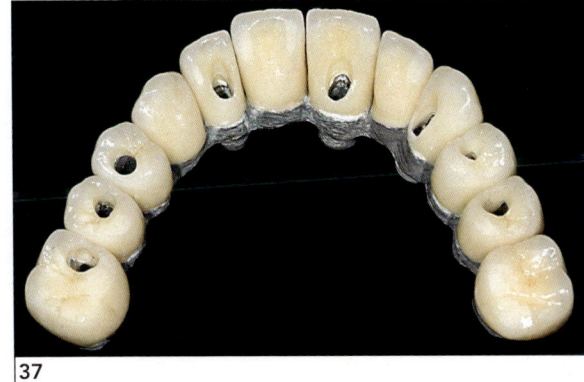

37

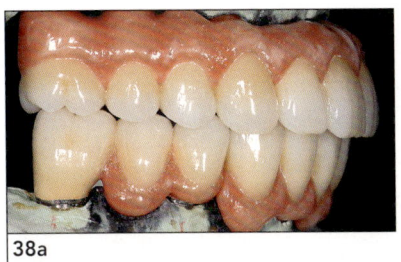

38a

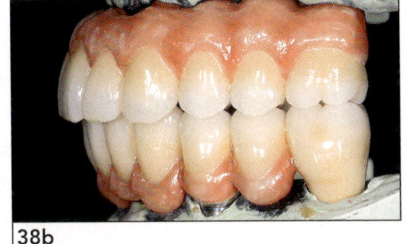

38b

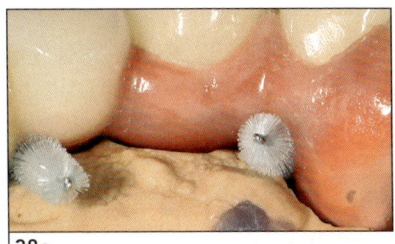

38c

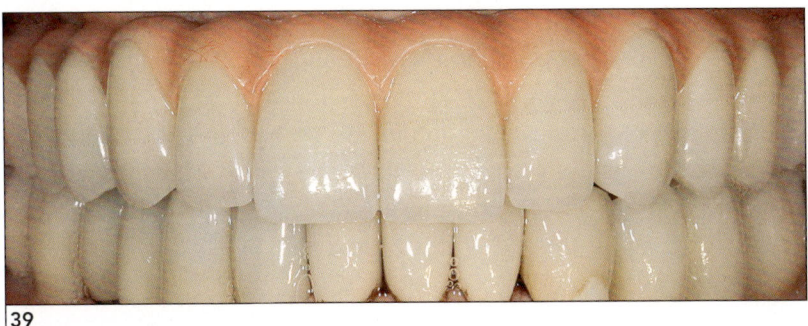

39

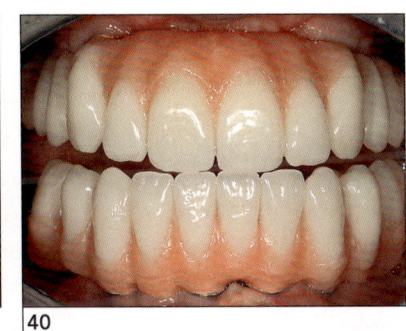

40

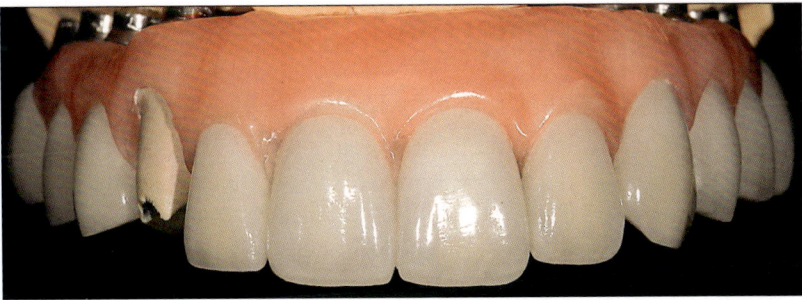

Fig 41 Definitive maxillary porcelain restoration, which required one crown (canine) to be cemented postdelivery. (Ceramist: Dr Dario Adolfi.)

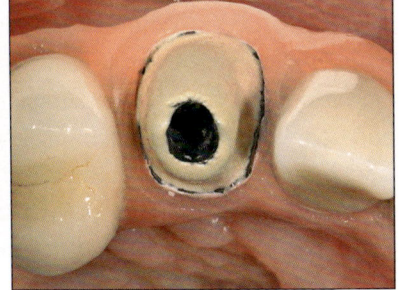

Fig 42 Occlusal view of the framework after delivery and prior to cementation of the canine crown. This framework design exhibits limited retrievability.

This type of restoration can also be designed with limited retrievability by placing the screw access holes within the confines of the crown. To remove the framework, the screw channel must be accessed by grinding through the porcelain, or the crown can be cemented with a nonhardening cement to allow for removal (Figs 40 to 42). Unless the screw channel undermines the porcelain and puts it

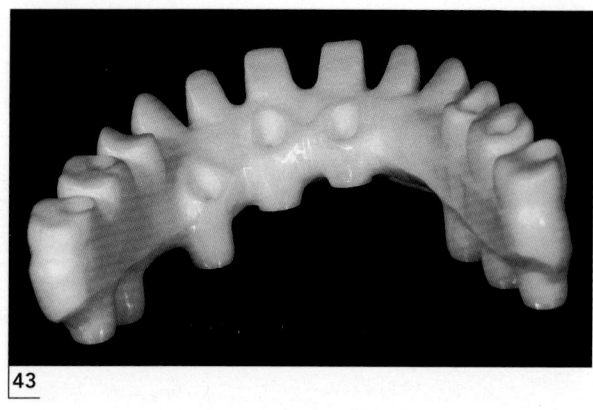

43

Fig 43 Framework milled from one piece of zirconium oxide. (Ceramist: Mr Ernst A. Hegenbarth.)

at risk for fracture, it is advisable to carry the screw channel though the occlusal surface for easy access. With all-ceramic crowns, obliteration of the access hole can be accomplished predictably with composite materials without impairing the esthetic result.

State-of-the-Art Implant-Supported Full-Arch Restorations

Currently, the most technologically advanced fixed implant-supported full-arch prosthesis is the Procera Implant Bridge Zirconia (Nobel Biocare), with individual pressed or layered porcelain for the teeth and pink porcelain for the tissue portions of the framework.

The process is very similar to the previous laboratory protocols. When fabricating a zirconium framework, factors that need to be addressed include length of cantilevers (maximum one tooth) and connector height. Also, to benefit from the superior soft tissue compatibility of zirconium, the areas in contact with the residual ridge are left in machined zirconium oxide and are not veneered with porcelain.

After the framework has been duplicated and cut back as previously described, it is inspected for adequate bulk and sufficient connector strength. Then it is scanned and milled from one piece of zirconium oxide (Fig 43). After the machining process, the framework is tried in to verify the fit and occlusal relationships. The technician has the choice of either building the crowns directly with the appropriate porcelain on the zirco-

nium oxide (NobelRondo Zirconia, Nobel Biocare) or fabricating zirconium copings for individual crown fabrication, which are cemented onto the framework at a later stage. In some cases, both techniques can be used on the same framework. The soft tissue portion of the framework is veneered with gingival ceramic (Fig 44). The result is a beautiful, strong, and well-fitting full-arch restoration (Figs 45 and 46). If individual crowns were used on the framework, any porcelain fracture in the future can be handled as a simple single-crown replacement, which prevents facing a catastrophic failure that may require re-fabricating the entire prosthesis.

CONCLUSIONS

With today's advances in dental materials and technology, numerous options are available to fabricate implant-supported full-arch restorations. CAD/CAM implant planning, implant placement, and framework fabrication have increased the predictability of outcomes while reducing patient discomfort and treatment time. Well-fitting screw-retained frameworks fabricated using titanium or zirconium oxide are readily available and exhibit sufficient fit and strength. Material selection should be based on each patient's esthetic demands and financial considerations. Techniques exist that not only provide esthetics and function in the present, but also anticipate fractures of porcelain in years to come by providing solutions for repair.

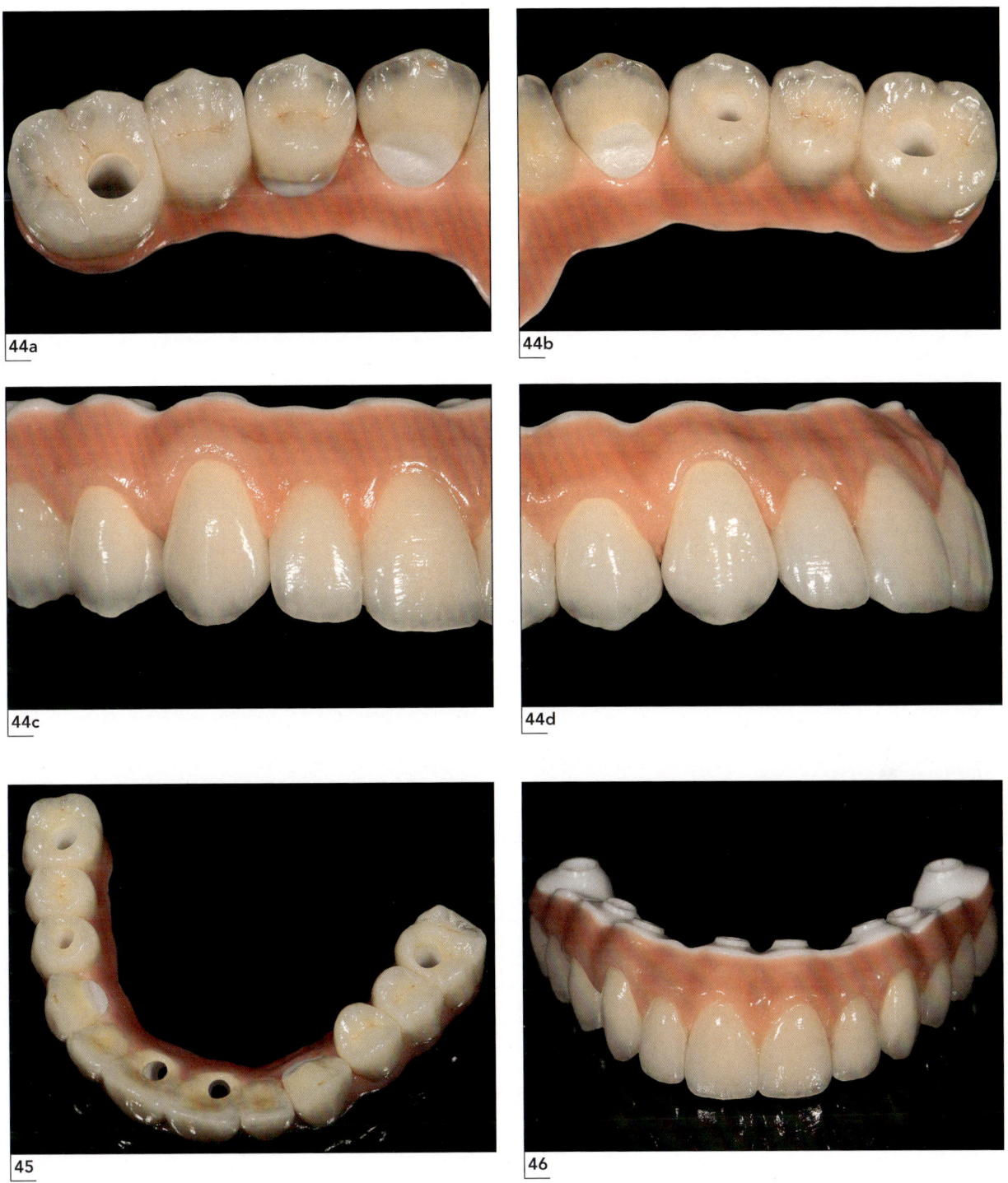

Figs 44a to 44d Zirconium framework veneered with gingival ceramic. The canines and right first premolar are individual crowns to cover screw access holes.

Fig 45 Occlusal view of the definitive prosthesis with screw access holes at the canine and right first premolar covered by single crowns.

Fig 46 Frontal view of the definitive prosthesis.

The machined, screw-retained titanium framework supporting acrylic resin or composite teeth and processed with acrylic resin offers predictable, esthetic results at a good financial value. Patients that require a more lifelike appearance of their teeth should select individual all-ceramic crowns luted to a titanium framework. The most advanced technique for restoring full-arch implant cases—the Procera Implant Bridge Zirconia with single crowns and pink porcelain—is the most pleasing restoration esthetically, but is also the most costly. Explaining these choices to patients and helping them choose the best solution is ultimately the great challenge.

ACKNOWLEDGMENTS

The authors would like to thank Ernst A. Hegenbarth, Germany, and Dr Dario Adolfi, Brazil, for their great technical skill and expertise in providing some of the restorations presented in this article.

REFERENCES

1. Adell R, Lekholm U, Rockler B, Brånemark PI. A 15-year study of osseointegrated implants in the treatment of the edentulous jaw. Int J Oral Surg 1981;10:387–416.

2. Branemark PI. Osseointegration and its experimental background. J Prosthet Dent 1983;50:399–410.

3. Sahin S, Cehreli MC. The significance of passive framework fit in implant prosthodontics: Current status. Implant Dent 2001;10:85–92.

4. Carr AB. Comparison of impression techniques for a five-implant mandibular model. Int J Oral Maxillofac Implants 1991;6:448–455.

5. Carr AB, Stewart RB. Full-arch implant framework casting accuracy: Preliminary in vitro observation for in vivo testing. J Prosthodont 1993;2:2–8.

6. Lorenzoni M, Pertl C, Penkner K, Polansky R, Sedaj B, Wegscheider WA. Comparison of the transfer precision of three different impression materials in combination with transfer caps for the Frialit-2 system. J Oral Rehabil 2000; 27:629–638.

7. Roberts WE. Bone dynamics of osseointegration, ankylosis, and tooth movement. J Indiana Dent Assoc 1999; 78:24–32.

8. Ma T, Nicholls JI, Rubenstein JE. Tolerance measurements of various implant components. Int J Oral Maxillofac Implants 1997;12:371–375.

9. Assif D, Fenton A, Zarb G, Schmitt A. Comparative accuracy of implant impression procedures. Int J Periodontics Restorative Dent 1992;12:112–121.

10. Assif D, Marshak B, Schmidt A. Accuracy of implant impression techniques. Int J Oral Maxillofac Implants 1996; 11:216–222.

11. Assif D, Nissan J, Varsano I, Singer A. Accuracy of implant impression splinted techniques: Effect of splinting material. Int J Oral Maxillofac Implants 1999;14:885–888.

12. Holst S, Blatz MB, Bergler M, Goellner M, Wichmann M. Influence of impression material and time on the 3-dimensional accuracy of implant impressions. Quintessence Int 2007;38:67–73.

13. Heshmati RH, Nagy WW, Wirth CG, Dhuru VB. Delayed linear expansion of improved dental stone. J Prosthet Dent 2002;88:26–31.

14. Finger W. Effect of the setting expansion of dental stone upon the die precision. Scand J Dent Res 1980;88: 159–160.

15. Morey EF. Dimensional accuracy of small gold alloy castings. Part 1. A brief history and the behaviour of inlay waxes. Aust Dent J 1991;36:302–309.

16. Davis DR, Nguyen JH, Grey BL. Ring volume/ring liner ratio and effective setting expansion. Int J Prosthodont 1992;5:403–408.

17. Bridger DV, Nicholls JI. Distortion of ceramometal fixed partial dentures during the firing cycle. J Prosthet Dent 1981;45:507–514.

18. Rubenstein JE, Ma T. Comparison of interface relationships between implant components for laser-welded titanium frameworks and standard cast frameworks. Int J Oral Maxillofac Implants 1999;14:491–495.

19. Zoidis PC, Winkler S, Karellos ND. The effect of soldering, electrowelding, and cast-to procedures on the accuracy of fit of cast implant bars. Implant Dent 1996;5:163–168.

20. Karl M, Taylor TD, Wichmann MG, Heckmann SM. In vivo stress behavior in cemented and screw-retained five-unit implant FPDs. J Prosthodont 2006;15:20–24.

21. Hebel KS, Gajjar RC. Cement-retained versus screw-retained implant restorations: Achieving optimal occlusion and esthetics in implant dentistry. J Prosthet Dent 1997;77:28–35.

22. Michalakis KX, Hirayama H, Garefis PD. Cement-retained versus screw-retained implant restorations: A critical review. Int J Oral Maxillofac Implants 2003;18:719–728.

23. Atwood DA. Reduction of residual ridges: A major oral disease entity. J Prosthet Dent 1971;26:266–279.

24. Atwood DA, Coy WA. Clinical, cephalometric, and densitometric study of reduction of residual ridges. J Prosthet Dent 1971;26:280–295.

25. Bahat O, Fontanesi RV, Preston J. Reconstruction of the hard and soft tissues for optimal placement of osseointegrated implants. Int J Periodontics Restorative Dent 1993;13:255–275.

26. Cornell DF, Wöhrle PS. The altered framework design: Aesthetic full-arch implant supported restorations with predictable fit. [Proceedings of the Quintessence Symposium, 1992, Berlin, Germany].

27. Schnitman PA. Dental implants. State of the art, state of the science. Int J Technol Assess Health Care 1990;6: 528–544.

28. Misch CE. Contemporary Implant Dentistry, ed 2. St. Louis: CV Mosby, 1999.

29. van Steenberghe D, Molly L, Jacobs R, Vandekerckhove B, Quirynen M, Naert I. The immediate rehabilitation by means of a ready-made final fixed prosthesis in the edentulous mandible: A 1-year follow-up study on 50 consecutive patients. Clin Oral Implants Res 2004;15:360–365.

30. Van Steenberghe D. Interactive imaging for implant planning. J Oral Maxillofac Surg 2005;63:883–84.

31. Sanna AM, Molly L, van Steenberghe D. Immediately loaded CAD-CAM manufactured fixed complete dentures using flapless implant placement procedures: A cohort study of consecutive patients. J Prosthet Dent 2007; 97:331–339.

32. Rocci A, Martignoni M, Gottlow J. Immediate loading in the maxilla using flapless surgery, implants placed in predetermined positions, and prefabricated provisional restorations: A retrospective 3-year clinical study. Clin Implant Dent Relat Res 2003;5 Suppl 1:29–36.

33. Schnitman PA, Wöhrle PS, Rubenstein JE, DaSilva JD, Wang NH. Ten-year results for Brånemark implants immediately loaded with fixed prostheses at implant placement. Int J Oral Maxillofac Implants 1997;12:495–503.

34. van Steenberghe D, Naert I, Andersson M, Brajnovic I, Van Cleynenbreugel J, Suetens P. A custom template and definitive prosthesis allowing immediate implant loading in the maxilla: A clinical report. Int J Oral Maxillofac Implants 2002;17:663–670.

35. Guerrero ME, Jacobs R, Loubele M, Schutyser F, Suetens P, van Steenberghe D. State-of-the-art on cone beam CT imaging for preoperative planning of implant placement. Clin Oral Investig 2006;10:1–7.

36. van Steenberghe D, Glauser R, Blomback U, et al. A computed tomographic scan-derived customized surgical template and fixed prosthesis for flapless surgery and immediate loading of implants in fully edentulous maxillae: A prospective multicenter study. Clin Implant Dent Relat Res 2005;7 suppl 1:S111–S120.

37. Malo P, Nobre Mde A, Petersson U, Wigren S. A pilot study of complete edentulous rehabilitation with immediate function using a new implant design: Case series. Clin Implant Dent Relat Res 2006;8:223–232.

38. Malo P, Rangert B, Nobre M. "All-on-Four" immediate-function concept with Brånemark System implants for completely edentulous mandibles: A retrospective clinical study. Clin Implant Dent Relat Res 2003;5 Suppl 1:2–9.

39. Wöhrle PS, Levin RP. Implant marketing: Cost effective implant dentistry. Implant Soc 1996;6:6–8.

40. Balmer S, Mericske-Stern R. Implant-supported bridges in the edentulous jaw. Clinical aspects of a simple treatment concept [in German]. Schweiz Monatsschr Zahnmed 2006;116:728–739.

41. Parel SM. The single-piece milled titanium implant bridge. Dent Today 2003;22:96–99.

42. Jemt T, Back T, Petersson A. Precision of CNC-milled titanium frameworks for implant treatment in the edentulous jaw. Int J Prosthodont 1999;12:209–215.

43. Riedy SJ, Lang BR, Lang BE. Fit of implant frameworks fabricated by different techniques. J Prosthet Dent 1997; 78:596–604.

44. Ortorp A, Jemt T. Clinical experiences of computer numeric control-milled titanium frameworks supported by implants in the edentulous jaw: A 5-year prospective study. Clin Implant Dent Relat Res 2004;6:199–209.

45. Larsson C, Holm L, Lovgren N, Kokubo Y, Von Steyern PV. Fracture strength of four-unit Y-TZP FPD cores designed with varying connector diameter. An in-vitro study. J Oral Rehabil 2007;34:702–709.

46. Kokubo Y, Tsumita M, Sakurai S, Torizuka K, von Steyern PV, Fukushima S. The effect of core framework designs on the fracture loads of all-ceramic fixed partial dentures on posterior implants. J Oral Rehabil 2007;34:503–507.

47. Mitrani R, Vasilic M, Bruguera A. Fabrication of an implant-supported reconstruction utilizing CAD/CAM technology. Pract Proced Aesthet Dent 2005;17:71–78.

PRECISION IN DENTAL ESTHETICS

CLINICAL AND LABORATORY PROCEDURES

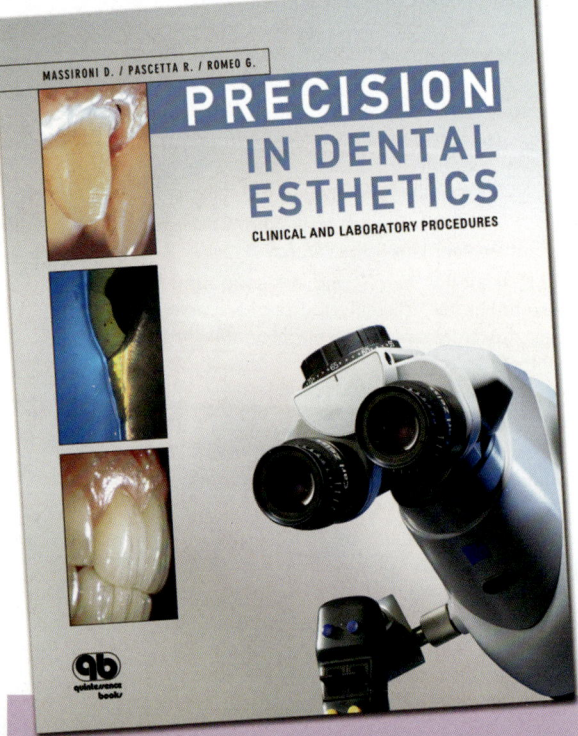

Domenico Massironi, Romeo Pascetta, Giuseppe Romeo

Achieving a favorable esthetic and functional prosthetic outcome requires progression through an intricate sequence of clinical steps. The first section of this beautifully illustrated, highly practical book guides the dental practitioner through each of these steps in the treatment of various common clinical situations. The second part addresses the technical and esthetic aspects of dental laboratory techniques, covering precision in metals and new and conventional ceramics as well as the esthetic realization of prosthetic devices, including diagnostic waxups, communication with patients and clinicians, color matching, and the fabrication of ceramic restorations. Throughout the book, the authors advocate a philosophy emphasizing close clinician-technician collaboration and cooperation, and they are strong proponents of the use of the microscope in most dental procedures.

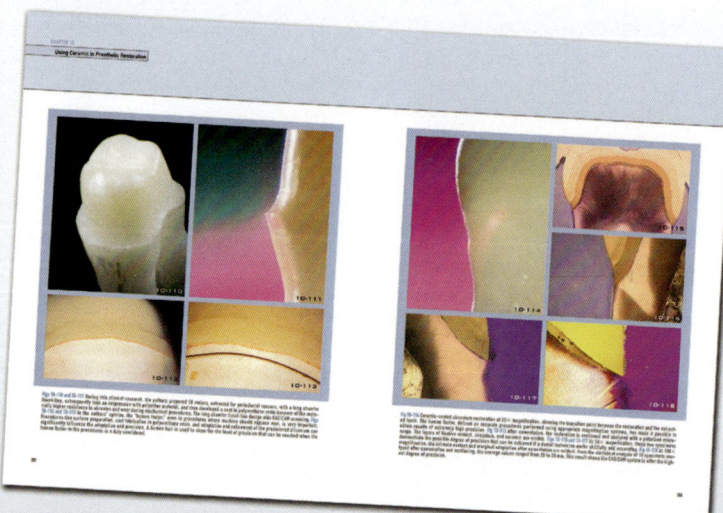

464 pp; 1,331 illus (mostly color); ISBN 1-85097-163-3; US $278

CONTENTS

1. Managing the Treatment Plan with the Prosthetic Team
2. Magnification Systems Used in Dentistry
3. Tooth Preparation for Complete Crowns
4. Finish Line Designs for Complete Crown Preparations
5. Repositioning and Completing the Finish Line with Oscillating Instruments
6. Technical Considerations for Soft Tissue Retraction
7. Clinical Considerations for Provisional Prostheses
8. Technical Considerations for Provisional Prostheses
9. Custom Impression Trays and Impression Materials
10. Laboratory Procedures
11. Using Ceramic in Prosthetic Restoration
12. Esthetic Considerations for Ceramic Restorations
13. Cementation *(with Federico Ferraris)*

CURRENT CLINICAL AND TECHNICAL PROTOCOLS FOR SINGLE-TOOTH IMMEDIATE IMPLANT PROCEDURES

Iñaki Gamborena, DMD, MSD, FID[1]
Markus B. Blatz, DMD, PhD[2]

Loss of a single tooth and its replacement with an implant-supported restoration in the esthetic zone present several challenges when optimal function and esthetics are the goals.[1-3] Immediate placement of dental implants into fresh extraction sockets limits overall treatment time and offers some esthetic and functional advantages.[4] A recent systematic review of the scientific evidence supports immediate implant placement as a safe procedure when certain guidelines are followed.[5] Immediate provisionalization or restoration of such implants provides additional benefits to the pa-tient in terms of appearance, chewing ability, and overall length of treatment.[4] A provisional removable appliance in the form of a denture or retainer is avoided.[4] The existing evidence supports the immediate restoration of dental implants after insertion and reports clinical success rates comparable to traditional multistep protocols.[6] Numerous publications have reported excellent success with these treatment options and discussed diagnostic, surgical, and technical parameters more or less independently from each other.

This article presents a comprehensive approach to optimize functional and esthetic results with immediate implant placement and immediate restoration by blending surgical, technical, and restorative steps into one successful protocol.

[1]Clinical Assistant Professor, Department of Preventive and Restorative Sciences, University of Pennsylvania School of Dental Medicine, Philadelphia, Pennsylvania, USA; Private Practice, San Sebastian, Spain.

[2]Professor of Restorative Dentistry and Chairman, Department of Preventive and Restorative Sciences, University of Pennsylvania School of Dental Medicine, Philadelphia, Pennsylvania, USA.

Correspondence to: Dr Iñaki Gamborena, Resurecccion mª de azkue, 6 20018 San Sebastian, Spain. E-mail: gambmila@telefonica.net

CASE SELECTION

The driving philosophy behind current implant/restorative protocols is *preservation*. The preservation of existing and intact oral structures

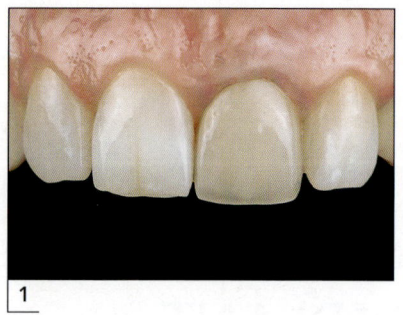
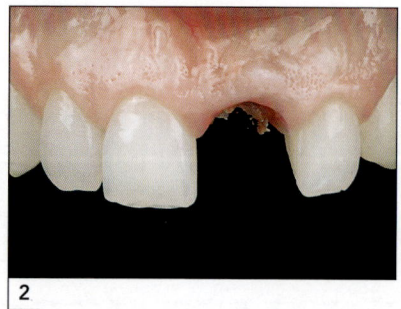
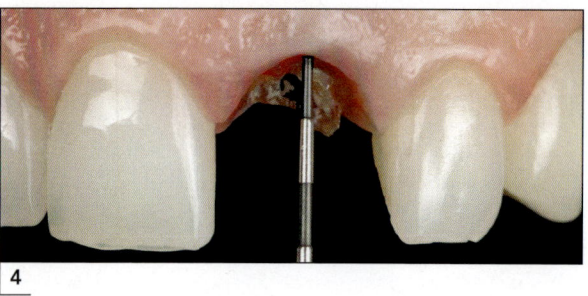

Figs 1 to 3 Initial situation with a failing maxillary left central incisor in a 44-year-old patient.

Figs 4 and 5 Buccal and interproximal bone sounding.

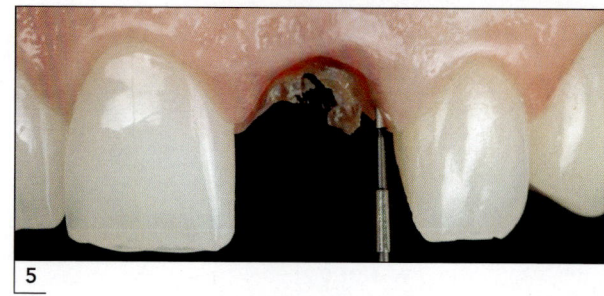

requires a sensitive and conservative treatment approach. Careful case selection and comprehensive treatment planning are essential for final success. The following parameters must be present in each tooth for optimal clinical success with immediate implant placement:

1. Normal dentogingival complex (3 mm from the free gingival margin to the bone crest on the buccal aspect and 4.5 mm interproximally)
2. Tooth position centered with the buccolingual bone plates and normal orientation within the arch
3. Medium to thick gingival biotype

Figures 1 to 3 show the initial intraoral situation of a 44-year-old patient with a failing maxillary left central incisor. The parameters above were verified preoperatively via thorough examination and bone sounding (Figs 4 and 5).

SURGICAL PROTOCOL

Atraumatic tooth extraction is the first and one of the most critical steps of immediate implant placement. Even small periotomes—typically forced between the alveolar bone and the root of the tooth—may damage vital structures and compromise healing. One recommended technique for atraumatic extraction is to hollow out the tooth with rotating instruments and remove remaining tooth fragments from the inside. Commercial products such as the Easy X-TRAC system (ATitan Instruments, Hamburg, NY) allow for atraumatic extraction without damaging instruments and rotary movements, minimize loss of bone and soft tissue, reduce posttraumatic swelling, and provide excellent conditions for immediate implant placement (Figs 6 and 7). Preparation of the implant bed (osteotomy) with the recommended sequence of bone drills should

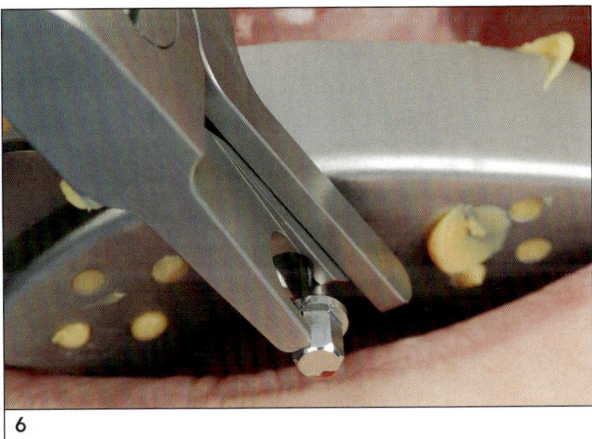

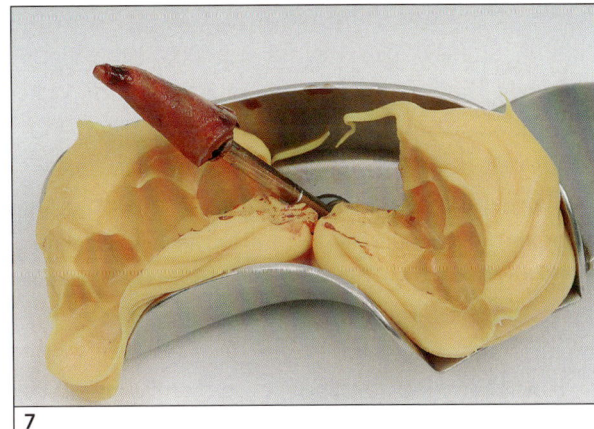

Figs 6 and 7 Araumatic tooth extraction using the Easy X-TRAC system.

Fig 8 Palatal osteotomy for optimal implant positioning and angulation.

Fig 9 A tapered dental implant is placed immediately after tooth extraction with a flapless surgical procedure.

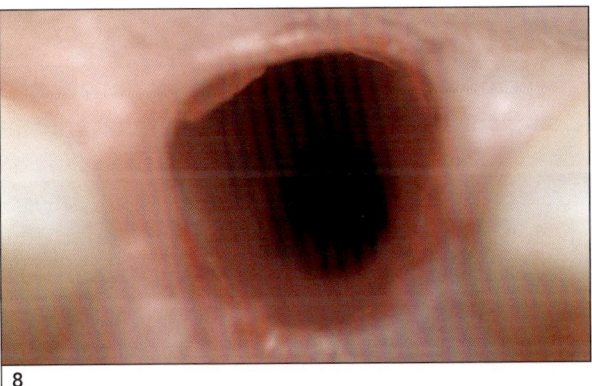

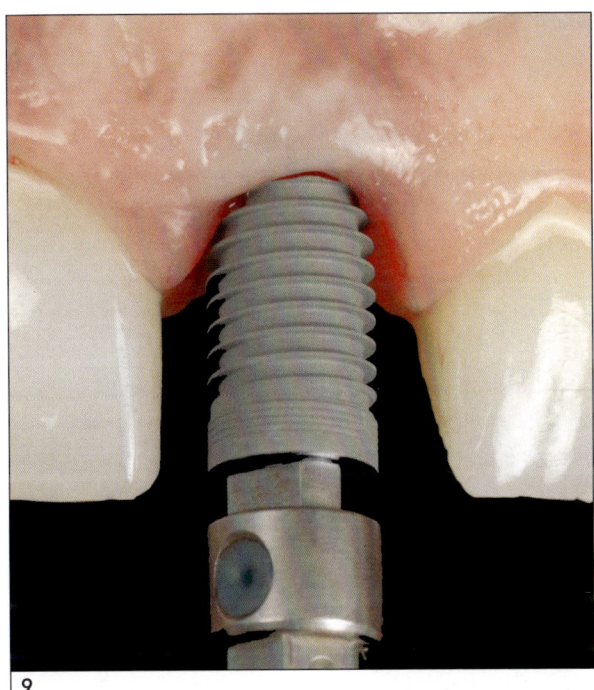

start on the palatal aspect of the extraction socket when an anterior tooth is immediately replaced. It is a common error to start the osteotomy with the bur centered in the alveolus. During drilling, the bur is typically displaced toward the less resistant bony wall, which, in most cases, is the buccal wall. Such displacement causes the implant to be either positioned too far buccally or angulated unfavorably, which makes final restoration more difficult and sometimes even impossible. For an ideal osteotomy, the

drills should be placed along the palatal wall of the extraction socket to achieve a final implant location centered between the incisal edge and cingulum of the prospective tooth. The diameter of the selected implant should be as close as possible to the cervical alveolar diameter of the extracted root. Figure 8 shows the palatal osteotomy in the present case. A NobelReplace Select Tapered Groovy implant (5 × 13 mm, Nobel Biocare, Göteborg, Sweden) was placed in the extraction socket of the central incisor (Fig 9). A bone substitute material (eg, Bio-Oss, Osteo-health, Shirley, NY) may be placed in the gaps between the implant and alveolar bone to avoid resorption. Condensation of the bone filling material can be simplified by attaching a narrower healing abutment to the implant, for example, by attaching a regular-platform abutment to a wide-platform implant. This increases visibility and ensures that bone filling particles are not trapped in the implant-abutment connection.

It was planned to connect a definitive prefabricated abutment to the implant immediately after surgery. In such cases, it is key to ensure proper orientation of the implant and its connection interface to facilitate correct orientation of the prefabricated abutment and provisional restoration. The trilobe connection and indicator marks of the NobelReplace Select implant provide simple references; one of the lobes should be oriented toward the buccal aspect. This configuration allows some prosthetic components to be prepared preoperatively and transferred easily to the patient's mouth.

RESTORATIVE PROTOCOL

It is recommended to insert the final implant abutment as soon as possible after implant placement, preferably on the same day. This will avoid repetitive mutilation of the fragile peri-implant soft tissue collar, which occurs whenever abutments are removed or inserted. Abutment disconnections and reconnections compromise the mucosal barrier and result in a more "apically" positioned zone of connective tissue, thus leading to marginal bone resorption.[10]

Implant abutments made from zirconium oxide ceramic provide sufficient strength, excellent biologic response, and superior esthetic properties.[7,8] The white color of zirconia ceramic abutments prevents grayish discoloration of peri-implant soft tissues. It is also beneficial in the event of postoperative soft tissue recession, which seems unavoidable in immediate implant protocols.[9] A

metal alloy abutment would possibly be exposed and severely compromise the esthetic outcome of the restoration. Two aspects that may limit the amount of bone and soft tissue recessions are delicate atraumatic handling during all clinical procedures (eg, avoiding dis- and reconnections of implant abutments) and a thick tissue biotype.

Prefabricated Zirconia Abutments

For the aforementioned reasons, a customized definitive zirconia abutment that does not need to be removed again should be inserted immediately after implant placement. One option is to scan and fabricate a customized abutment (eg, Procera Zirconia Abutment, Nobel Biocare) before the surgery based on the diagnostic waxup. Another option is to insert and customize a prefabricated abutment at the time of surgery. The NobelReplace Procera Esthetic Abutment Kit (Nobel Biocare) includes an assortment of prefabricated zirconia abutments that can be selected, inserted, and prepared chairside. The prefabricated zirconia abutments feature a removable internal implant connection (NobelReplace Select). The selection kit is organized by the size of the implant connection as narrow platform (NP), regular platform (RP), and wide platform (WP). The abutments are available in various diameters, finish-line heights, and angulations. Abutment designs and dimensions were developed based on average values from the Procera software network. Finish-line heights range from 1.5 to 2 mm. Since the implant should ideally be placed about 3 mm below the free gingival margin, the abutment with the 2-mm finish-line height is often used for chairside preparation. Abutment selection is simplified by measuring the mesiodistal width of the original root in the preoperative periapical radiograph. The measurement should be taken at the most coronal part of the portion of the root that is left within the dentogingival complex. The abutment should support the surrounding tissue and clinical crown in the transmucosal area in the same manner as the natural tooth.

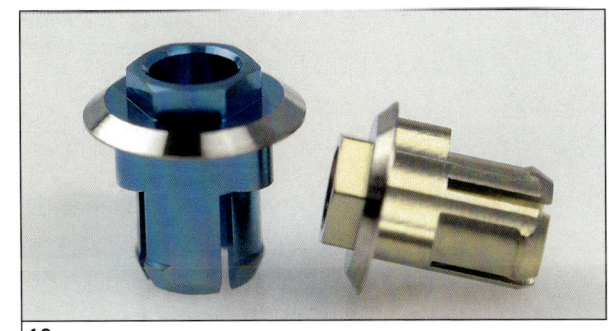

Fig 10 Platform-shifting adapters for the Replace Select trilobe internal connections were used to convert RP implants to NP abutments *(right)* and WP implants to RP abutments *(left)*.

Platform Shifting

There is increasing evidence that supports the concept of platform switching. This concept refers to the connection of restorative components with smaller diameters to implant platforms with larger diameters. The positive effects of platform switching were discovered by coincidence when an implant manufacturer introduced wide-diameter implants.[11] Initially, prosthetic abutments with matching diameters were not available; therefore, smaller-diameter abutments were used, causing circumferential horizontal discrepancies. When radiographs of these restorations were taken and examined 5 years postoperatively, the crestal bone lateral to the implants appeared to respond differently from what is typically observed with same-sized implant-abutment components: There was significantly less crestal bone loss.[12] The authors concluded that this was caused by the inward shift of the implant-abutment junction. The inflammatory cell infiltrate was repositioned and confined within a 90-degree area that was not directly adjacent to the crestal bone. In addition, a biomechanical analysis by Maeda et al[13] demonstrated a shift of the stress concentration area away from the cervical bone/implant interface. In a recent prospective clinical trial, Huerzeler et al[14] found that platform-switched abutments caused significantly less crestal bone resorption. These and other authors reason that the reduced crestal bone loss has a positive effect on the peri-implant soft tissue and, ultimately, the esthetic outcome.[14–16] Esthetic predictability makes platform switching a preferred concept for immediate placement/restoration protocols. However, although the existing evidence is encouraging, more clinical data with various implant systems are needed.

Platform switching may be performed simply by using prosthetic components that have smaller diameters at the connection interface than the supporting implants, provided that the connecting interfaces have the same dimensions. Otherwise, special components such as the recently introduced platform-shifting adapters (Nobel Biocare) must be used. These platforming-shifting adapters are designed for Replace Select trilobe internal connections and convert RP and WP implants to NP and RP abutments, respectively (Fig 10). At the same time, they switch internal connection (trilobe) implants to external hex platforms.

Chairside Abutment Selection and Preparation

When measured on the preoperative radiograph (Fig 11), the mesiodistal width of the failing root was 6.6 mm. An RP abutment with a width of 6.7 mm and a 2-mm finish-line height was selected from the NobelReplace Procera Esthetic Abutment Kit (Figs 12 and 13). The original connection was removed from the zirconia abutment. The adapter that converts WP implants to RP abutments was attached to the abutment and both were screwed onto the WP implant (NobelReplace Tapered Groovy). Care was taken to orient and align the

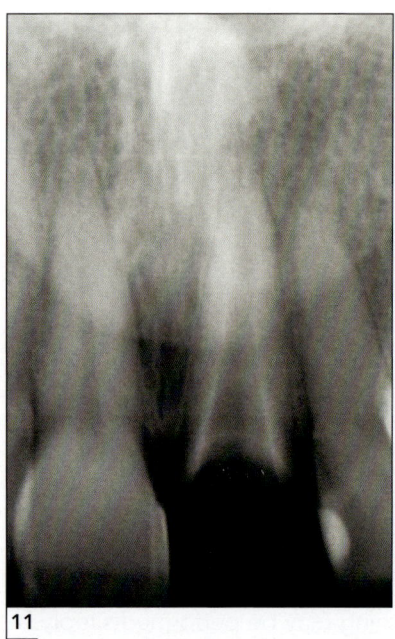

Fig 11 Mesiodistal width of coronal aspect of the root was measured on the preoperative periapical radiograph to select the abutment with the closest diameter.

Fig 12 Prefabricated zirconia abutment kit offers various diameters, angulations, and finish-line heights.

Fig 13 Chairside selection of a prefabricated zirconia abutment with the same diameter as the extracted tooth.

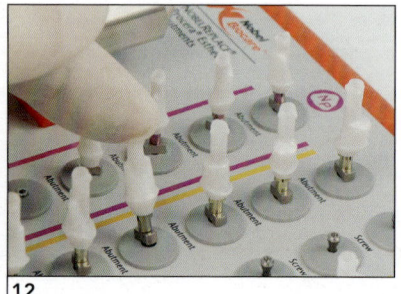

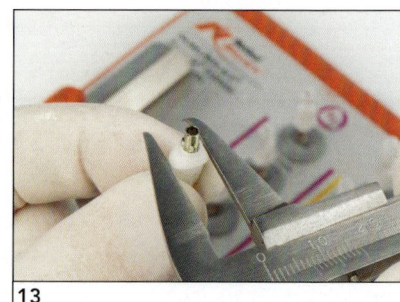

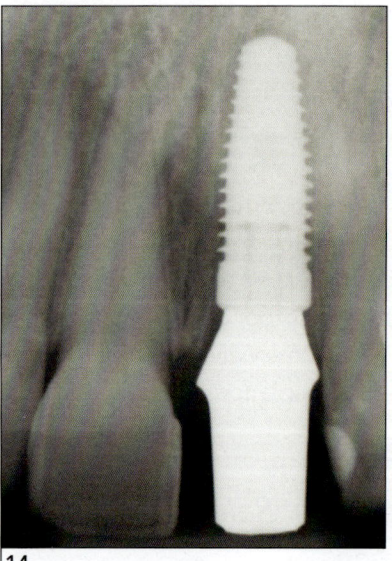

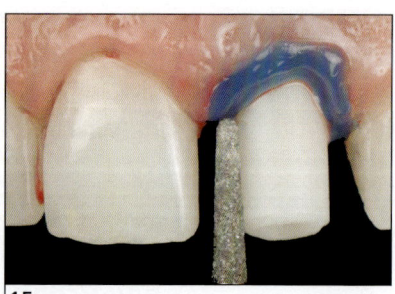

Fig 14 Radiograph used to verify fit and proper seating of the prefabricated zirconia abutment.

Fig 15 Intraoral preparation of the prefabricated zirconia abutment. Block-out material is used to avoid penetration of zirconia particles into the gap between the abutment and free gingival margin.

connection and abutment so that the buccal aspect of the abutment coincided with one of the lobes of the implant connection. Proper adaptation was verified with a periapical radiograph (Fig 14). The radiopacity of the zirconia abutment allows for evaluation of the crestal bone and its proximity to the diverging abutment for adequate preparation. After verification of proper seating, three silicone matrices (Zetalabor laboratory high-precision condensation silicone, Zhermack, Badia Polesine, Italy) made from a diagnostic waxup were used for anatomic abutment modifications and provisional shell orientation. The abutment was prepared with diamond burs at a high speed with copious water. A light-curing resin barrier was applied to seal the gap between the free gingival margin and zirconia abutment and to avoid penetration of zirconia particles into the fresh extraction socket during preparation (Fig 15). Final preparation was verified with the silicone indices (Figs 16 to 18) to ensure adequate space for the final restoration. The screw access hole in the abutment

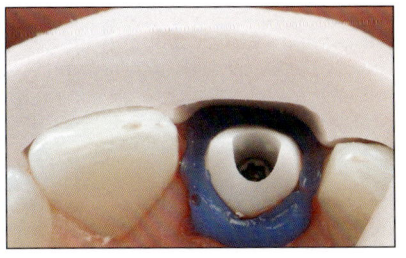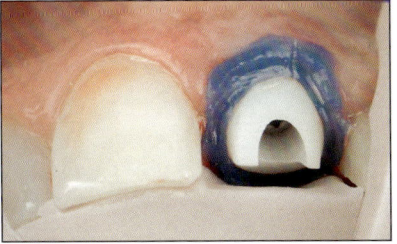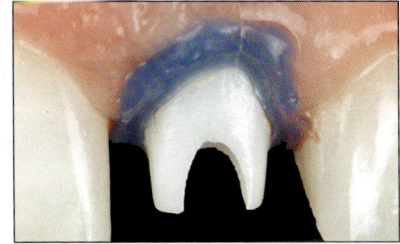

Figs 16 to 18 Silicone matrix of the diagnostic waxup used to verify an adequate preparation. This ensures adequate space for the definitive restoration.

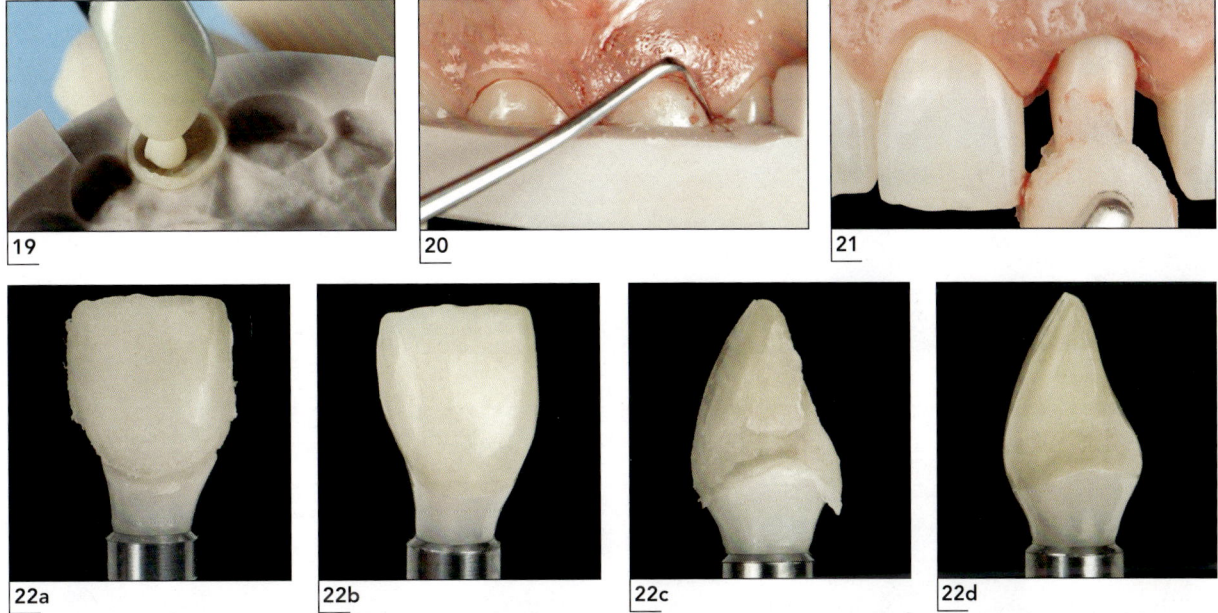

Figs 19 to 21 The provisional crown was prefabricated in the laboratory with a silicone matrix of the diagnostic waxup. The crown is then relined chairside with self-curing acrylic resin and a silicone matrix to ensure exact positioning.

Figs 22a to 22d Anterior and buccolingual views of the provisional crown before (*a and c*) and after (*b and d*) recontouring. Note the subgingival concavitiy for improved tissue proliferation. Only minor adjustments were necessary, indicating an optimal implant position.

was sealed with Fermit (Ivoclar Vivadent, Amherst, NY), and a separating agent (petroleum jelly) was applied to the abutment.

Provisional Restoration

It is recommended to fabricate the provisional restoration from the diagnostic waxup before the surgical appointment to simplify the clinical procedure and limit chairside treatment time. The silicone matrix ensured that the provisional crown was properly oriented. The crown was hollowed out

and relined (Figs 19 and 20) with a self-curing acrylic material (Temporary Bridge Resin, Dentsply Caulk, Milford, Delaware). Excess acrylic resin was carefully removed (Fig 21) to maintain the desired emergence profile. The provisional crown and abutment were removed from the implant after complete setting of the acrylic resin and connected to a laboratory analog for finishing and polishing. Excess acrylic resin flashes were trimmed carefully to preserve the original shape and emergence profile. Only minimal adjustments were necessary in this case, indicating optimal implant placement and location (Figs 22a to 22d). A separating agent was

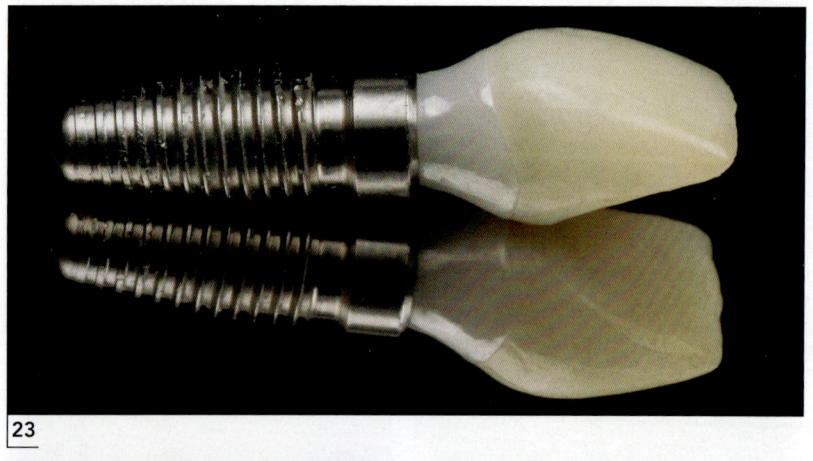

23

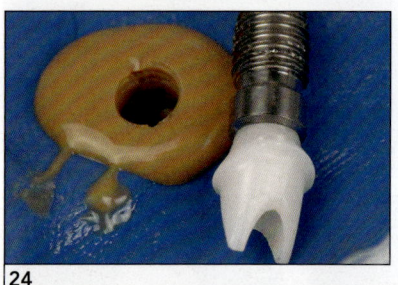

24

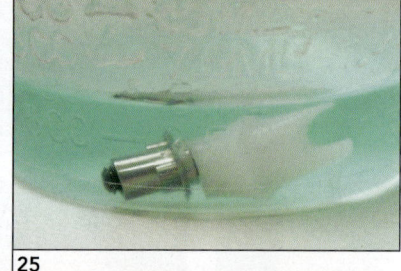

25

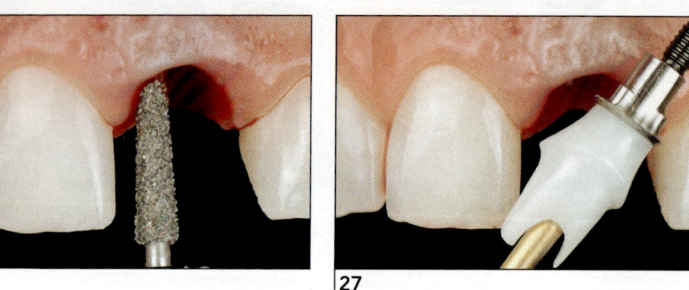

26

27

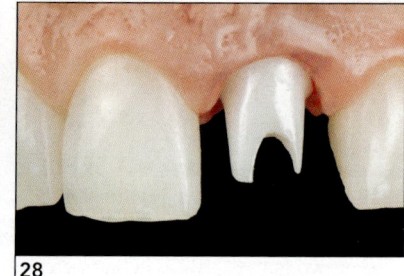

28

Fig 23 Finalized provisional crown. Note the platform shift and subgingival concavitiy with increasing diameter toward the coronal aspect of the abutment to full contour at the transmucosal level.

Fig 24 Final impression of the customized prefabricated abutment for fabrication of the definitive crown.

Fig 25 The abutment was disinfected in 2% glutaraldehyde for 5 minutes before final insertion.

Fig 26 Refreshing the sulcular epithelium with a diamond bur before abutment connection.

Fig 27 Platform shift adapter and zirconia abutment.

Fig 28 Zirconia abutment in place, demonstrating adequate tissue support.

again applied to the abutment, and small remaining gaps were filled with acrylic resin to optimize the emergence profile and create a smooth transition between the abutment and provisional crown. Complete curing of the acrylic resin was ensured by placing the relined crown in a pressure pot with hot water for 5 minutes. Silicone diamond disks and water/pumice slurry were used for final polishing (Fig 23). The customized prefabricated zirconia abutment was also highly polished with silicone diamond disks and pumice to minimize bacterial colonization.[17] A final impression was made from the abutment before returning it to the mouth (Fig 24). This impression is necessary for fabrication of the definitive restoration and eliminates the need for future disconnection of the abutment from the im-

plant. It also negates the need for a final impression with the abutment in place, which would typically require tissue retraction. The screw access hole was filled with Fermit (Ivoclar Vivadent), and the impression was carried out with the double-mix impression technique (Virtual VPS putty base, regular set and extra light–body fast set, Ivoclar Vivadent). All prosthetic parts in contact with tissues were placed in a glutaraldehyde solution of 2% for 5 minutes for disinfection (Fig 25). The sulcular epithelium was refreshed with a diamond bur (Fig 26). Figure 27 depicts the WP-RP platform-shifting adapter connected to the abutment. The abutment was screwed on the implant with a torque of 35 Ncm and thoroughly rinsed with water (Fig 28). The provisional restoration was then cemented with

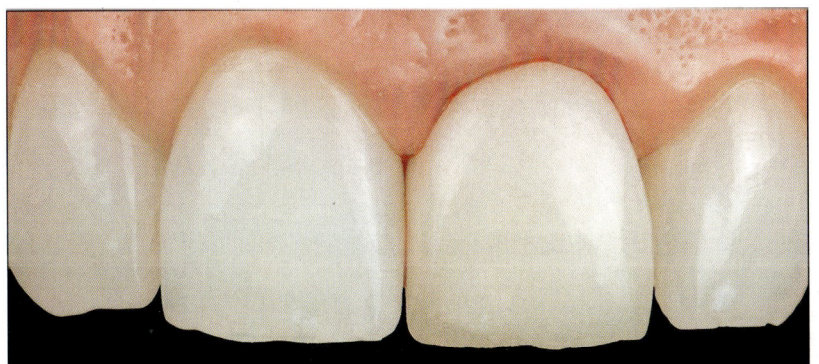

Fig 29 Postoperative labial view of the immediate provisional crown supported by the prefabricated zirconia abutment and immediately placed implant at the left central incisor site.

Fig 30 Postoperative radiograph. Note the level of crestal bone.

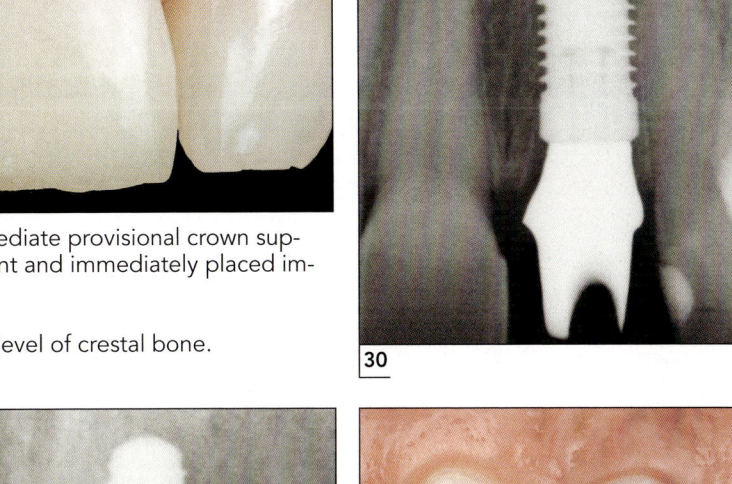

Figs 31 to 33 Intraoral and radiographic views 6 months after surgery. The abutment placed at the time of surgery is not removed in order to avoid disturbance of the fragile peri-implant soft tissue.

Figs 34a and 34b Occlusal views of the preoperative (a) and 6-month postoperative (b) situation. The customized prefabricated zirconia abutment provides adequate tissue support.

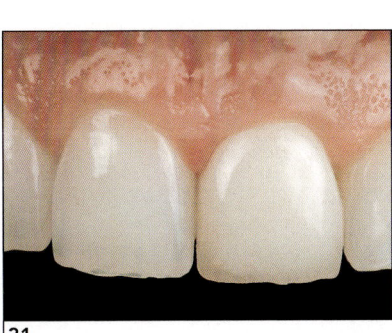

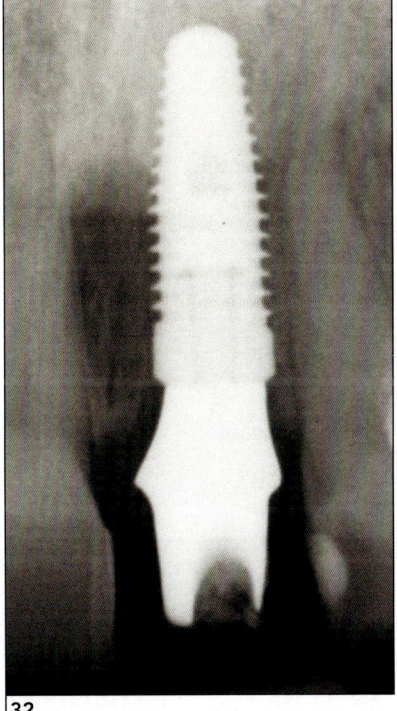

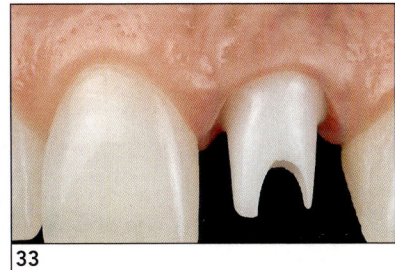

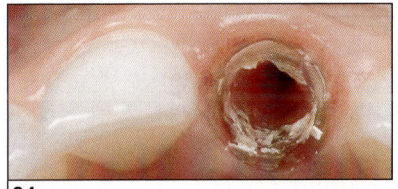

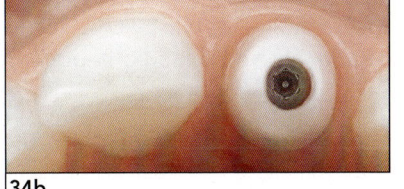

temporary cement (Temp-bond NE, Kerr, Orange, California, USA). The cement was applied with a thin brush to minimize excess. Functional and esthetic parameters were verified after removal of excess cement (Fig 29) and radiographic examination (Fig 30). The absence of occlusal contacts on the provisional crown during excursions was verified with articulating film. Follow-up visits were scheduled for 15 days, 1 month, 2 months, 3 months, and 6 months later.

Final Restoration

All relevant parameters were re-evaluated 6 months after implant placement and provisionalization. Wound healing and soft tissue integration were ideal, and radiographic evaluation revealed positive bone remodeling (Figs 31 to 33). Figures 34a and 34b provide a comparison of tissue support between the original situation and the prepared Procera Esthetic abutment (Nobel Biocare).

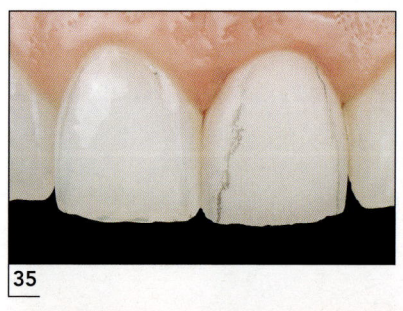

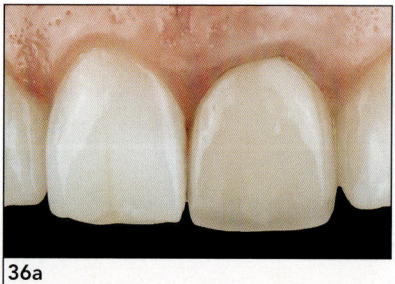

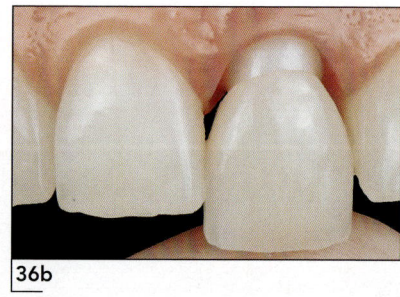

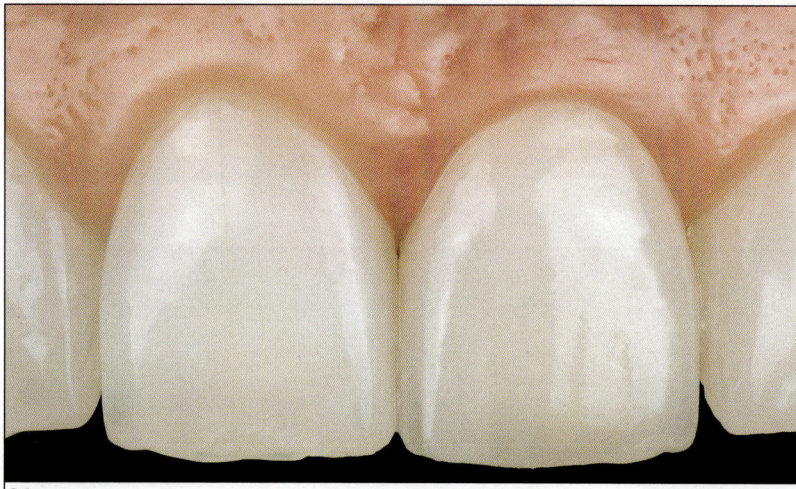

Fig 35 Try-in of definitive crown at the bisque-bake stage.

Figs 36a to 36c Labial views of the initial situation (a) and try-in (b) and cementation (c) of the definitive crown.

A master cast was fabricated from the impression of the abutment and scanned with the Procera Forte scanner (Nobel Biocare) for the fabrication of a 0.4-mm Procera Alumina coping (Nobel Biocare). A pick-up impression was made with the double-mix technique (Virtual VPS putty base, regular set and extra light–body fast set) to finalize the Procera Alumina Crown. The 0.4-mm translucent coping was preheated to 1,000°C for 15 minutes to create a whitish appearance. Conventional porcelain layering techniques were then applied to finalize shape and color. These parameters, the interproximal contacts, and the occlusion were verified and adjusted at the bisque-bake try-in (Fig 35). The dramatic esthetic improvement from the initial situation to try-in and final insertion of the definitive restoration is shown in Figs 36a to 36c. Final cementation was performed with adhesive resin (RelyX Unicem transparent, 3M ESPE, St Paul, MN). Ultimate fit, osseous implant integration, and bone support were verified with a periapical radiograph (Fig 37).The intraoral initial situation compared to the final result is shown in Figs 38a and 38b. A follow-up evaluation 2 years postoperatively revealed stable conditions (Figs 39 and 40). Figure 41 demonstrates the esthetic integration of the definitive restoration in the patient's smile.

CONCLUSION

Immediate surgical and restorative protocols facilitate superior esthetic and functional success. However, strict guidelines for atraumatic intervention and preservation of existing anatomic structures must be carefully followed. This article presented a comprehensive treatment approach and discussed current immediate procedures based on the existing scientific evidence. The sequential surgical, technical, and restorative techniques were blended into one successful protocol, which was demonstrated with a clinical case report.

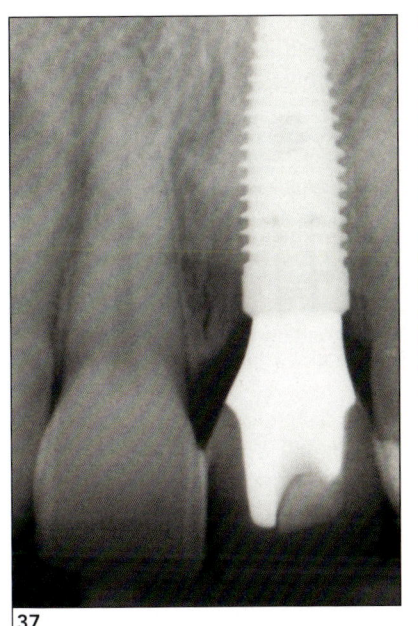

37

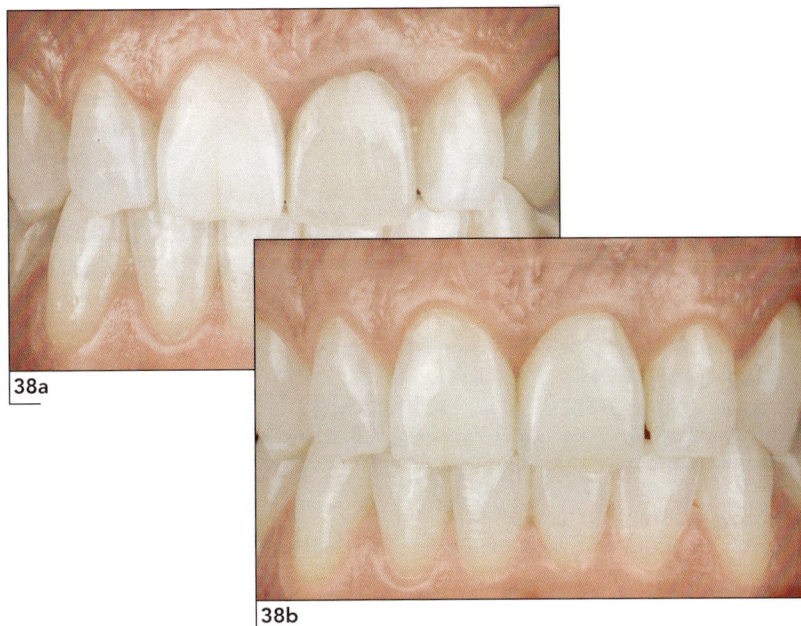

38a

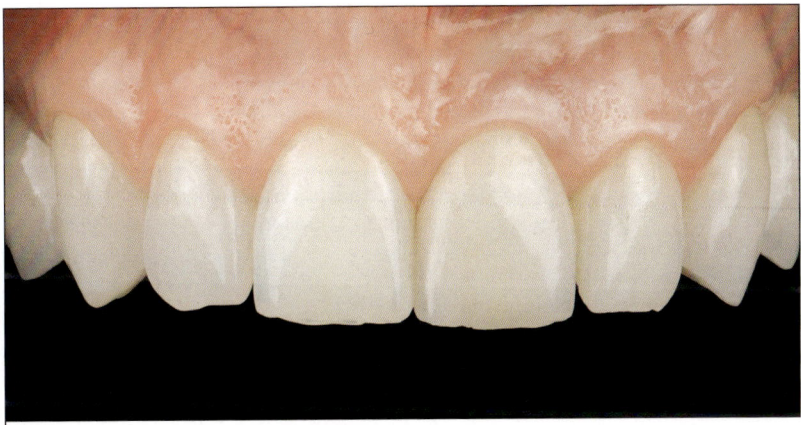

38b

Fig 37 Radiograph of the definitive crown after cementation. Note the crestal bone level.

Figs 38a and 38b Labial views of the preoperative (a) and postoperative (b) situation.

Figs 39 and 40 Two-year postoperative intraoral and radiographic situation.

Fig 41 Final extraoral view showing excellent esthetic integration.

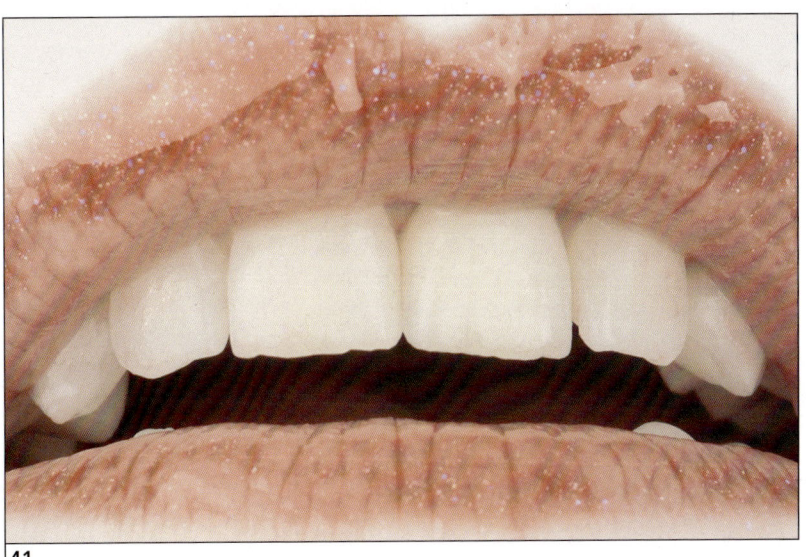

39

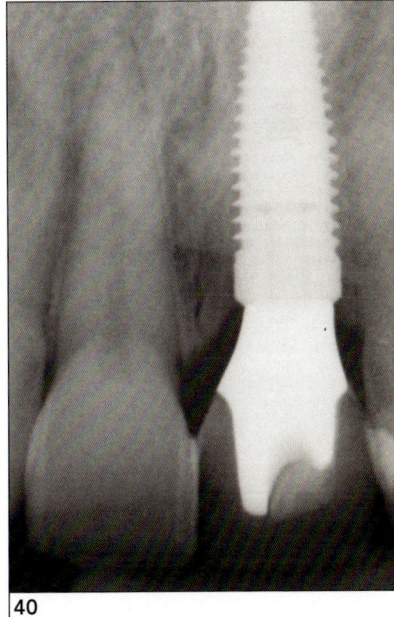

40

41

ACKNOWLEDGMENT

The authors thank Mr Iñigo Casares for the beautiful porcelain work featured in the case presentation.

REFERENCES

1. Gamborena I, Blatz MB. Transferring the emergence profile of single-tooth implant restorations. Quintessence Dent Technol 2004;27:119–132.

2. Sadan A, Blatz MB, Salinas TJ, Block M. Single-implant restorations: A contemporary approach for achieving a predictable outcome. J Oral Maxillofac Surg 2004;62:73–81.

3. Sadan A, Blatz MB, Bellerino M, Block M. Prosthetic design considerations for anterior single-implant restorations. J Esthet Restor Dent 2004;16:165–175.

4. Barone A, Rispoli L, Vozza I, Quaranta A, Covani U. Immediate restoration of single implants placed immediately after tooth extraction. J Periodontol 2006;77:1914–1920.

5. Esposito MA, Koukoulopoulou A, Coulthard P, Worthington HV. Interventions for replacing missing teeth: Dental implants in fresh extraction sockets (immediate, immediate-delayed and delayed implants). Cochrane Database Syst Rev 2006;18:CD005968.

6. Esposito M, Grusovin MG, Willings M, Coulthard P, Worthington HV. Interventions for replacing missing teeth: Different times for loading dental implants. Cochrane Database Syst Rev 2007;18:CD003878.

7. Glauser R, Sailer I, Wohlwend A, Studer S, Schibli M, Schärer P. Experimental zirconia abutments for implant-supported single-tooth restorations in esthetically demanding regions: 4-year results of a prospective clinical study. Int J Prosthodont 2004;17:285–290.

8. Jung RE, Sailer I, Hämmerle CH, Attin T, Schmidlin P. In vitro color changes of soft tissues caused by restorative materials. Int J Periodontics Restorative Dent 2007;27:251–257.

9. Grunder U, Gracis S, Capelli M. Influence of the 3-D bone-to-implant relationship on esthetics. Int J Periodontics Restorative Dent 2005;25:113–119.

10. Abrahamsson I, Berglundh T, Lindhe J. The mucosal barrier following abutment dis/reconnection. An experimental study in dogs. J Clin Periodontol 1997;24:568–572.

11. Blatz MB, Strub JR, Gläser R, Gebhardt W. Use of wide-diameter and standard-diameter implants to replace molars: Two case presentations. Int J Prosthodont 1998;11:356–363.

12. Lazzara RJ, Porter SS. Platform switching: A new concept in implant dentistry for controlling postrestorative crestal bone levels. Int J Periodontics Restorative Dent 2006;26:9–17.

13. Maeda Y, Miura J, Taki I, Sogo M. Biomechanical analysis on platform switching: Is there any biomechanical rationale? Clin Oral Implants Res 2007;18:581–584.

14. Huerzeler M, Fickl S, Zuhr O, Wachtel HC. Peri-implant bone level around implants with platform-switched abutments: Preliminary data from a prospective study. J Oral Maxillofac Surg 2007;65:33–39.

15. Baumgarten H, Cochetto R, Testori T, Meltzer A, Porter S. A new implant design for crestal bone preservation: Initial observations and case report. Pract Proced Aesthet Dent 2005;17:735–740.

16. Gardner DM. Platform switching as a means to achieving implant esthetics. A case study. N Y State Dent J 2005;71:34–37.

17. Scotti R, Kantorski KZ, Monaco C, Valandro LF, Ciocca L, Bottino MA. SEM evaluation of in situ early bacterial colonization on a Y-TZP ceramic: A pilot study. Int J Prosthodont 2007;20:419–412.

NONMETAL POSTS: HOW DO THEY FARE IN DAILY DENTISTRY?

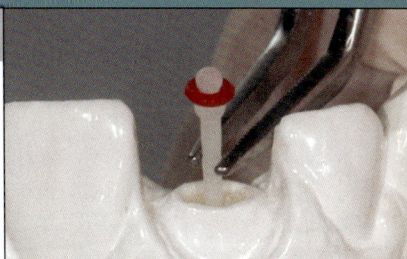

Stefan J. Paul, PD, Dr Med Dent[1]

The increasing use of high-translucency ceramics for fixed prosthodontics suggests that light-conducting nonmetal post systems should be considered for endodontically treated teeth that require crown therapy. The main objective of the post is to increase retention for the core material and to distribute occlusal stresses along the remaining interface with the tooth structure[1-3]; use of a nonmetal post would prevent the grayish appearance of the marginal gingiva that occurs due to unfavorable light reflection from a dark post.

Current recommendations for post placement include minimal removal of existing tooth substance, placement of a post only if more then 50% of tooth substance is lost, use of the narrowest post diameter possible, and avoidance of cantilevered prostheses on abutment teeth.[4-7]

Glass fiber–reinforced composite resin posts and ceramic posts are the major alternative post options if esthetic qualities are required, with one-appointment direct buildup cores being most popular. Alternatively, ceramic posts can be combined with a ceramic core in an indirect procedure.

There are divergent opinions concerning the properties of the post/core materials used in post-and-core restorations. Some authors advocate a modulus of elasticity for posts similar to that of dentin,[8-11] while others believe that high-stiffness posts provide greater longevity.[11,12] Both theories remain widely untested in clinical trials. Of the direct-placement materials, amalgam scores well in strength, high stiffness, and dimensional stability. However, amalgam also has significant disadvantages, such as discoloration of tooth structure from corrosion products, which preclude its use in anterior teeth. Composite resins have high flexural strength, while glass ceramics are more suitable for buildups in the anterior dentition.[13]

[1]Private practice, Zürich, Switzerland.

Correspondence to: Dr Stefan J. Paul, Stadelhoferstrasse 33, 8001 Zürich, Switzerland. E-mail: office@drpaul.ch

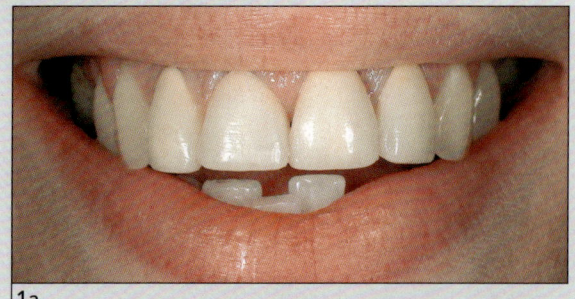

1a

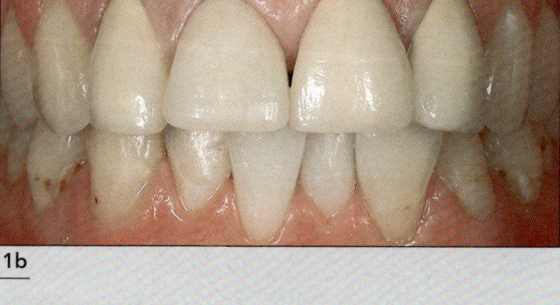

1b

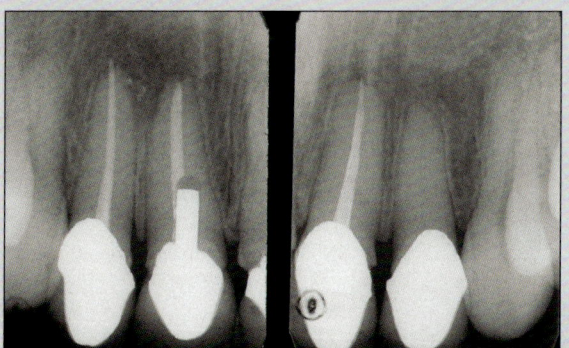

2

Fig 1a Initial smile displaying unsatisfactory restorations.

Fig 1b Close-up view of the four maxillary crowns that needed replacement and the crowding in the mandibular anterior segment.

Fig 2 Initial radiograph of the maxillary incisors.

ZIRCONIUM OXIDE POSTS

Zirconium oxide ceramics generally provide superior physical properties, biocompatibility, and excellent esthetics. The inherent high flexural strength of zirconia makes it useful not only for crowns, fixed partial dentures, and implant abutments, but also for posts. In dental applications, zirconium oxide ceramics are used mostly in a tetragonal crystalline phase that is partially stabilized with yttrium oxide, providing flexural strength greater than 1,000 MPa. This makes zirconia suitable also as post material, and zirconia posts are available today in cylindrically, as well as conically, shaped designs.

In terms of surface quality, zirconia posts with slightly roughened finishes are preferred for good micromechanical retention to adhesive cements. While zirconia posts provide excellent radiographic opacity, the reported strength becomes a significant disadvantage if the post later needs to be retrieved. The likelihood of endodontic reintervention therefore needs to be considered. Clinical long-term success, however, appears to be excellent for adhesively cemented zirconia posts with direct composite buildups.[14]

Case Presentation

A 30-year-old female patient presented with crowns on the four maxillary anterior incisors that she wanted replaced. Smile analysis revealed inadequate crown length, surface texture, and shade (Fig 1a) of the four maxillary anterior restorations. In addition, an unequal zenith position of the central incisors and crowding of the mandibular anterior dentition were noted (Fig 1b). The radiographic examination (Fig 2) revealed prior endodontic treatment on three of the teeth

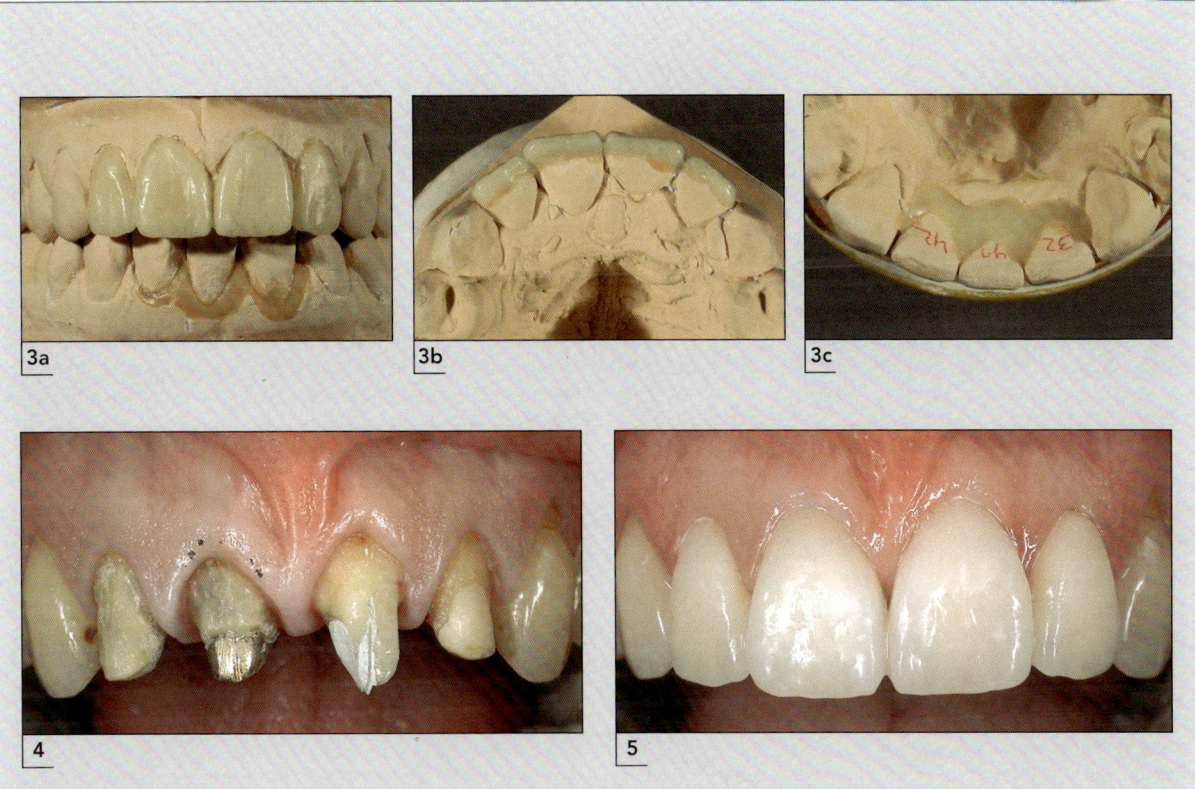

Fig 3a Diagnostic waxup for the four maxillary incisors.

Fig 3b Occlusal view of waxup showing archwise positioning of the maxillary anterior teeth.

Fig 3c Diagnostic elimination of the crowding in the mandibular anterior segment.

Fig 4 Tooth display after removal of existing crowns showing indicative marks on the marginal gingiva of the right central incisor prior to crown lengthening.

Fig 5 Temporization according to the diagnostic waxup.

(right central, right lateral, and left lateral incisors) with a post on the left central. The left canine did not demonstrate the typical lumen for nerve tissue but reacted with normal vitality during the clinical examination.

A facebow transfer, clinical images, and facial and smile analysis were transferred to the dental laboratory. Based on this information, a diagnostic waxup was made to visualize improved crown length and width (Fig 3a), as well as archwise positioning and inclination (Fig 3b) of the four restorations. The crowding of the mandibular anterior teeth would be resolved by elimination of

one incisor and subsequent realignment of the mandibular anterior teeth (Fig 3c).

After approval by the patient, the four maxillary anterior restorations were removed. The metal post of the right central incisor was removed and zirconia posts were luted adhesively into the canals of both central incisors. The left central incisor received a composite buildup without using a post. Crown lengthening was performed on the right central incisor to level the zenith point with the left central (Fig 4). Provisional restorations were placed based on the diagnostic waxup (Fig 5).

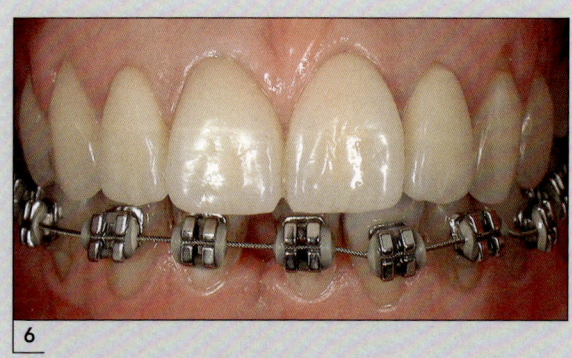

Fig 6 During soft tissue maturation, orthodontic treatment was carried out in the mandible.

Fig 7 Soft tissue maturation prior to impression taking.

Fig 8 Try-in of the treatment waxup.

Fig 9 Final glass-ceramic crowns.

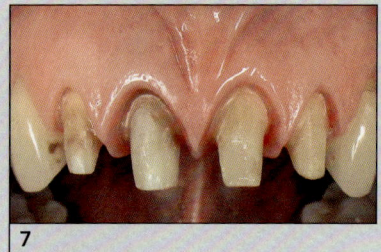

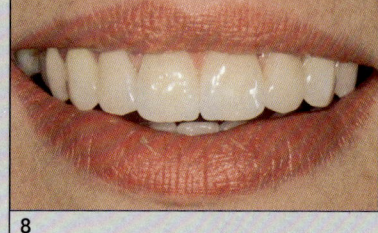

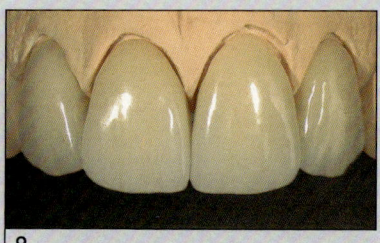

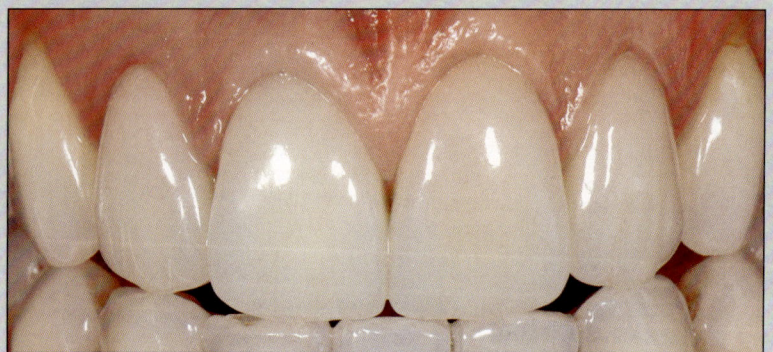

Fig 10 Immediately after final adhesive cementation, the four maxillary restorations show a satisfactory match with the adjacent dentition.

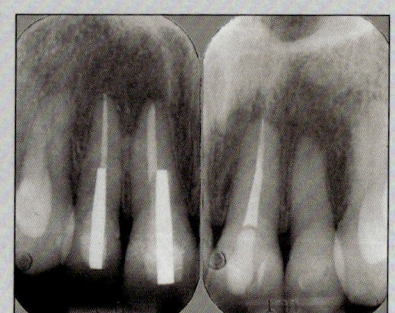

Fig 11 Radiograph after final cementation.

Orthodontic treatment was carried out to align the mandibular anterior teeth after extraction of one incisor (Fig 6).

After maturation of the maxillary gingival tissues (Fig 7), impressions were made and a treatment waxup was tried in (Fig 8). Respective corrections were made where necessary and four glass-ceramic crowns were fabricated (Fig 9).

After final cementation, the four glass-ceramic crowns showed an excellent match with the adja-cent and opposing dentition in terms of shade, re-flection lines, and surface texture (Fig 10). The post-and-core retreatment was checked radio-graphically, particularly to verify the zirconia post in the right central incisor, as the initial metal post in that tooth had shown some misalignment (Fig 11). Excellent integration with the marginal tissues was achieved, maintaining the high scallop of the papillae. Color and texture of the marginal tissues of two of the nonvital teeth (right central and left

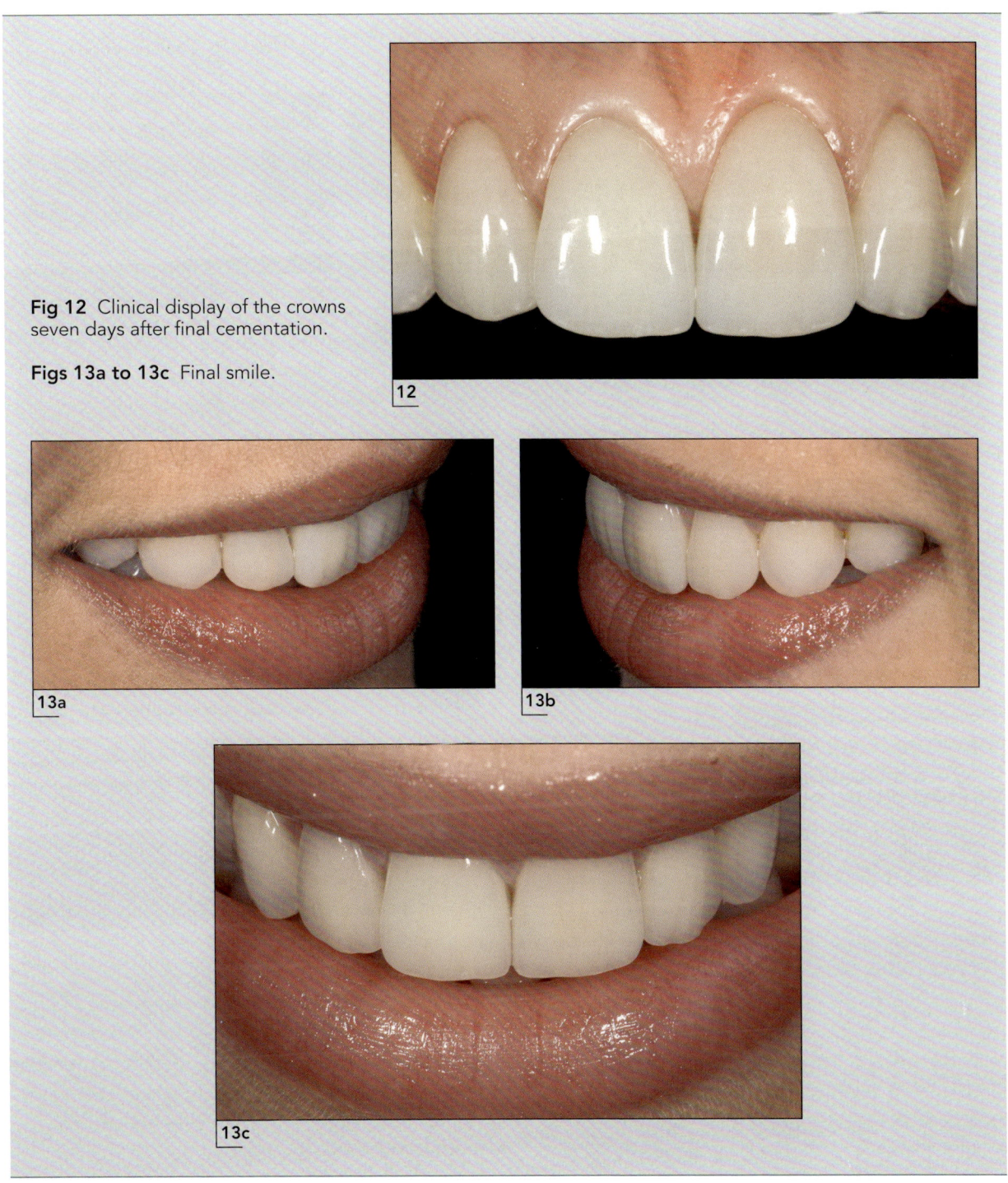

Fig 12 Clinical display of the crowns seven days after final cementation.

Figs 13a to 13c Final smile.

lateral incisors) matched those of the vital tooth (left canine) perfectly. The marginal gingiva of the left central incisor still appeared slightly grayish due to the persisting discoloration of the underly-ing root substance (Fig 12). The four maxillary restorations portrayed an optimal enhancement of a natural smile (Figs 13a to 13c).

CASE PRESENTATION

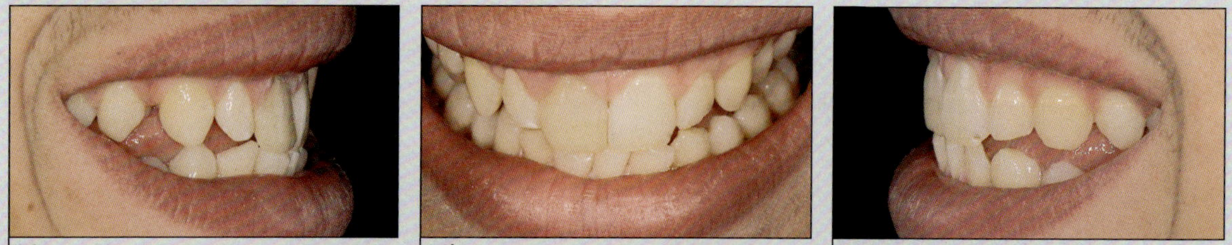

Figs 14a to 14c Initial discoloration of patient's maxillary right central incisor.

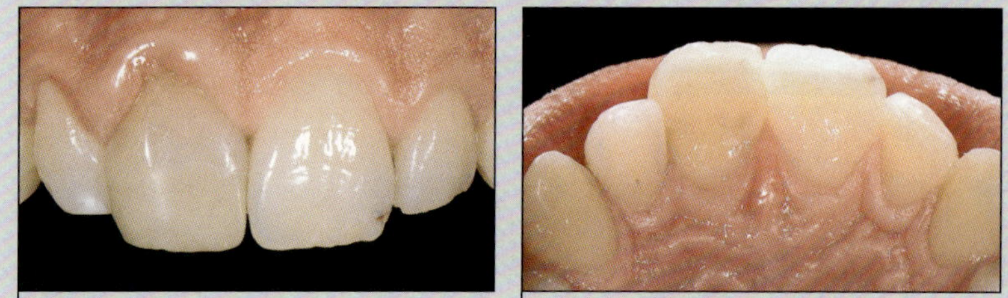

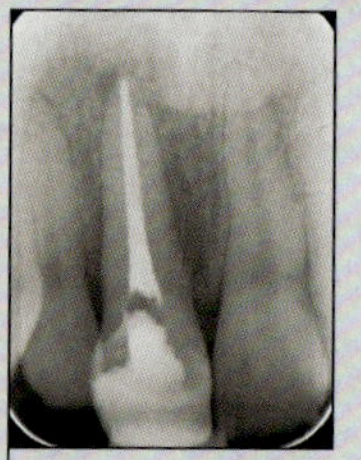

Figs 15a and 15b Close-up of discolored tooth for examination of horizontal fracture line.

Fig 16 Radiograph of previous root canal treatment.

GLASS-FIBER POSTS

In a recent meta-analysis,[15] glass-fiber posts were compared to metal and ceramic posts. Custom-cast post systems showed higher failure loads than prefabricated glass-fiber posts and ceramic posts. Failure modes were significantly more favorable with prefabricated glass-fiber posts compared to prefabricated or custom-cast metal post systems.

These results, although derived mainly from in vitro studies, coupled with those of other in vitro studies,[16–18] indeed suggest that glass-fiber posts provide good clinical utility; clinical data also support this finding.[19] Whereas the radiographic opacity of glass-fiber posts needs improvement, the retrievability in case of a fracture or an endodontic emergency is excellent. Unfortunately, clinical long-term results are not yet available for glass-fiber post systems. Extrapolation of the favorable in vitro data to the clinical outcome must be carefully considered.

Case Presentation

A 19-year-old male patient requested an esthetic improvement of his maxillary right central incisor (Figs 14a to 14c). Upon clinical examination, a horizontal fracture line was detected about 4 mm above the labial zenith point of the tooth (Figs 15a and 15b). In addition, the mesiodistal width of the tooth measured 1 mm less than the respective width of the left central incisor. Zenith points were at similar levels. The radiographic examination revealed an excellent previous root canal treatment (Fig 16).

Placement of a glass-fiber post with subsequent crowning using an all-ceramic restoration was favored over an internal bleaching procedure with post placement alone. The patient gave his consent to this treatment option. Shade was determined in a conventional manner by use of a standardized shade guide (Fig 17). The glass-fiber post was placed (Fig 18), and the post position

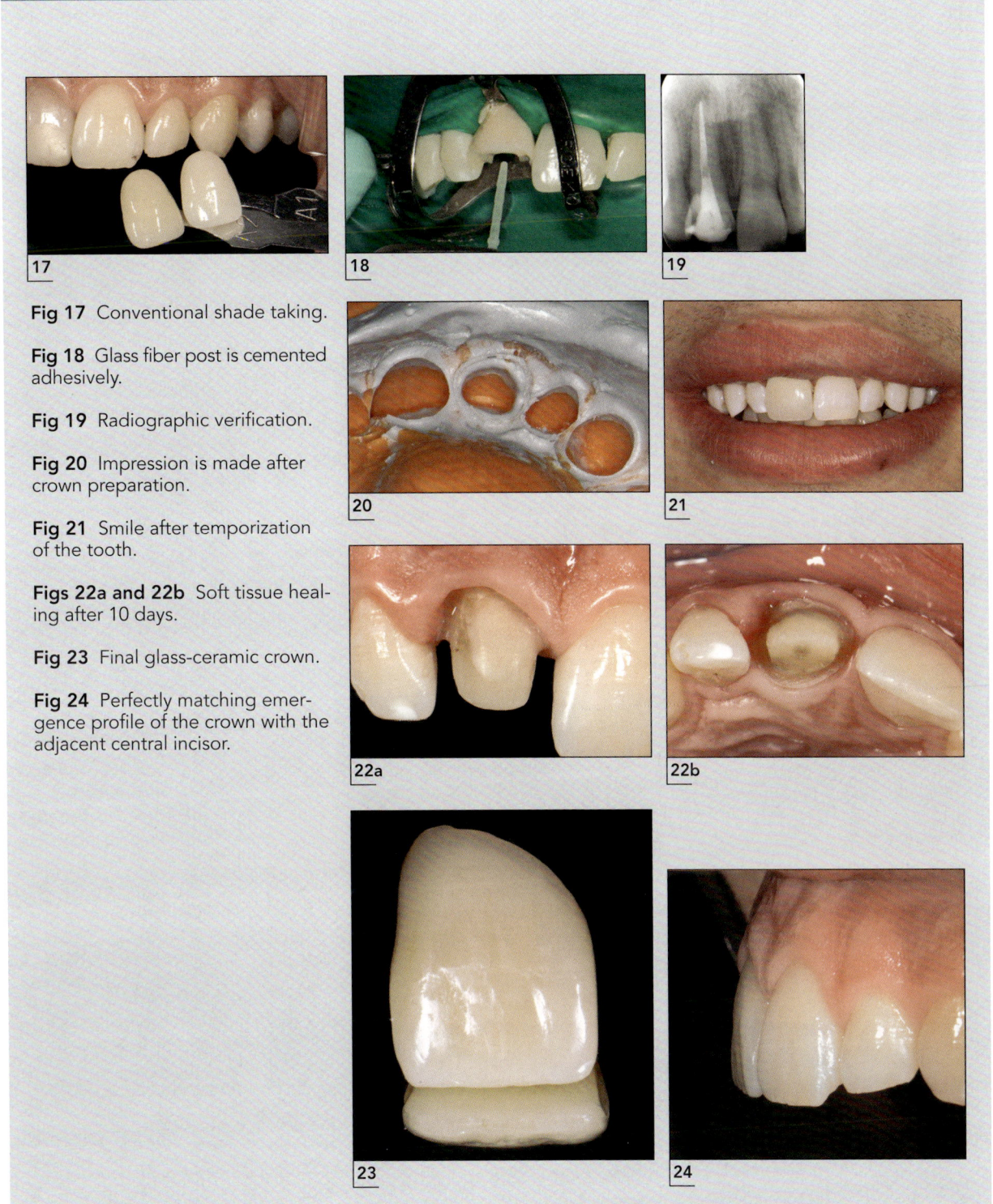

Fig 17 Conventional shade taking.

Fig 18 Glass fiber post is cemented adhesively.

Fig 19 Radiographic verification.

Fig 20 Impression is made after crown preparation.

Fig 21 Smile after temporization of the tooth.

Figs 22a and 22b Soft tissue healing after 10 days.

Fig 23 Final glass-ceramic crown.

Fig 24 Perfectly matching emergence profile of the crown with the adjacent central incisor.

was verified radiographically after adhesive cementation of the post in the root canal (Fig 19).

An impression was made (Fig 20), and a provisional restoration placed (Fig 21). The marginal soft tissues displayed satisfactory healing 10 days later (Figs 22a and 22b). The glass-ceramic crown created offered an emergence profile that satisfactorily matched the adjacent central incisor (Figs 23 and 24).

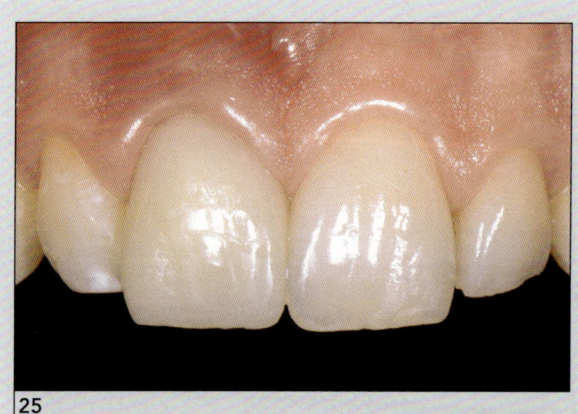

25

Fig 25 Immediately after adhesive cementation, the glass-ceramic crown on the right central incisor matches well with the adjacent incisor, except for value, which is too low.

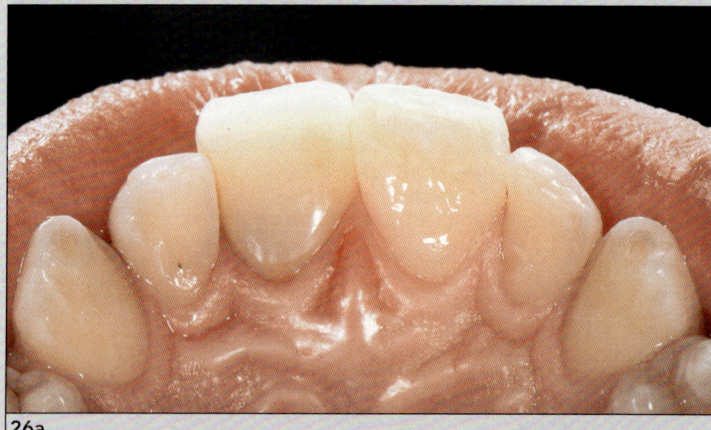

26a

Figs 26a and 26b Seven days later, soft tissue adaptation and color match are very satisfactory.

Fig 27 Final radiograph reveals an excellent marginal fit.

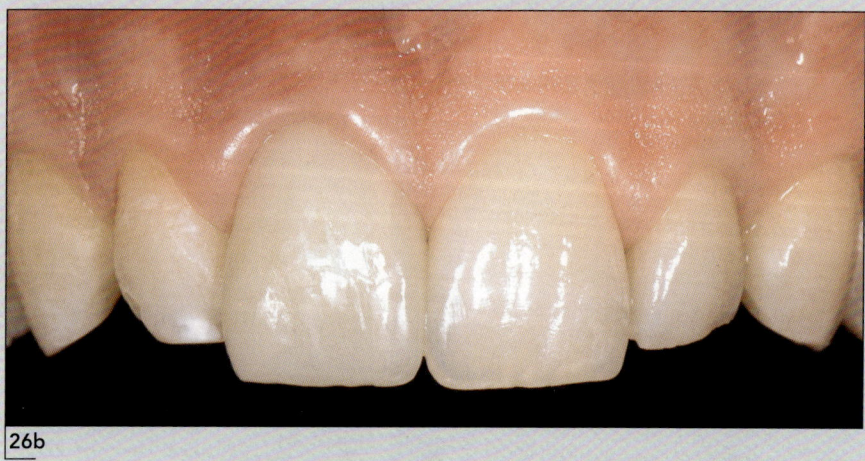

26b

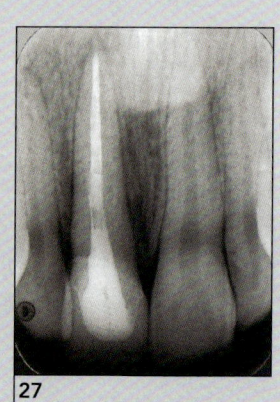

27

Immediately after final adhesive cementation, the glass-ceramic crown displayed acceptable length-to-width ratio, surface texture, and reflection lines that matched the adjacent incisor. The zenith point and the position of the central papilla were satisfactory. However, value was a bit too low (Fig 25).

The adjacent natural teeth had rehydrated 7 days after final delivery of the crown, displaying good color match with the restored tooth (Figs 26a and 26b). An excellent marginal fit was confirmed in the radiograph (Fig 27).

CONCLUSION

Zironia and glass-fiber post systems can be considered equal with respect to the final esthetic result. Although in vitro data of these two post systems show controversial results, zirconia post systems do offer some clinical evidence of long-term success. Clinicians must therefore be prudent when deciding which post system to use in an endodontically treated tooth until further clinical evidence is available.

ACKNOWLEDGMENTS

The author wishes to express his gratitude to the ceramists, Nicola Pietrobon, Zürich, and Martin Lampl, Bregenz Dornbirn, for contributing the excellent all-ceramic restorations.

REFERENCES

1. Sorensen JA, Martinoff JT. Intracoronal reinforcement and coronal coverage: A study of endodontically treated teeth. J Prosthet Dent 1984;51:780–784.

2. Caputo AA, Standlee JP. Restoration of endodontically treated teeth. In: Biomechanics in Clinical Dentistry. Chicago: Quintessence, 1987:185–203.

3. Nathanson D, Ashayeri N. New aspects of restoring the endodontically treated tooth. Alpha Omegan 1990;83: 76–80.

4. Randow K, Glantz PO. On cantilever loading of vital and non-vital teeth. An experimental clinical study. Acta Odontol Scand 1986;44:271–277.

5. Christensen GJ. Posts, cores and patient care. J Am Dent Assoc 1993;124:86–90.

6. Torbjörner A. Treatment management. Posts and cores. In: Karlsson S, Nilner K, Dahl BL (eds). A Textbook of Fixed Prosthodontics. Stockholm: Gothia, 2000:173–186.

7. Fernandes AS, Dessai GS. Factors affecting the fracture resistance of post-core reconstructed teeth: A review. Int J Prosthodont 2001;14:355–363.

8. Assif D, Oren E, Marshak BL, Aviv I. Photoelastic analysis of stress transfer by endodontically treated teeth to the supporting structure using different restorative techniques. J Prosthet Dent 1989;61:535–543.

9. Hornbrook DS, Hastings JH. Use of a bondable reinforcement fiber for post and core build-up in an endodontically treated tooth: Maximizing strength and esthetics. Pract Periodont Aesthet Dent 1995;7:33–42.

10. Rudo DN, Karbhari BM. Physical behaviors of fiber reinforcement as applied to tooth stabilization. Dent Clin North Am 1999;43:7–35.

11. Anusavice KJ. Dental ceramic and metal ceramics. In: Okabe T, Takahashi S (eds). Transactions of the International Congress on Dental Ceramics, South Carolina, 1989. Academy of Dental Materials, 1989:159–172.

12. Scherrer SS, deRijk WG. The fracture resistance of all-ceramic crowns on supporting structures with different elastic moduli. Int J Prosthodont 1993;6:462–267.

13. Sorensen JA, Ahn SG, Berge HX, Edelhoff D. Selection criteria for post and core materials in the restoration of endodontically treated teeth. In: Transactions of the Conference on Scientific Criteria for Selecting Materials and Techniques in Clinical Dentistry, Siena, Italy, September 2001. Academy of Dental Materials, 2001:67–84.

14. Paul SJ, Werder P. Clinical sucess of zirconium oxide posts with resin composite or glass-ceramic cores in endodontically treated teeth: A 4-year retrospective study. Int J Prosthodont 2004;17:524–528.

15. Fokkinga WA, Kreulen CM, Vallittu PK, Creugers NHJ. A structered analysis of in vitro failure loads and failure modes of fiber, metal, and ceramic post-and-core systems. Int J Prosthodont 2004;17: 476–482.

16. Stricker EJ, Göhring TN. Influence of different posts and cores on marginal adaptation, fractures resistance, and fracture mode of composite resin crowns on human mandibular premolars. An in vitro study. J Dent 2006;34: 326–335.

17. Goracci C, Sadek FT, Fabianelli A, Tay FR, Ferrari M. Evaluation of the adhesion of fiber posts to intraradicular dentin. Oper Dent 2005;30:627–635.

18. Naumann M, Preuss A, Rosentritt M. Effect of incomplete crown ferrules on load capacity of endodontically treated maxillary incisors restored with fiber posts, composite build-ups, and all-ceramic crowns: An in vitro evaluation after chewing simulation. Acta Odontol Scand 2006; 64:31–36.

19. Grandini S, Goracci C, Tay FR, Grandini R, Ferrari M. Clinical evaluation of the use of fiber posts and direct resin restorations for endodontically treated teeth. Int J Prosthodont 2005;18:399–404.

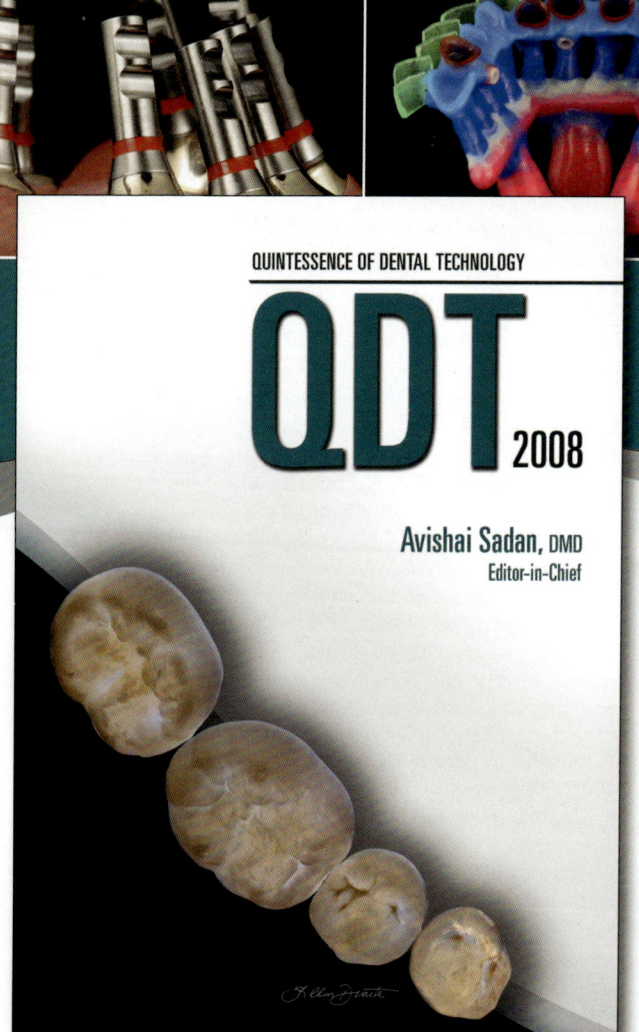

QUINTESSENCE OF DENTAL TECHNOLOGY

QDT 2008

Avishai Sadan, DMD
Editor-in-Chief

This annual publication features original articles on the year's newest materials, concepts, and laboratory techniques from the world's masters in dental technology and esthetic dentistry. Offered again this year as a hardbound edition to stand up to years of use.

QDT 2008 (Vol 31): 192 pp; 711 color illus;
*ISBN 978-0-86715-486-3; **US $80***

Quintessence of Dental Technology 2008
Editor: Avishai Sadan

CONTENTS

Also Available:

QDT 2007 (Vol 30)
224 pp; 900 color illus;
ISBN 978-0-86715-472-6; **US $80**

QDT 2006 (Vol 29)
200 pp; 700 color illus;
ISBN 978-0-86715-459-7; **US $76**

Quintessence Publishing Co, Inc, 4350 Chandler Drive, Hanover Park, IL 60133
Phone (630) 736-3600 • **Fax** (630) 736-3633
E-mail: service@quintbook.com • **Website:** www.quintpub.com

NEW HORIZONS IN ESTHETIC IMPLANTOLOGY

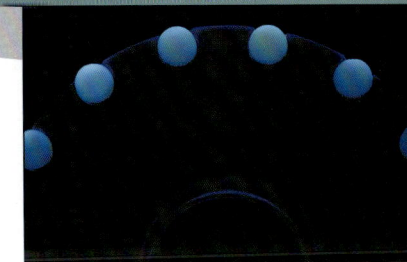

Luc Rutten, MDT[1]
Patrick Rutten, MDT[1]

No area of dentistry is as highly interdependent with dental technology as prosthodontics. Successful dental restorations are usually the result of close interdisciplinary cooperation between dental clinicians and technicians. Recently, dental technology underwent a shift in paradigm. A few years ago, craftsmanship was the focus of a technician's daily work. Issues such as brilliant natural layering techniques, precision of the margins, accuracy of the framework, and position and number of occlusal contact points were the primary focus. In short, technicians focused on the technical details. Today, this perspective has changed, expanding beyond the technical details, though these still remain important. The technician's work is now guided by the growing esthetic demands of the modern patient.

The true challenge does not lie only in ceramic layering, but also in bringing pink and white esthetics into harmony. Given this challenge, it is natural that the need for cooperation between the clinician and dental technician has intensified. A good team is distinguished by silent cooperation. The treatment concept is known to all and is well-structured. The communication channels are clear and functional.

The healthy appearance of the gingiva is a crucial issue. The fabrication of individual abutments, the gingiva-supporting formation of pontics, and the contouring of soft tissue by the controlled shaping of prosthesis elements are just a few examples of the greater demands placed on modern technology. In this context, metal-free restorations are becoming increasingly important. Modern computer-aided design/computer-assisted manufacture (CAD/CAM) technologies are finally able to ensure consistent quality and precision of all-ceramic constructions. The authors have long become accustomed to using a monitor in the workplace and routinely use all-ceramic CAD frameworks.

[1]Master Dental Technician, Dental Team BVBA, Tessenderlo, Belgium.

Correspondence to: Mr L. Rutten and Mr P. Rutten, Dental Team BVBA, Neerstraat 167, B-3980 Tessenderlo, Belgium. E-mail: dental.team@scarlet.be, www.dentalteam.be

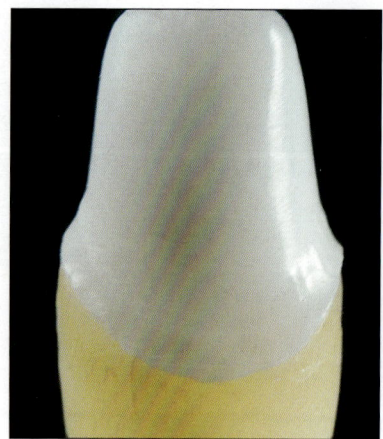 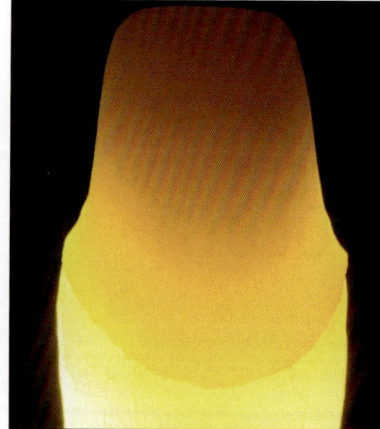

Figs 1a and 1b Scanned zirconium coping under natural *(a)* and transmitted *(b)* light.

ZIRCONIUM DIOXIDE

Zirconium dioxide is one of the highest-performance ceramics in dental technology. This material has excellent mechanical properties combined with bright color and semitranslucency, thus offering dental technicians an extraordinary array of options for fabricating all-ceramic restorations. The option to process this material using Procera 3D-CAD technology (Nobel Biocare, Göteborg, Sweden) makes it possible to break through the previous limitations of all-ceramic restorations while achieving sophisticated esthetic results.

The flexural strength of zirconium dioxide is approximately 1,200 MPa. This guarantees excellent long-term behavior and clinical success rates. The coefficient of thermal expansion (CTE) for a zirconium framework is around 10.5, which is ideal when the veneering ceramic has a somewhat lower CTE (approximately 9.0). Zirconium copings feature excellent fit and a dense, pore-free structure. Mechanical surface treatments, such as sandblasting and grinding with diamond burs, can critically stress the zirconium framework. This may lead to crack propagation or late fissure formation. Thermal treatment is recommended to reverse potential phase transformations. It is sufficient to fire the material at 1,000°C for a holding time of 15 minutes.

Zirconium copings have a white color (Fig 1a). *White* usually sets off alarm bells, since it is considered synonymous with opacity. Under transmitted light, however, semitranslucency is evident in alumina copings, and this is promising (Fig 1b). The light transmittance property of zirconium is 48%, whereas that of alumina is 72%. The refractive index of light is 1.67 for natural enamel, 1.8 for alumina, and 1.5 for ceramic. The refractive index of light of zirconium is 2.3. *Refraction* is the bending of light that occurs when light passes from one transparent material to another.

The optical conditions of metal are unfavorable. Metal blocks 100% of the light, preventing it from being transported into the gingiva and papillae. The advantage of semitranslucent material is that it completely masks discolorations or metal abutments and has no negative effects on the color of the veneer. Thus, semitranslucency is an extremely advantageous characteristic.

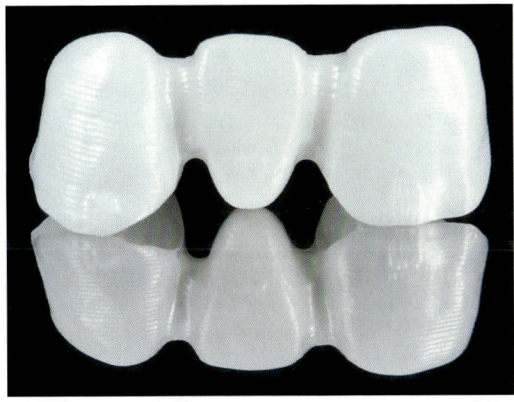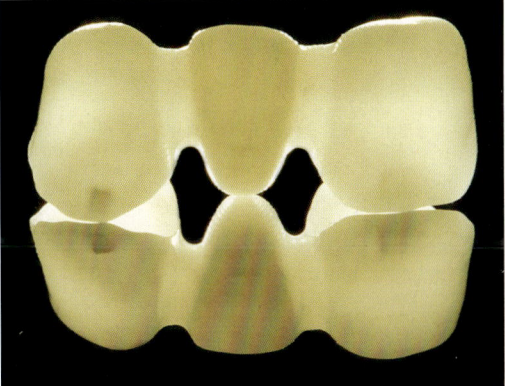

Figs 2a and 2b Zirconium restoration under natural (*a*) and transmitted (*b*) light.

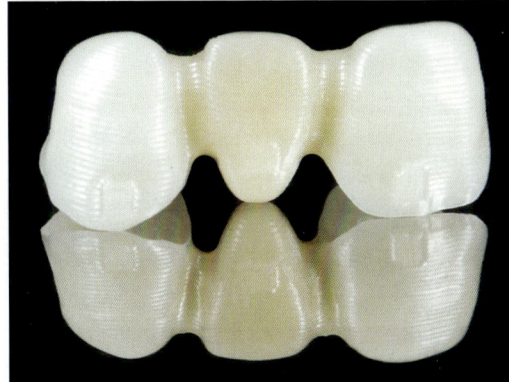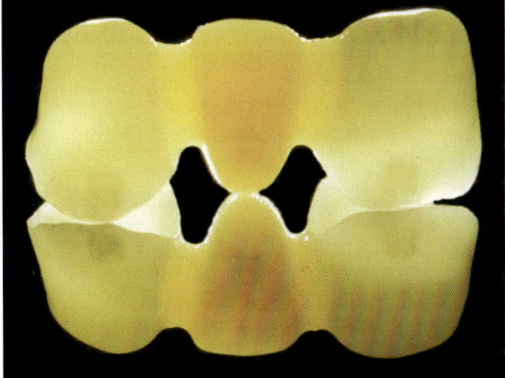

Figs 3a and 3b Alumina restoration under natural (*a*) and transmitted (*b*) light.

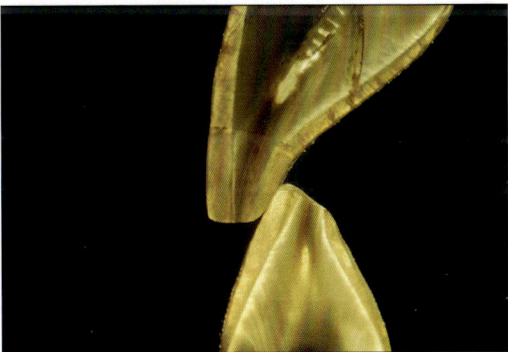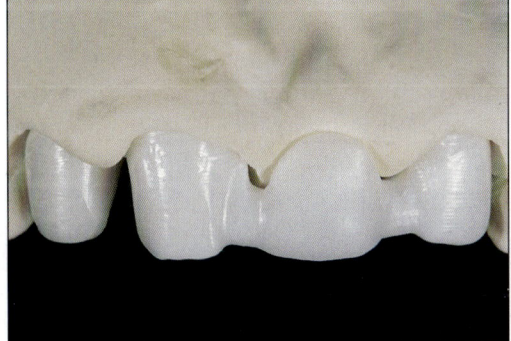

Fig 4 Cross sections of natural teeth under back light.

Fig 5 Due to its white color, zirconium is an ideal material for porcelain buildup.

Observe the differences between a zirconium prosthesis and an alumina prosthesis in normal daylight (Figs 2a and 3a) and transmitted light (Figs 2b and 3b). Both materials exhibit semitranslucency, which is ideal to fabricate natural-looking restorations. Alumina clearly has a warmer chroma than zirconium. This warmer saturation is also evident in natural teeth under transmitted light (Fig 4).

Due to its bright color (Fig 5), zirconium has a very high value. *Value* or *brightness* is the dimension of a color that represents its similarity to one of a series of achromatic colors, ranging from very dim (dark) to very bright (dazzling). In other words, value is the percentage of white in a certain color. More white means a higher value, while less white means a lower value.

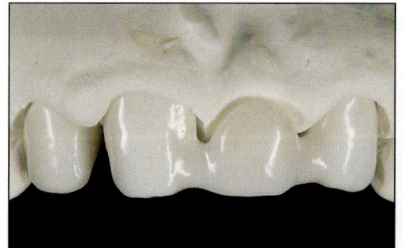

Fig 6 Liners can be used to modify the brightness of zirconia.

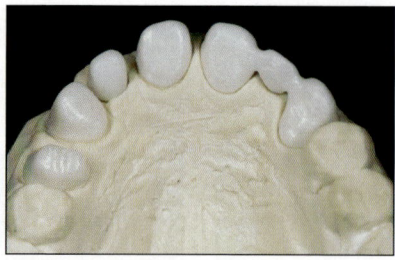

Fig 7 Unprepared zirconium restoration. Note the lack of saturation.

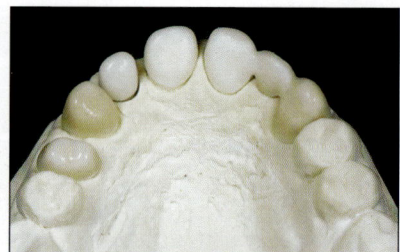

Fig 8 Zirconium restoration after the chroma has been controlled using liners.

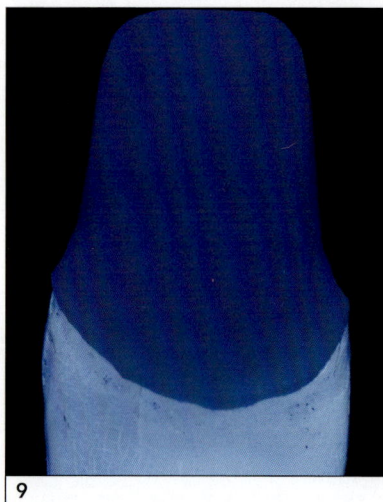

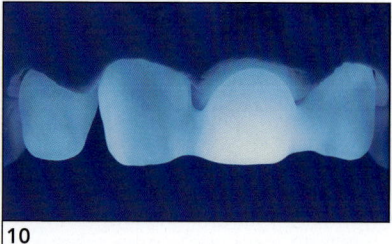

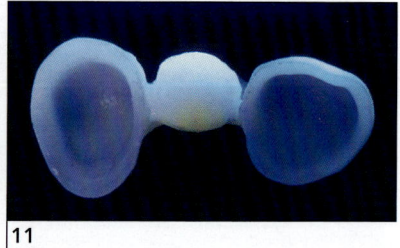

Fig 9 Under ultraviolet light, zirconium copings show a dark shadow.

Fig 10 Fluorescent effects brighten the zirconium framework and improve light conduction.

Fig 11 Even the basal surface of the pontic is covered with fluorescent shoulder material.

The chroma of zirconium is zero because of its very white and bright color (Fig 6). *Saturation* or *chroma* refers to the intensity of a specific hue. A highly saturated hue has a vivid, intense color, while a less saturated hue appears more muted. In other words, saturation is the percentage of a neutral substance (eg, water) in a certain color. More of a neutral substance in a certain color means less saturation. To communicate efficiently between the dental practice and dental laboratory, it is important that all parties understand these terms and their importance in tooth selection.

Figure 7 shows a "naked" unprepared restoration, with an extremely high brightness and no saturation at all. What steps should now be taken, considering that canines almost always have a higher chroma? First, a prewash or thin layer of dentin is applied. This prewash bonder application and firing step facilitates a strong bond between the framework and layering porcelain. The second step is to layer fluorescent shoulder ceramic over the entire framework. For the canines and posterior region, fluorescent shoulder porcelain with higher saturation is used (Fig 8). This technique optimizes light transmittance.

Under ultraviolet light, zirconium copings produce an undesirable dark shadow (Fig 9). To retain the appearance of vital gingiva, strong luminosity is required, even under ultraviolet light. Thus, the zirconium coping is shortened or the scanner is activated in "short-scan" mode. *Fluorescence* is the capability of a body to receive radiation at one wavelength and emit radiation at another wavelength. Short-wave ultraviolet light (ie, black light), which is visible to the human eye, is part of daylight. When it makes contact with a natural tooth, it passes through the enamel, penetrates

Fig 12 Zirconium makes it possible to fabricate increasingly large restorations.

Fig 13 The connectors between the crowns and pontics should be at least 2 × 3 mm.

Figs 14a to 14c Three-dimensional model of the zirconium restoration.

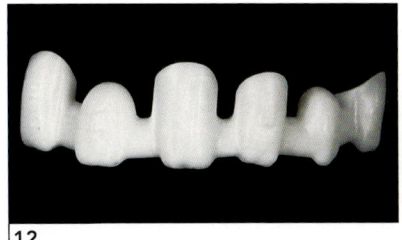

12

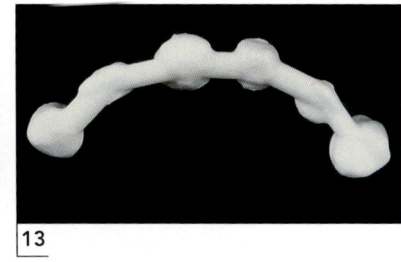

13

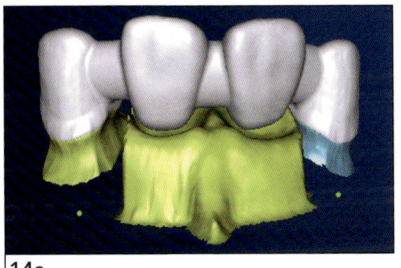

14a

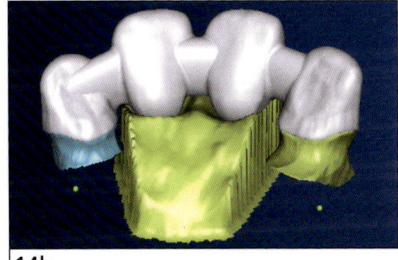

14b

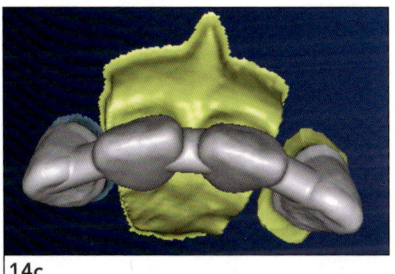

14c

the dentin, and is then reflected (Fig 10). To obtain identical optical characteristics, highly fluorescent shoulder material is fired onto the basal area of the pontics (Fig 11). The shoulder ceramic has slightly higher color saturation than the basic shade of the restoration and masks the underlying cervical shadows of the framework.

This material opens many doors for esthetic implantology. Large fixed prostheses and even full-mouth prostheses can now be fabricated (Fig 12). The connections to the pontics are designed as large as possible; nevertheless, there is still sufficient space to allow for anatomic shaping and contouring and natural staining. According to the manufacterer, the connection should be at least 6 mm² (2 × 3 mm) (Fig 13).

COMPUTER-AIDED PONTIC DESIGN

The indications for zirconium fixed restorations are basically the same as for alumina fixed restorations; however, the performance of this ceramic is markedly greater and offers patients more security and confidence. Ceramic materials are the materials of the future, and all-ceramic materials such as zirconium will likely replace metal in many cases.

The dies for the restoration are scanned in exactly the same way as for a single crown, although this is only possible in a Procera Forte scanner (Nobel Biocare). The scanning procedure is carried out automatically. The software will automatically check if all prosthesis components are present. The restoration can then be viewed from all sides on the computer monitor (Figs 14a to 14c). The data can then be transmitted electronically to Sweden.

Modern prosthetic rehabilitation requires extensive knowledge and clinical experience from different dental specialities and related disciplines. Teamwork is necessary even when treating smaller cases with ovate pontics. After healing of a modified connective tissue graft (site development), the tissue bed can be prepared for ovate pontics using

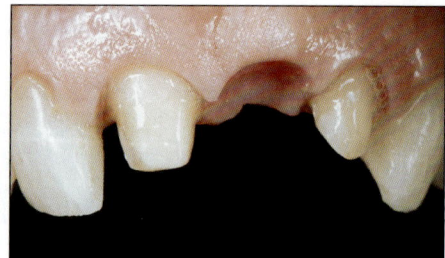
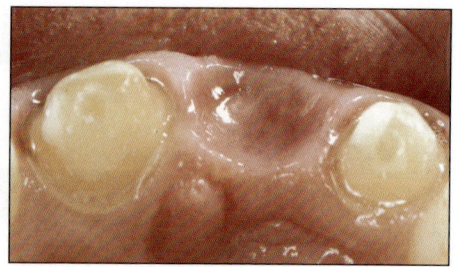

Figs 15a and 15b After the connective tissue graft, a ball-shaped diamond bur was used to modify the gingiva for the ovate pontic.

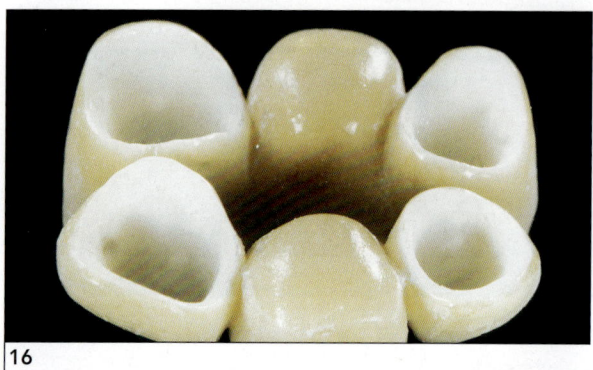

Fig 16 The basal surface of the ovate pontic must be mechanically polished and smoothed.

Fig 17 Finished zirconium restoration on the master cast.

Fig 18 Definitive zirconium restoration showing a natural-looking emergence profile.

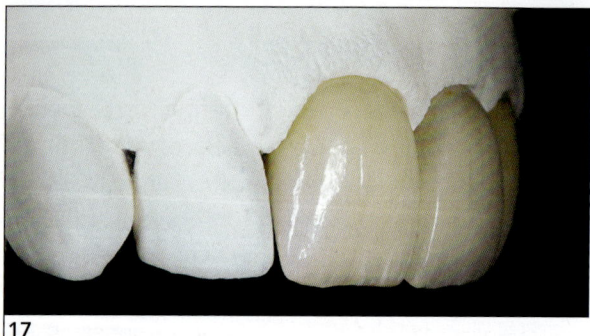
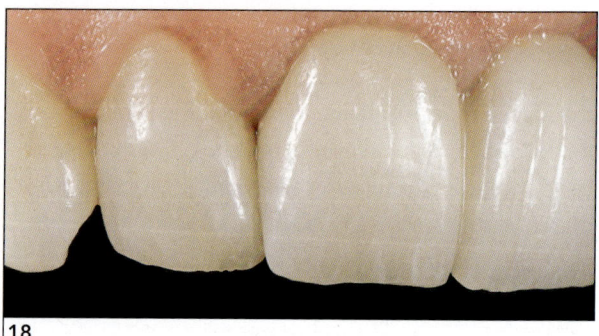

a ball-shaped diamond bur (Figs 15a and 15b). It is the job of the dental technician to transfer the impressions to the cast and grind the cast selectively at the pontic area. This ensures sufficient support of the gingiva. In addition, the basal surface of the pontic is mechanically polished and smoothed (Fig 16). The pontics may appear to be too long; however, since the convex pontic is seated 1 to 1.5 mm into the gingiva, this appearance will vanish once the restoration is placed on the cast (Fig 17).

For the definitive restoration shown in Fig 18, a vast amount of experience was required to satisfactorily restore this anterior space with a three-unit fixed prosthesis. Even with all of this experi-

ence, detailed diagnosis and treatment planning were still indispensable. Prosthodontists and dental technicians must work together closely from the beginning, because any wrong step has an immediate consequence. In this case, harmony was restored with the natural adjacent teeth. The pontic's emergence profile was not much different from that of the natural situation. Note the correct value and somewhat warm chroma in this restoration. There is a lot of controversy and skepticism about the use of zirconium dioxide; however, as is evident in this restoration, it is perfectly possible to control the value and chroma.

CASE 1 (Figs 19 to 42)

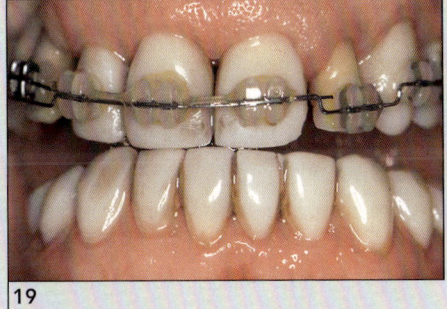

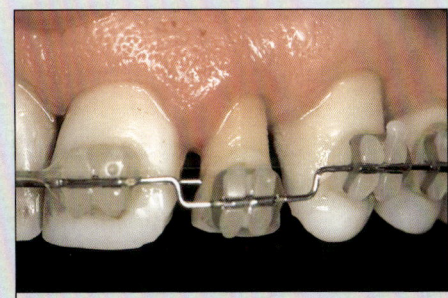

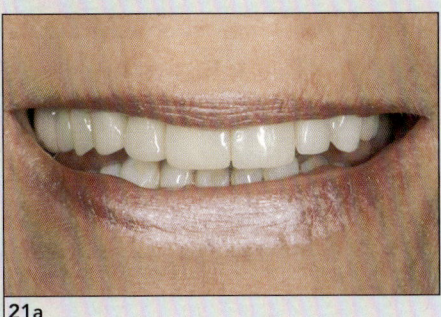

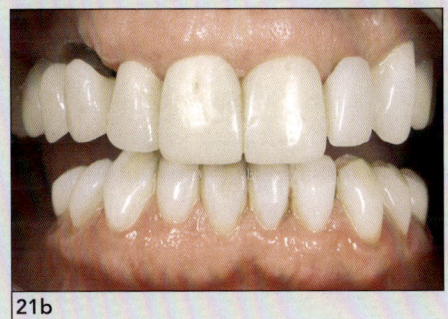

Fig 19 Initial situation.

Fig 20 Extrusion of the lateral incisor.

Fig 21a and 21b Laboratory-made provisional crowns incorporated the first esthetic and functional changes.

CASE REPORTS

The treatment of periodontally involved cases is gaining increasing importance in dental practice. These cases require close cooperation among the periodontist, orthodontist, prosthodontist, and dental technician. In the following case reports, comprehensive and esthetically challenging cases will be introduced. For all patients, the chosen material for the copings and abutments was zirconium dioxide.

Case 1

Figure 19 shows an anterior view of the initial situation. The esthetic and periodontal problems are obvious. Clinical analysis revealed the entire range

of esthetic problems, including flared anterior teeth with diastema (missing central papilla), an uneven gingival margin, and wide embrasure spaces emphasized by the triagular tooth shape.

Careful treatment planning is necessary to restore severely esthetically and functionally compromised dentition. Following a second evaluation of the esthetic situation, the periodontist decided to extrude the lateral incisor (Fig 20). Next, the lateral incisor was extracted and an implant was placed.

Provisional restorations were used to restore the vertical dimension of occlusion. Laboratory-made diagnostic provisional crowns quickly mollify the anxious patient and incorporate the first esthetic and functional changes (Figs 21a and 21b). In the mandible, laminate veneers were planned to improve the esthetics.

First, the cast was analyzed in the articulator (Fig 22). This is the initial step of good treatment planning in the lab. The bipupillary line was used as a guide to determine the correct horizontal line of the maxillary incisal edges. To obtain an optimal width-length ratio between the anterior crowns, a diagnostic waxup was fabricated. This showed the ideal situation in terms of both function and esthetics. Procera zirconium crowns on natural dies and customized abutments were used. It is recommended to fabricate the custom abutments with casting resin rather than wax. Abutments made with casting resin are more stable and will not break when the abutment is screwed in and out. A waxed-up abutment is more fragile.

The abutments were milled into shape. Thanks to the soft gingival mask, it was possible to remove the stable resin abutments from the cast without any problems. The abutments were mounted on the scanner's appropriate holder (Fig 23), and the screw access hole was sealed with wax. After finishing, the data were transmitted to the closest Procera production center (Nobel Biocare).

When fabricating individual abutments, good communication between the periodontist/prosthodontist and dental technician regarding the emergence angles and soft tissue support is required. If the implants are placed in the proper positions, selecting and designing an appropriate abutment is not problematic. In general, the desired position of the crown margin should be 0.5 mm below the gingiva at the labial side and level with the gingiva at the lingual and palatal sides. If the crown margin is lower, the prosthodontist will have difficulty visualizing and trimming any excess cement or composite. A qualified dental technician should be aware of this when designing the abutments.

It is important that there be sufficient space from the labial side for the crown and veneering material. There must be at least 0.5 mm between the desired margin of the abutment and the gingiva. If there is inadequate space, the gingiva will shift in the apical direction, leading to an automatic discrepancy in the gingival tissue levels. It is important to create a periodontally friendly mar-

gin. Concave contouring and shaping of the abutment at the area below the preparation margin extending to the base of the implant should be carried out. The requisite preparation for long-term success is a shoulder preparation with rounded edges (Figs 24a and 24b).

The use of a biocompatible abutment material is advised for transmucosal soft tissue adhesion. Along with excellent tissue adhesion, zirconium brightens the gingiva due to its bright, white color. If the biotype is thin, the material underneath may shine through. In these cases, titanium abutments or cast abutments in an alloy would have a negative effect on the pink esthetics by creating a shadow or a grayish color at the gingiva.

To evaluate the paradigm shift in abutment design, Rompen et al[1] examined the effect of a concave transmucosal profile on the vertical stability of soft tissues at the facial aspect of dental implants (Curvy Abutment, Nobel Biocare). In a pilot phase, grooves were individually milled using a diamond bur into the concave subgingival area between the preparation margin and implant base (Figs 25a and 25b). This stabilized and promoted the soft tissue seal. Note that Curvy Abutments are available only in titanium.

In each phase, the silicone index of the waxup was used as a reference (Fig 26). The position of the zirconium crowns should be in relation to the desired tooth shape and size to ensure correct support of the ceramics. The framework was reduced approximately 2 mm incisally and 1.5 mm labially and lingually. The framework must be accurately dimensioned to prevent fracturing.

Correct implant placement allows for individually designed all-ceramic abutments on each implant. Thanks to the industrial-grade precision of CAD procedures, the all-ceramic crowns arrive with a cement gap (50 to 60 µm in width) that is consistently maintained between the prepared die or abutment and coping, providing 100% passive retention without friction. The computer-controlled precision of fit ensures that the cement gap is optimal (Fig 27).

Since all-ceramic materials such as alumina and zirconium have no fluorescence, it is important to

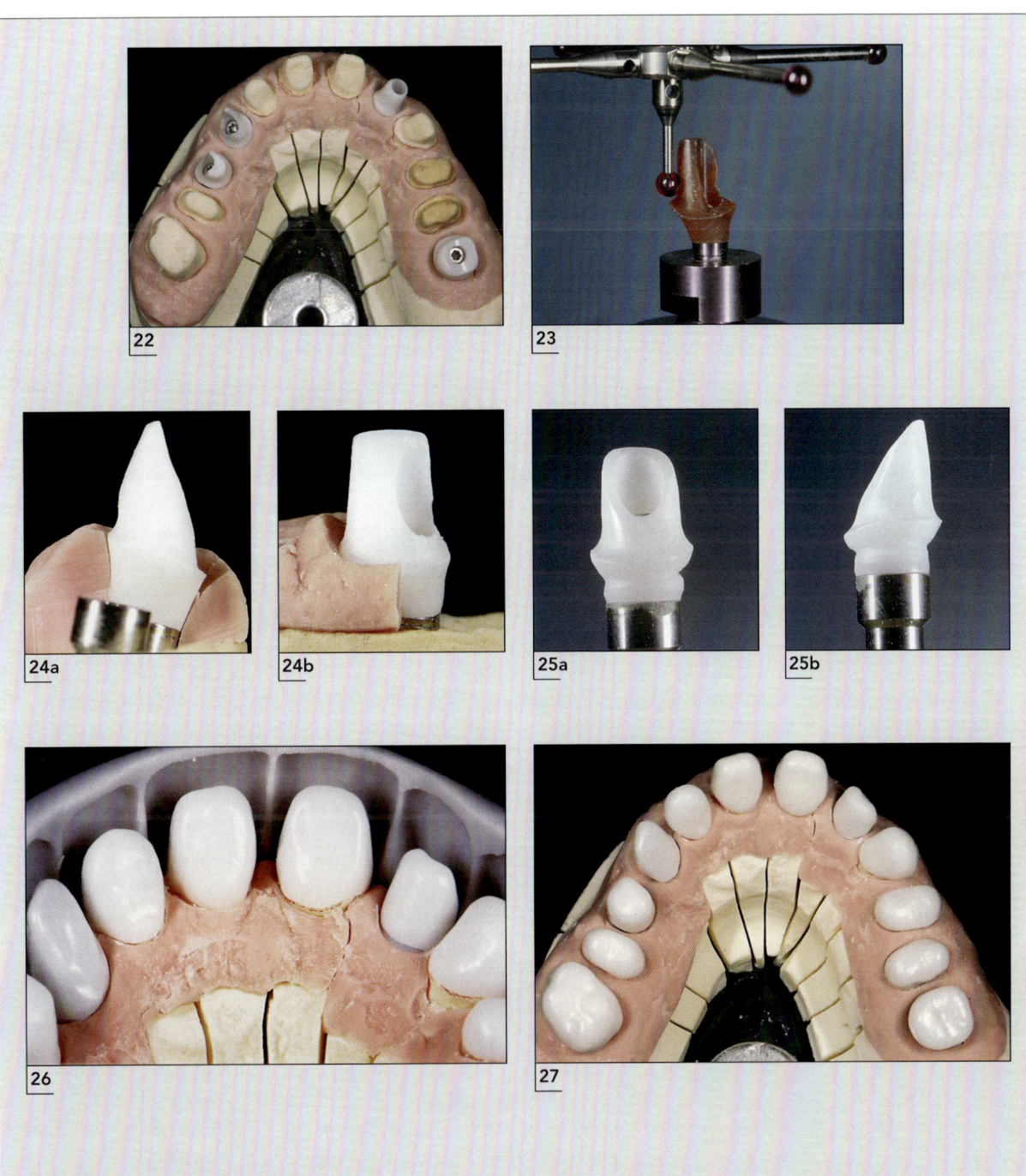

Fig 22 Master cast with the flexible removable gingival mask and all-ceramic custom abutments.

Fig 23 The custom abutments were scanned for data transmittal.

Figs 24a and 24b Sufficient space between the margin of the abutment and the gingiva is necessary for stability.

Figs 25a and 25b Abutment designed with a groove into the concave transmucosal profile.

Fig 26 Positioning of the zirconium crowns was controlled with a silicone index.

Fig 27 CAD procedures ensure precise and consistent cement gaps.

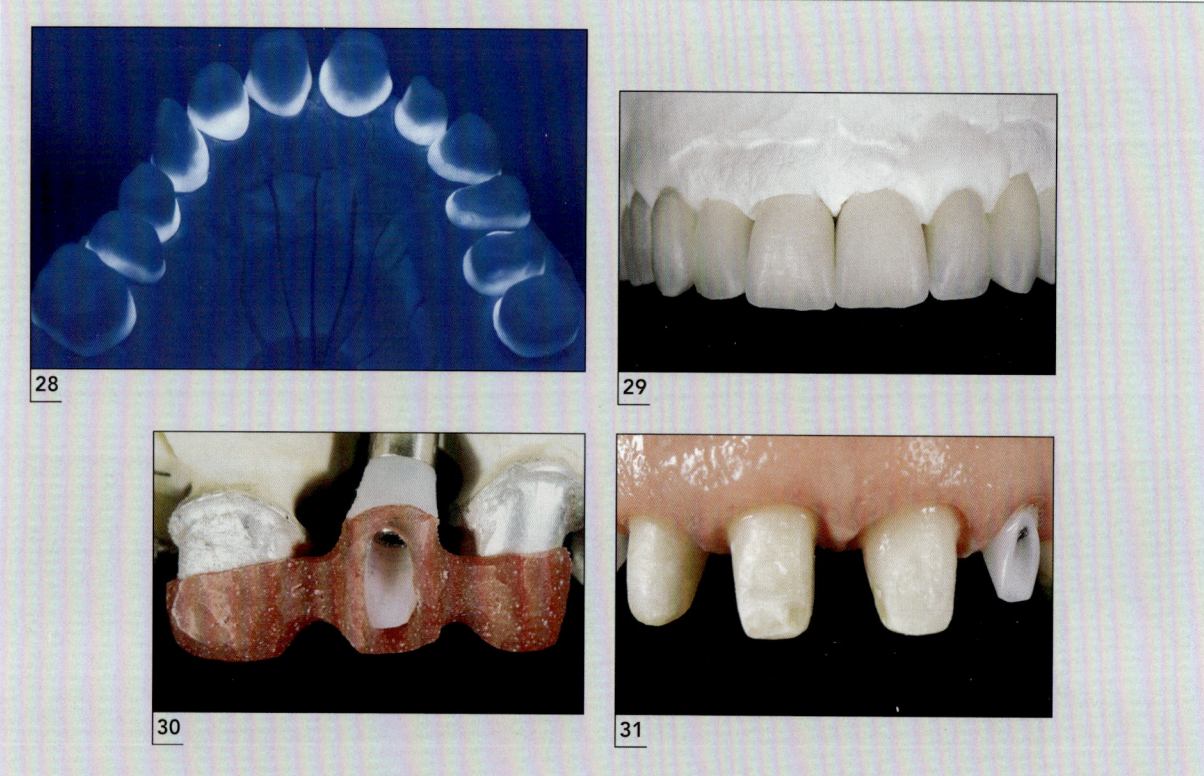

Fig 28 Under ultraviolet light, zirconium crowns produce a dark shadow, and fluorescent ceramic powders brighten up the cervical areas.

Fig 29 The contact surfaces of the crowns were controlled on an unsectioned master cast.

Fig 30 Acrylic key used to transfer the abutment in the mouth.

Fig 31 Individual zirconium abutment in place on the implant.

brighten the "critical" gingival zones to prevent shadows and improve light conduction. In ultraviolet light, the crowns produce a dark shadow, especially in the cervical area, which will affect the final esthetic result (Fig 28). Strong luminosity is needed to produce a vital-looking restoration. All-ceramic restorations cannot tolerate shadows.

The rubber-polished crowns were placed on the unsectioned master cast for fine adjustment of the marginal ridges and contact surfaces and to produce the final shape. The contact area between the crowns was particularly long, extending from the remaining papillae and nearly approaching the incisal edges. The contact surfaces of single crowns should always, without exception, be controlled on an unsectioned cast. The solid cast eliminates the die movement inherent in all sectioned

casts. In addition, the solid cast allows the crown to be designed within the context of the soft tissues. This produces correct line angles for elegant restorations and closed interdental spaces. Unesthetic black holes should not be tolerated. After bisque firing, the crowns were ready to be sent to the dental clinic on the master cast (Fig 29).

Using an acrylic key fabricated on the master cast by the dental technician, the abutment can be transferred in the patient's mouth quickly and easily (Fig 30). The acrylic key ensures the correct fit of the abutment on the implant. The connection was extended to the natural dies, and the screw access hole was open to screw the abutment on top of the implant.

Figure 31 shows the situation before try-in of the bisque-bake restorations. The hollow-neck

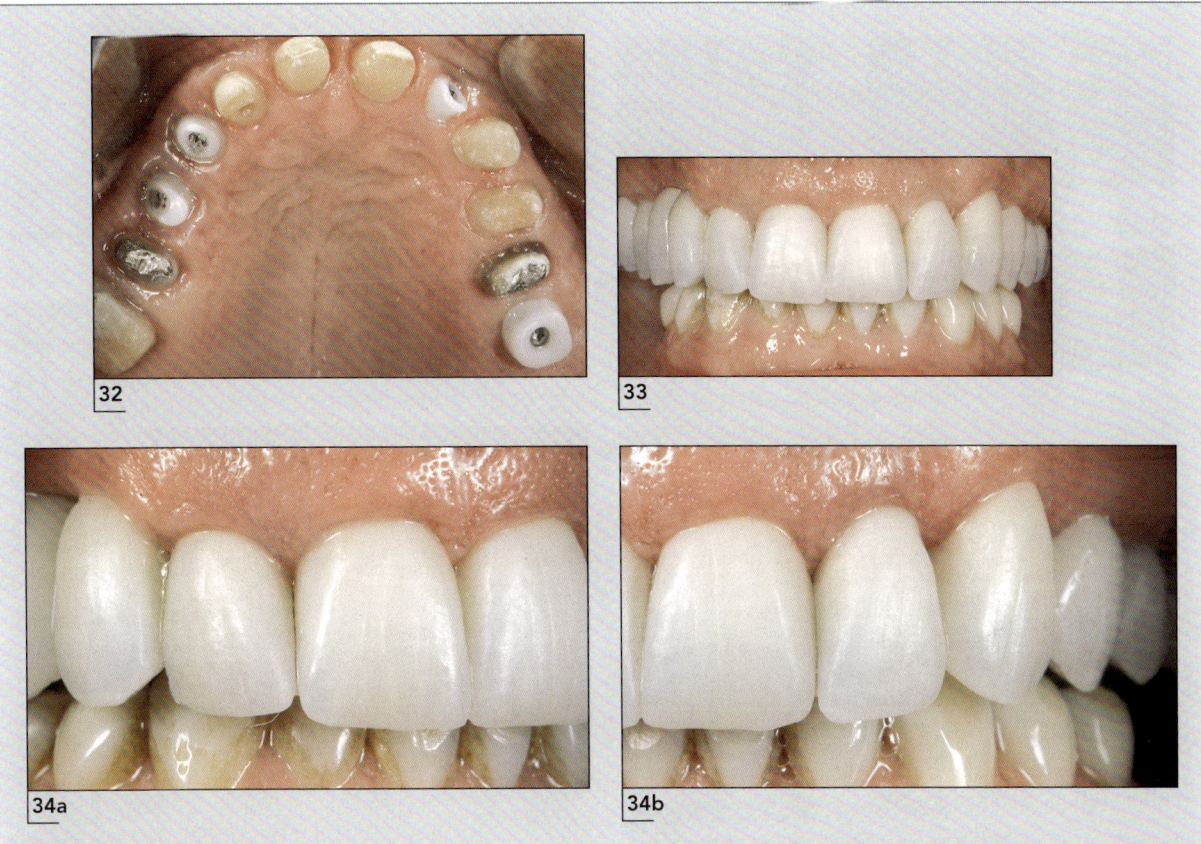

Fig 32 Occlusal view showing the custom abutments and natural tooth dies.

Fig 33 Try-in of the bisque-bake restoration.

Figs 34a and 34b The gingiva quickly adapted to the abutments and crowns.

preparation is perfect for an all-ceramic restoration. The preparation margin of the abutment defined in the lab was located slightly subgingival, approximately 0.4 to 0.5 mm from the labial side. With this type of preparation, the dental technician has sufficient space to design a corresponding margin. The technician can scan any type of preparation; however, copings tend to crack more with tangential preparations. Customers should be informed of this drawback.

Figure 32 shows the custom zirconium abutments and natural stumps prior to insertion of the crowns. The oral situation has been expertly prepared by the periodontist. Using a predefined torque of 35 Ncm, the prosthodontist placed the abutment onto the implant. Try-in of the bisque-bake crowns is highly recommended (Fig 33). Not

only does this allow the patient to evaluate the restoration, but it is also the ideal phase to adjust both the occlusal and interdental contact points and contact surfaces. On this topic, the authors recommend the work of Tarnow et al,[2] who described the relationship between the distance from the bony margin to the interdental contact point and the ability of the papillae to regenerate. In this case, the gingiva adapted quickly to the zirconium abutments and instantly made a visually healthy impression (Figs 34a and 34b).

One important question is whether the dental technician needs direct access to the patient for anterior crown reconstructions. The answer, of course, depends on the desired results. The authors prefer to see patients in the lab. This way, the shape and surface can be adjusted according

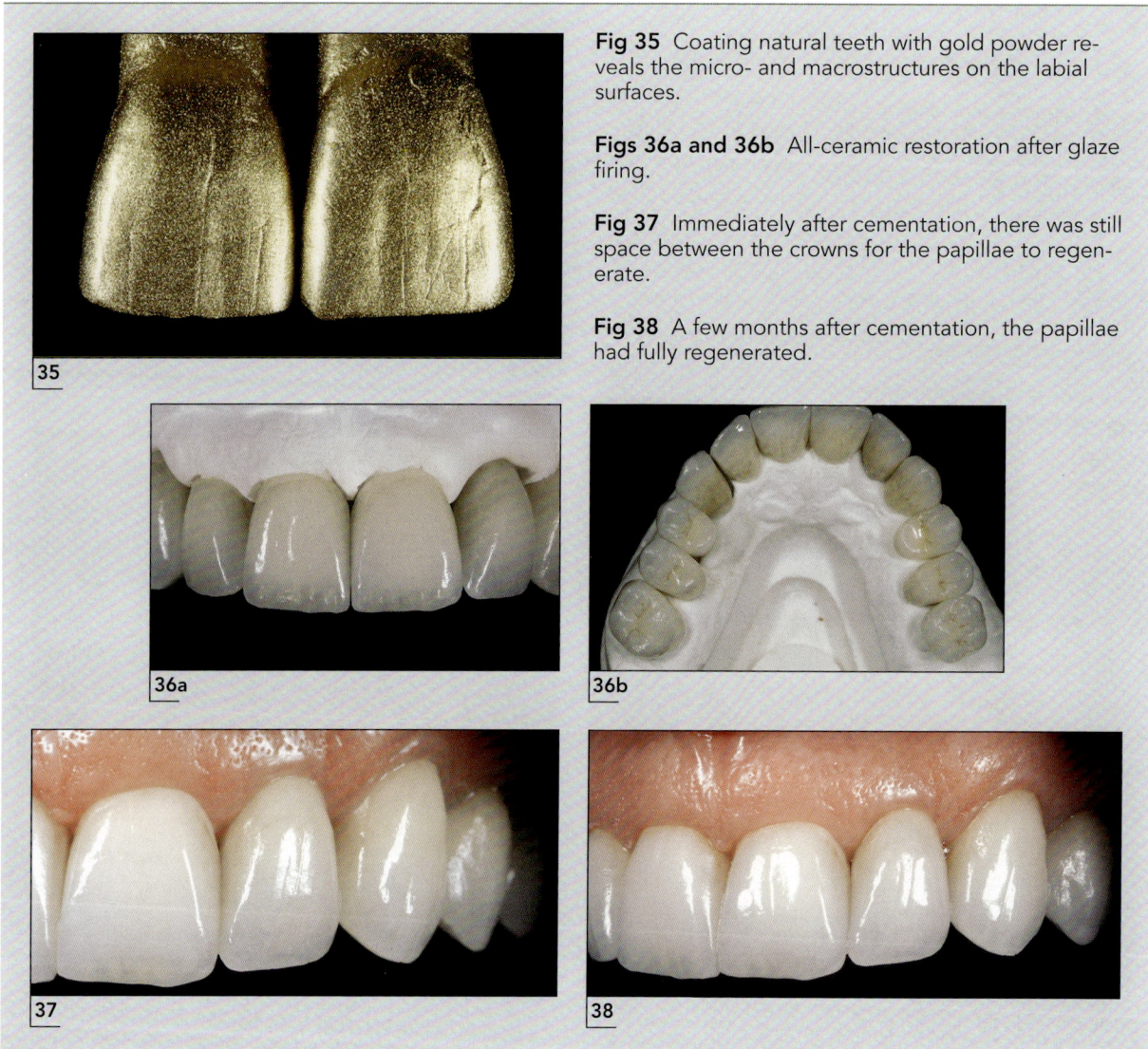

Fig 35 Coating natural teeth with gold powder reveals the micro- and macrostructures on the labial surfaces.

Figs 36a and 36b All-ceramic restoration after glaze firing.

Fig 37 Immediately after cementation, there was still space between the crowns for the papillae to regenerate.

Fig 38 A few months after cementation, the papillae had fully regenerated.

to the patient's wishes. Further, it is important for technicians to take many photographs to better understand the natural oral situation. For example, by viewing teeth coated with gold powder, new details can be discovered and incorporated into daily work (Fig 35). The vertical marks identify the grooves and ridges, which correspond to the microstructure. The macrostructure consists of fine horizontal growth lines.[3]

In this case, the layering was kept simple, relying instead on the effects created by the vitality in the incisal area and the harmony of the tooth shape. The crowns were separated by a delicate incisal triangle. The emergence profile turned out well, and the contact surfaces were ideal (Figs 36a and 36b). The overall layering, especially in the incisal area, was designed to be particularly lifelike. Ceramic stains should never be used in the incisal area, because they restrict the depth of reflection and light transmittance.

After placement of the restoration, there was still space between the crowns for the papillae to regenerate (Fig 37). Oral hygiene and regular checkups will ensure the long-term success of treatment and maintain the bone, periodontium, and teeth. After a few months, the papillae between the implant crown and the natural die were restored (Fig 38).

The emergence profile, ie, the natural physiologic profile of the crown emerging through the

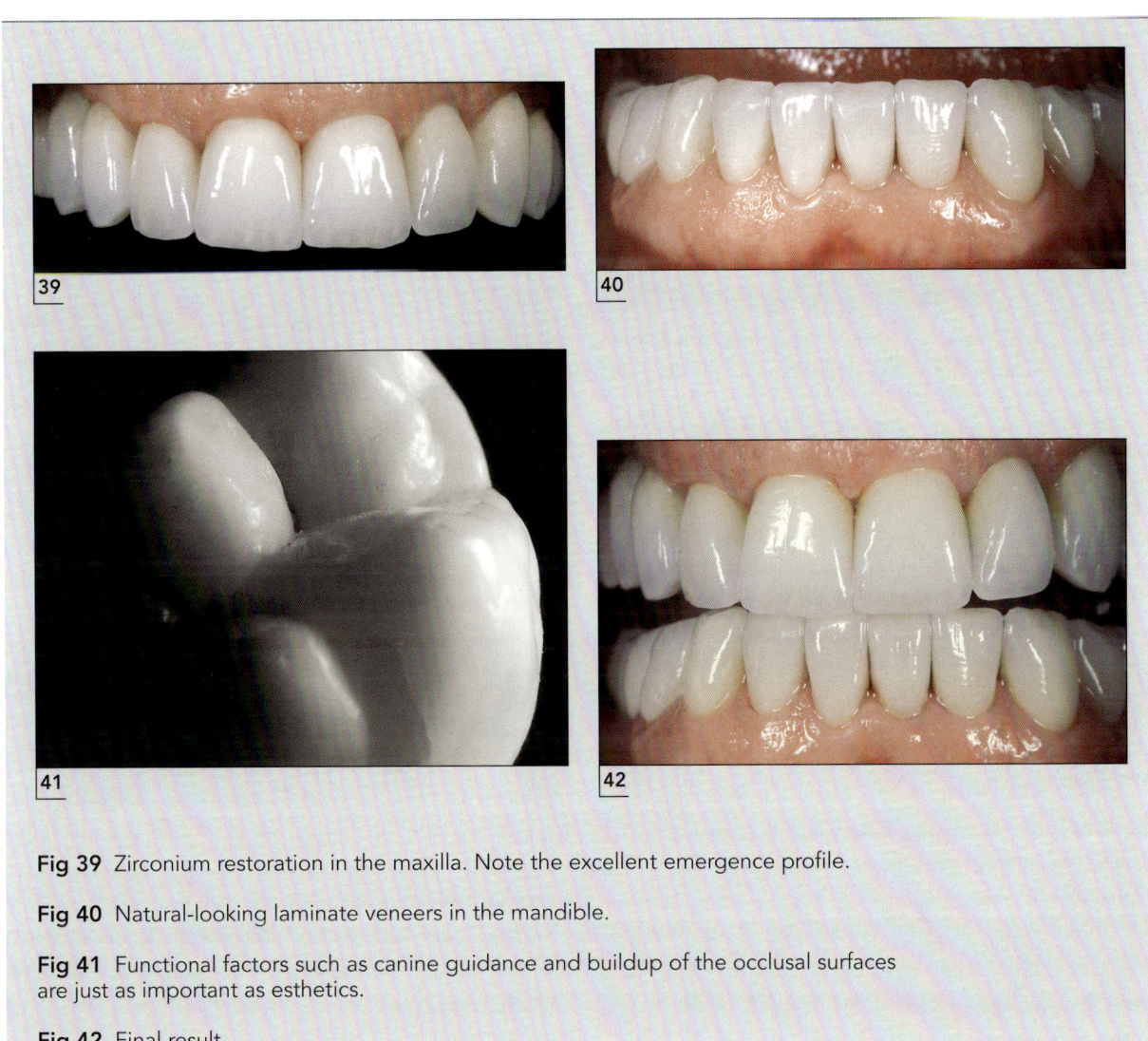

Fig 39 Zirconium restoration in the maxilla. Note the excellent emergence profile.

Fig 40 Natural-looking laminate veneers in the mandible.

Fig 41 Functional factors such as canine guidance and buildup of the occlusal surfaces are just as important as esthetics.

Fig 42 Final result.

gingiva, has a major influence on soft tissue regeneration. The best conditions for gingival and papillary healing is when the emergence profile is correct and the crown contours support the gingiva. The interdental contact surfaces shifted significantly in a cervical direction, sealing the interdental spaces and giving the restoration a natural appearance. Figure 39 shows the final result in the maxilla.

In the mandible, the prosthodontist used a minimally invasive preparation. Laminate veneers on refractory die material were fabricated. The same tooth shade that was used for the maxillary crowns was used for the mandibular laminate veneers, as well. This bright shade does not detract from the appearance, thus illustrating how shape trumps

shade. As is standard for laminate veneers, the gingiva was untouched and showed a pink and healthy appearance. Fourteen days after cementation, the gingival situation was healthy (Fig 40).

The functional requirements were met with classic anterior tooth guidance. The palatal surfaces guide the central incisors in protrusion. The posterior region discludes during canine guidance (Fig 41). The lengths of the maxillary central incisors differed to ensure even anterior tooth guidance. Esthetically, harmony between the pink and white esthetics transformed a good result into an outstanding result—one that could only be achieved with teamwork. The final result shows a natural, harmonious appearance (Fig 42).[4]

CASE 2 (Figs 43 to 59)

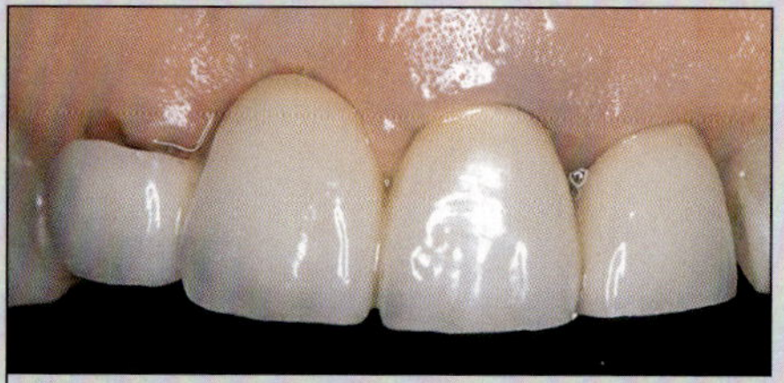

Fig 43 Initial situation with an existing porcelain-fused-to-metal restoration.

Figs 44a and 44b After extraction, two implants were placed at the lateral incisor sites.

Figs 45a and 45b Finished abutments on the gypsum master cast.

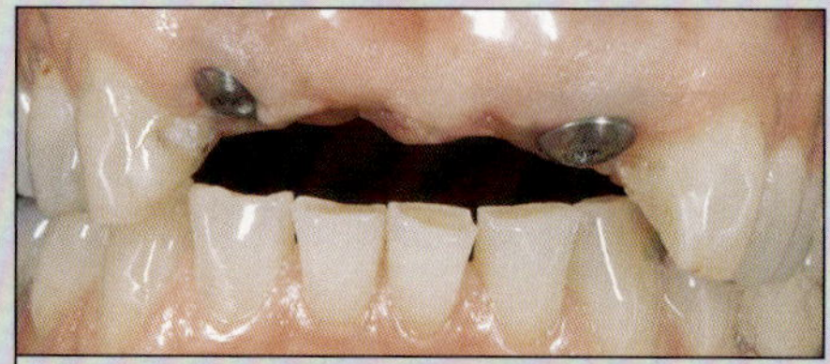

Case 2

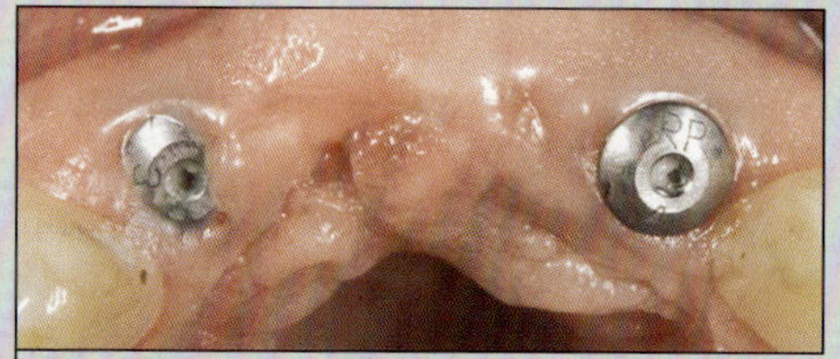

The patient presented with an inadequate porcelain-fused-to-metal prosthesis (Fig 43). The prosthesis was removed, and two implants were placed at the lateral incisor sites (Figs 44a and 44b). To achieve optimal esthetic design of the pontic area in cases with unfavorable initial conditions, measures should be taken to augment gingival tissue supply and condition the site. In general, the periodontist will harvest an approximately 0.8-mm-thick connective tissue graft from the palate.

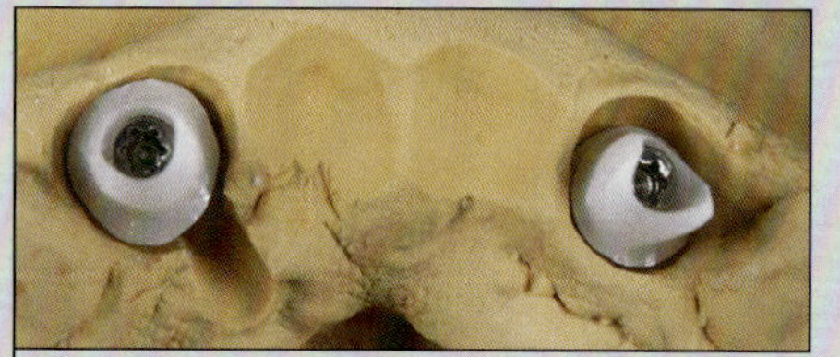

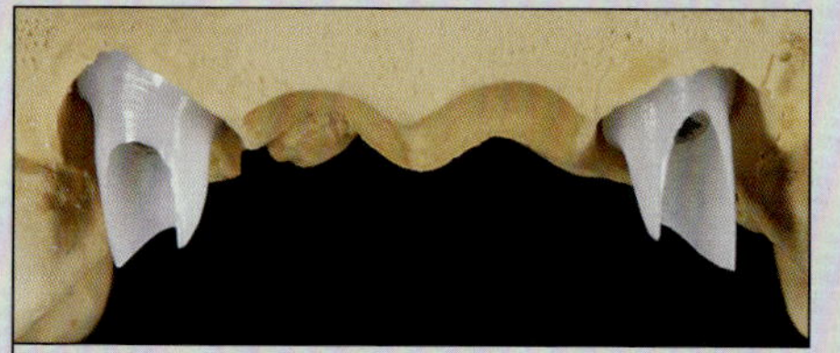

Before carrying out any modifications of the soft tissue, an impression was taken of the implants and poured in gypsum without the removable gingival mask. Often, gingival masks are too flexible and therefore reduce the stability of the restoration on the cast. The prosthodontist used a standard healing abutment and standard impression coping. This explains why the shape of the gingiva did not meet the requirements for a correct emergence profile. The extension of the planned cus-

tom abutments was traced. Figures 45a and 45b show occlusal and labial views of the finished abutments on the master cast. The shape of the abutment between the preparation of the margin and the implant base was concave to prevent the gingiva from being pressed in an apical direction.[5]

After scanning, the zirconium framework was designed using the Procera software (Nobel Biocare). The framework was immediately checked for an accurate fit (Fig 46). It is important to ensure that gingival support is provided in the pontic area. Otherwise, the tediously crafted gingival tissue architecture would quickly collapse. Next, selective grinding was performed on the pontic area of the second unsectioned master cast to prepare the shape for the ovate pontics.

Laminate veneers were planned for the canines and first premolar. Figures 47a and 47b show the silver galvanized dies on the master cast. In cases of combined implant and veneer treatment, it is important to choose an adequate cast system that allows the technician to make an exact copy of

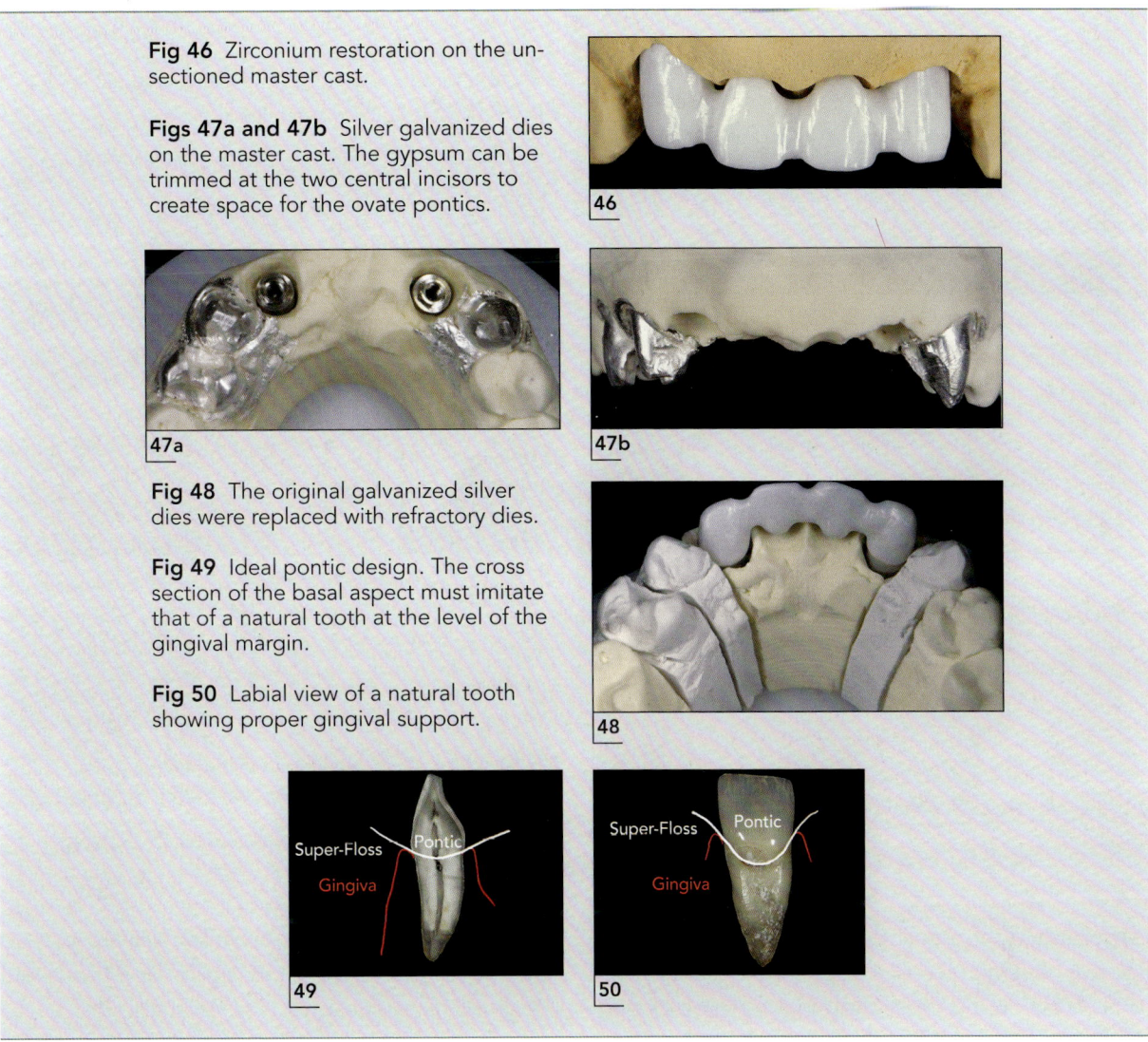

Fig 46 Zirconium restoration on the unsectioned master cast.

Figs 47a and 47b Silver galvanized dies on the master cast. The gypsum can be trimmed at the two central incisors to create space for the ovate pontics.

Fig 48 The original galvanized silver dies were replaced with refractory dies.

Fig 49 Ideal pontic design. The cross section of the basal aspect must imitate that of a natural tooth at the level of the gingival margin.

Fig 50 Labial view of a natural tooth showing proper gingival support.

the master die in refractory die material with ceramic pins. These ceramic pins guarantee a good overview while layering and an exact fit on the master cast before and after the firing procedure. Figure 48 shows the refractory dies with the all-ceramic restoration in place and ready for layering.[4]

An ovate pontic is an egg-shaped, convex component, which—after proper gingival tissue conditioning by the periodontist—can achieve compelling functional and esthetic results. For a dental technician, it is important to know how to create an ovate pontic. There is more to it than simply filling a gap. The pontic must approximate the cross section of a natural tooth at the level of the gingival margin. Figure 49 shows a lateral view of the basic design of an ovate pontic. Observing the emer-

gence profile of the pontic construction, it is clear that the gingiva and the pontic are in alignment. This should resemble the emergence profile of natural teeth as much as possible, ie, the pontic should appear to be growing out of the gingiva. The labial view of a natural tooth shows how the pontic should support the gingiva (Fig 50).[6] Depending on the circumstances, the egg-shaped site of the ovate pontic should extend aproximately 1 to 1.5 mm subgingival to the labial margin.

The basal surface and gingival tissue seal tightly, preventing food impaction. The convex ovate pontic is the most sensible shape for pontics in the anterior arch. Due to the convex shape, the patient can easily clean the basal surface of the ovate pontic with dental floss. The technician

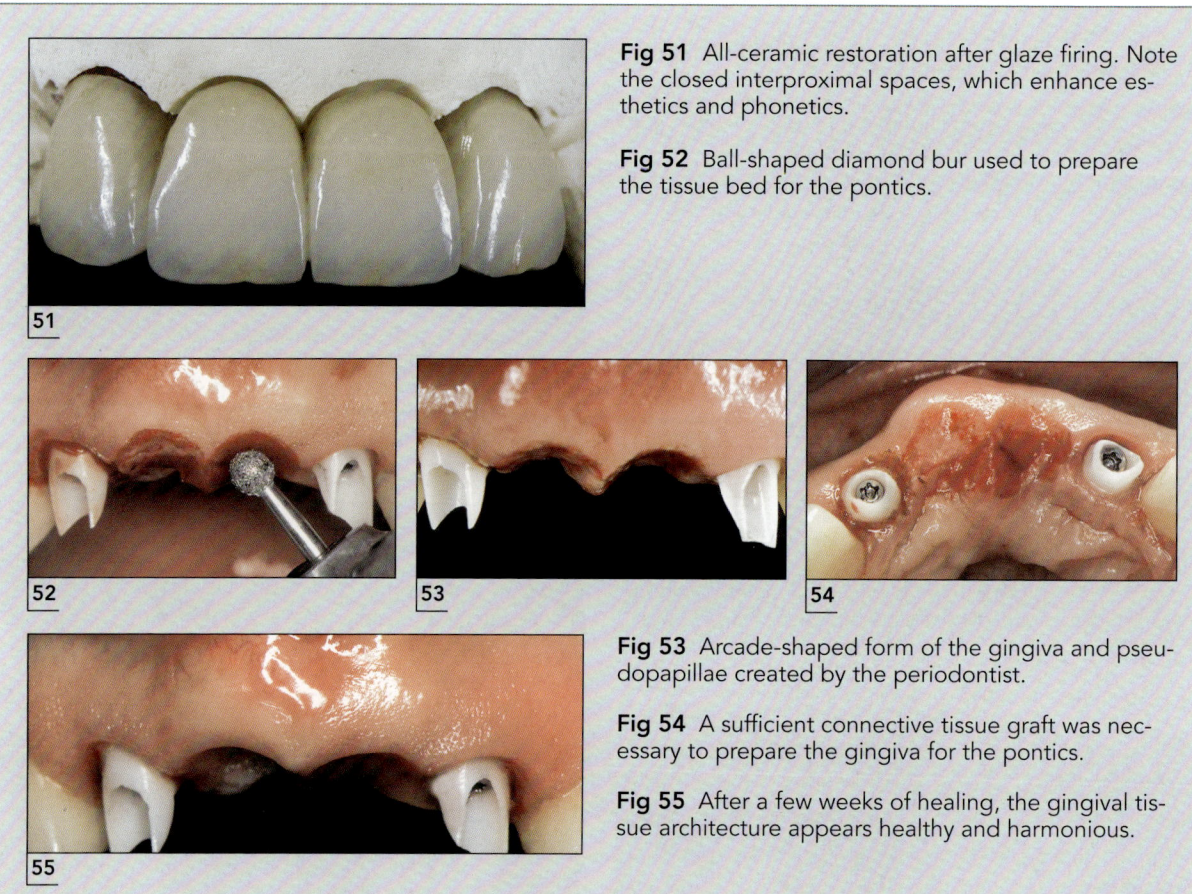

Fig 51 All-ceramic restoration after glaze firing. Note the closed interproximal spaces, which enhance esthetics and phonetics.

Fig 52 Ball-shaped diamond bur used to prepare the tissue bed for the pontics.

Fig 53 Arcade-shaped form of the gingiva and pseudopapillae created by the periodontist.

Fig 54 A sufficient connective tissue graft was necessary to prepare the gingiva for the pontics.

Fig 55 After a few weeks of healing, the gingival tissue architecture appears healthy and harmonious.

can promote the patient's hygiene efforts by giving the basal surface of the pontics a highly polished finish. In this case, the basal surfaces of the ovate pontics were mechanically polished with rubber polisher and diamond paste after the glaze firing. This creates a homogenous basal surface that prevents plaque buildup.

After glaze firing, the basal contact surfaces to the gingiva were optimized, the proximal contact surface to the adjacent laminate veneers were adjusted, and the glaze intensity of the restoration was adapted to the patient's natural teeth. These steps demand the technician's utmost attention. Any sloppiness here would endanger the elaborate preparations of the periodontist and jeopardize the final outcome. Ultimately, the pontics seemed to virtually grow out of the cast (Fig 51). The proximal spaces were essentially closed. Open proximal spaces are easier to clean but unacceptable from a phonetic and esthetic point of view.

After the all-ceramic abutments were placed on the implants, the periodontist's work will begin. The tissue bed was prepared for ovate pontics using a ball-shaped diamond bur. Automatically, the ovate pontic sites and pseudopapillae became clearly visible. The arcade-shaped contour of the gingiva and pseudopapillaes are the fruits of the periodontist's labor (Figs 52 to 54). After a few weeks, the gingival tissue architecture changed, and the gingiva had healed and stabilized. The gingival contour was harmonious, and epithelialization of the pontic sites—ie, the last phase of wound healing—had already begun (Fig 55).

What worked so well on the cast proved effective in situ: The definitive restoration was fitted tension-free and tried in without pressure. The tissue put up some resistance to the well-fitting pontic sites, but the restoration was pushed firmly into its final position (Fig 56). When modeling fixed prostheses, it

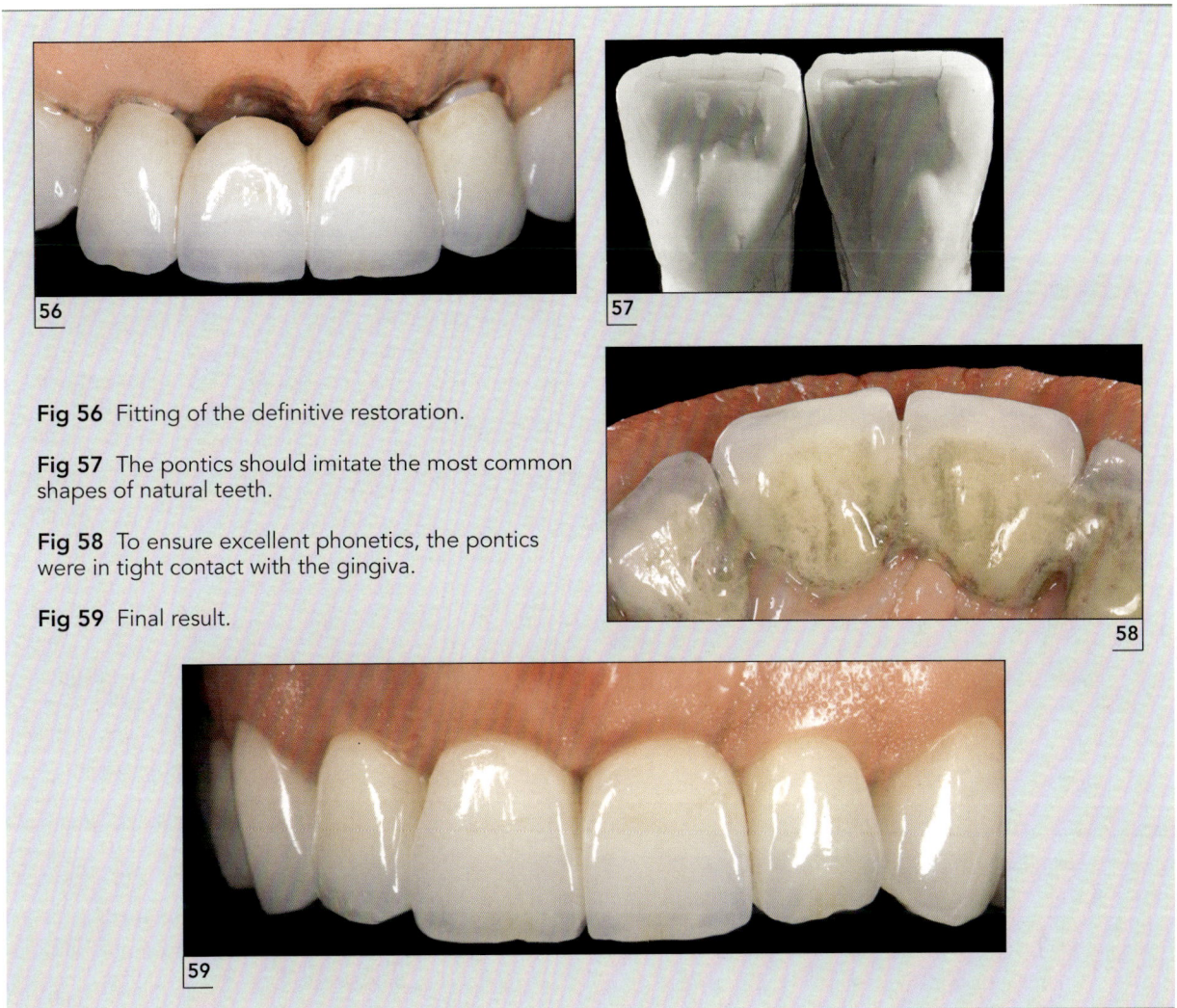

Fig 56 Fitting of the definitive restoration.

Fig 57 The pontics should imitate the most common shapes of natural teeth.

Fig 58 To ensure excellent phonetics, the pontics were in tight contact with the gingiva.

Fig 59 Final result.

may be preferable to adapt the maxillary restoration to the mandible. The palatal shape of the pontics, or of crowns in general, is important for proper function and phonetics. The functional surfaces are between the labial and palatal surfaces and have a sharp edge. They should be highly polished and adapted to the mandibular facets. It is paramount to imitate the shape of natural teeth (Fig 57). To achieve this result, the old adage applies: less is more. This is especially true for the palatal surface, which is responsible for phonetics.

The patient was particularly pleased with the palatal shape of the restoration. The restoration felt natural to the patient when she ran her tongue over it. The tight contact of the ovate pontics to the soft tissue creates an efficient barrier against air or saliva while speaking, thus preventing phonetic problems. Such results can be achieved only through skillful manipulation of the pontic base by an experienced periodontist and dental technician. The patient should feel no transition between the gingiva and pontic (Fig 58).

The restoration was pushed firmly into its final position. The pontics appeared to be growing naturally out of the gingiva. The egg-shaped convex surfaces supported the gingiva. The shape of the pontics was in harmony with the gingival architecture. The interproximal contact surfaces were shaped so as to prevent open interdental spaces. The overall esthetic result was successful and should be maintainable for a long time to come (Fig 59).

CASE 3 (Figs 60 to 76)

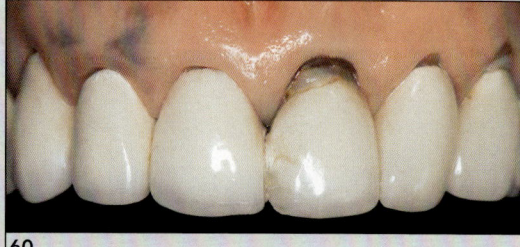

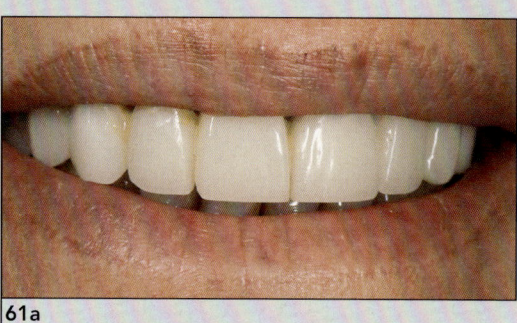

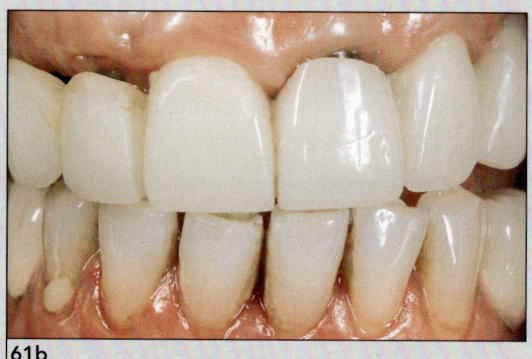

Fig 60 Initial situation with severe damage to the labial tissue and an existing porcelain-fused-to-metal restoration.

Figs 61a and 61b Provisional acrylic resin crowns were fabricated to restore the smile line and occlusal plane. The cervical profile of the restoration serves to further contour and condition the peri-implant soft tissue architecture.

Case 3

The patient presented with very poor oral conditions (Fig 60).[7] Because of the high degree of destruction, extraction of some teeth was unavoidable. The initial analysis revealed that the existing maxillary teeth could be retained after periodontal treatment. Clinical examination also revealed an amalgam tattoo at the right lateral incisor.

The maxilla required complete restoration with an all-ceramic reconstruction. As part of the full-mouth perioprosthetic rehabilitation, the patient received a laboratory-processed long-term provisional restoration for dental, periodontal, and occlusal pretreatment. Provisional crowns were fabricated to restore the correct smile line and occlusal plane (Figs 61a and 61b).

As is often the case in modern esthetic implantology, natural abutments were directly next to implants. This poses a special challenge to both the dentist and dental technician. The universal aim is to ensure the greatest mechanical stability while providing natural esthetics. Figure 62 shows the unsectioned master cast and custom abutments. The correct position of the abutment in relation to the desired tooth shape and dimension is based on the natural abutment. Because of the implants' labial axial alignment, the screw access hole was located toward the labial aspect (Fig 63a). From a palatal view, the abutments look just like natural prepared teeth (Fig 63b). A small slit was cut into the cast to check if the abutment was tightly seated on the cast.

The abutment had nearly the same dimensions as the prepared natural tooth (Figs 64a and 64b). The cast was once again sent back to the dentist so the pontic site could be reduced in preparation for the planned gingival tissue manipulation. No one can judge the oral situation better than the dentist. The dimensions of the custom abutments depend on the biotype of the gingiva. It goes without saying that in order to optimize the tooth size and length and improve the geometric distribution of the peri-implant space and crown, an optimized setup or waxup should be used for esthetically challenging situations. Additionally, it

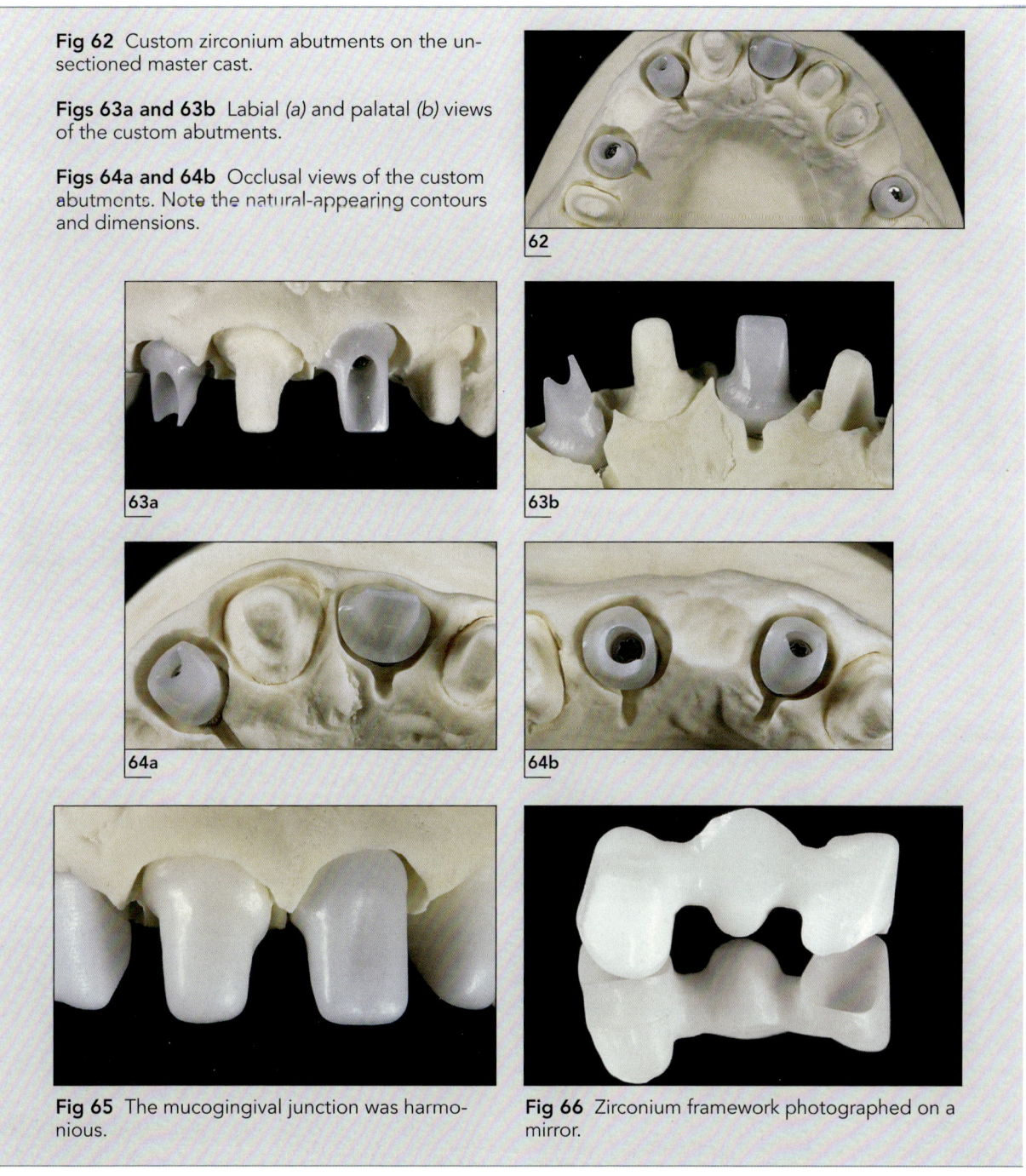

Fig 62 Custom zirconium abutments on the unsectioned master cast.

Figs 63a and 63b Labial (a) and palatal (b) views of the custom abutments.

Figs 64a and 64b Occlusal views of the custom abutments. Note the natural-appearing contours and dimensions.

62

63a

63b

64a

64b

Fig 65 The mucogingival junction was harmonious.

Fig 66 Zirconium framework photographed on a mirror.

is recommended to fabricate a labial and even a palatal silicone key from the setup or waxup.

Next, the zirconium restorations in the posterior area were scanned in the ususal manner. The margins were then perfectly adapted and reduced as necessary to leave sufficient space for the ceramic veneer. The zirconium crowns are mounted on the prepared teeth and custom abutments. The mucogingival junction was now harmonious (Fig 65).

After the cast was reduced, the framework was scanned using the Procera 3D-CAD software, and the data were transmitted electronically to Sweden. The form-fitting zirconium framework arrived at the lab a few days later (Fig 66). The thickness

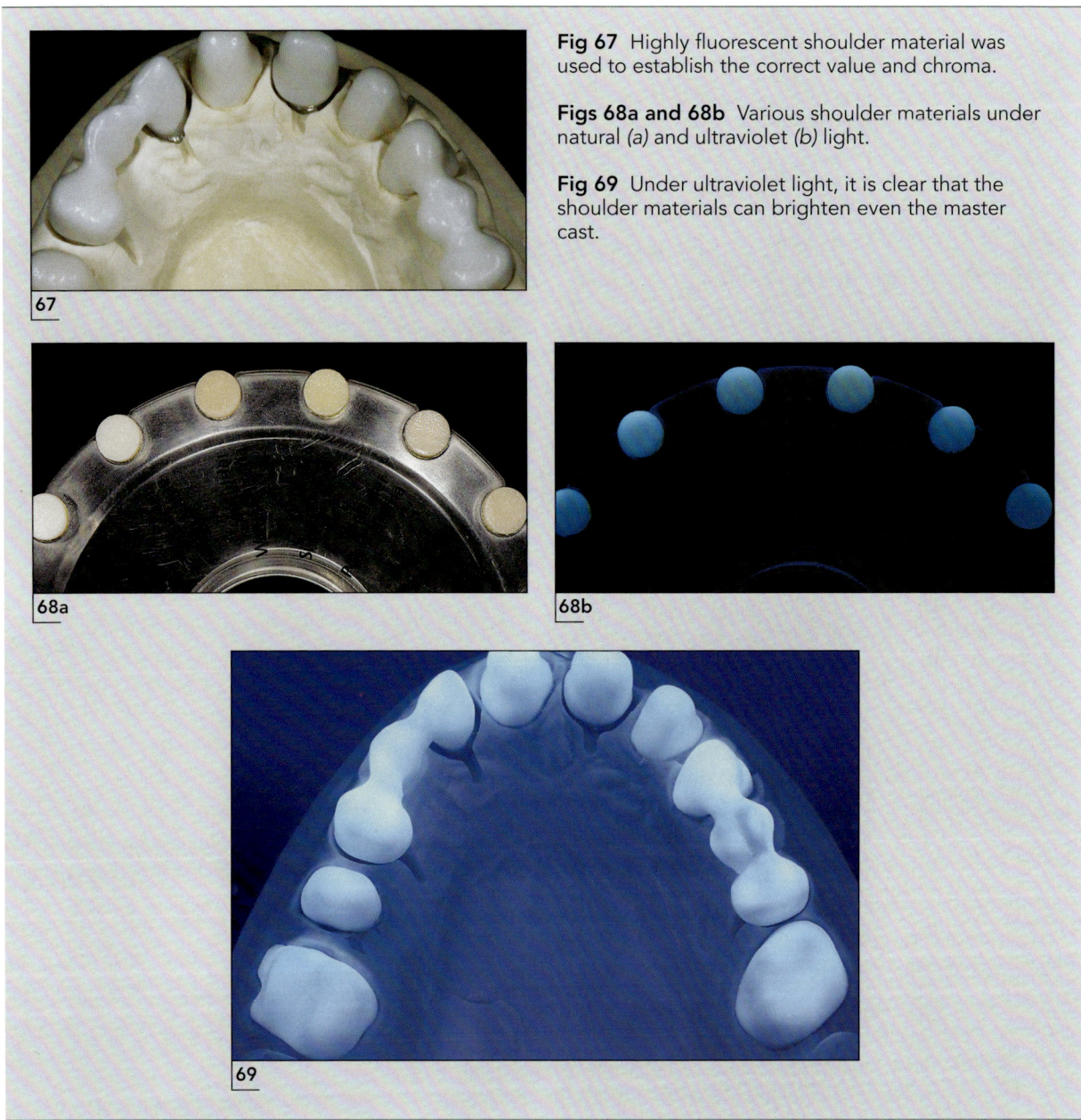

Fig 67 Highly fluorescent shoulder material was used to establish the correct value and chroma.

Figs 68a and 68b Various shoulder materials under natural *(a)* and ultraviolet *(b)* light.

Fig 69 Under ultraviolet light, it is clear that the shoulder materials can brighten even the master cast.

67

68a

68b

69

of the copings was 0.6 mm, which is sufficient to ensure long-term success. These frameworks are highly stable as long as the connecting points are dimensioned according to the manufacturer's specifications (6 mm²). The dimensions of the pontic were oriented with those of the left canine.

As already discussed, zirconium dioxide does not show any noteworthy fluorescence. To avoid an underlying shadow, especially in the cervical region, the restoration was covered with highly fluorescent shoulder material. The pontics were also covered with highly fluorescent material on the basal side (Fig 67). Figure 68a shows a few color pallets of highly fluorescent shoulder material with varying value and chroma. The effect of fluorescent material is especially striking when observed under ultraviolet light (Fig 68b). The fluorescent masses even brighten up the plaster cast (Fig 69).

The ultimate goal, of course, is to re-create the light dynamics of a natural tooth. Note that fluorescence is not required over the entirety of the restoration. The cross section of a natural tooth

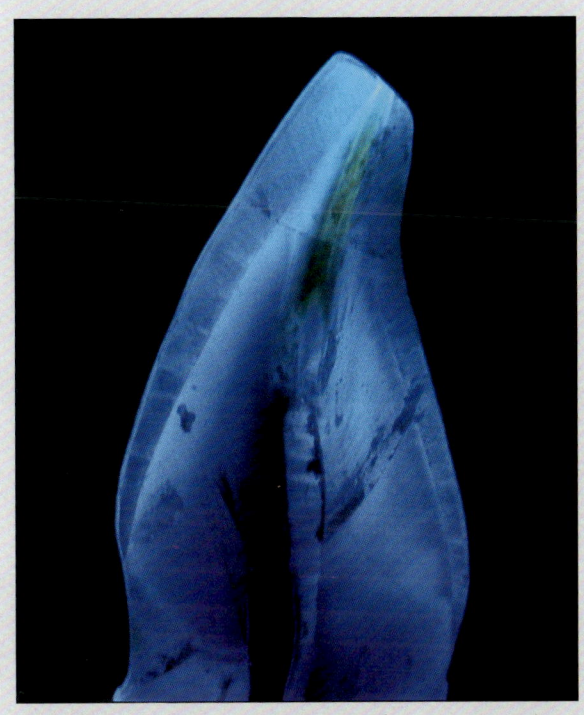 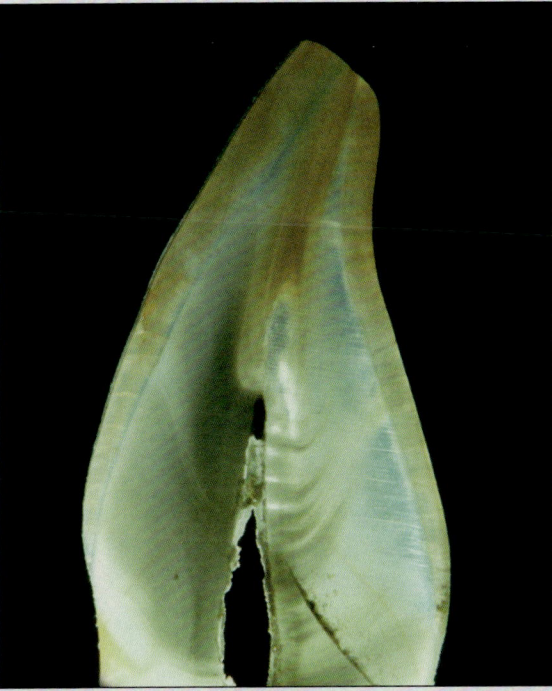

Figs 70a and 70b Cross section of a natural tooth under ultraviolet *(a)* and back *(b)* light.

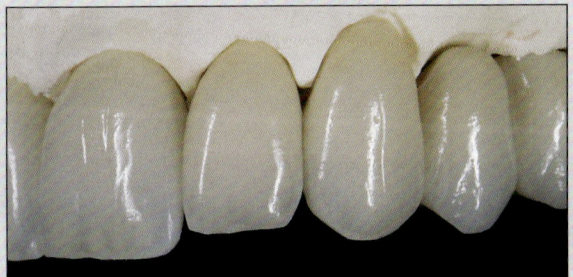 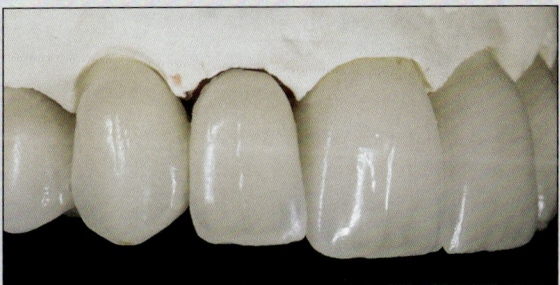

Figs 71a and 71b Ceramic crowns mounted on the master cast after layering.

shows that dentin in natural teeth has fluorescence, as do the mamelons located at the incisal edge (Fig 70a). The influence of the fluorescent natural dentin is higher in the cervical area, because the layer of natural enamel is thinner in this area. The enamel layer gets thicker at the incisal edge, and the influence of the fluorescent dentin is reduced.

Further, natural enamel shows an opalescent effect based on the interprismatic structure of the enamel (Fig 70b). The interprismatic structures of the enamel act like a spectrum filter, reflecting the short waves of light, ie, the blue waves. Long-wave orange-red light, on the other hand, penetrates the tooth enamel. The resultant blue-amber

effect is a primary component of the appearance of natural teeth. This explains the blue-gray gleam of enamel under incidental light. Under transmitted light, enamel shows a warm, orange shade.

After layering, the incisal area showed a natural appearance due to the fluorescent beige-orange mamelons and opalescent bluish-gray enamel (Figs 71a and 71b). The lateral incisors were somewhat more chromatic than the central incisors, and the canines showed a somewhat warmer chroma due to their structure. Final touch-ups were then carried out. In general, translucent materials should be used sparingly to prevent the loss of brightness and saturation. Nevertheless, translucent materials

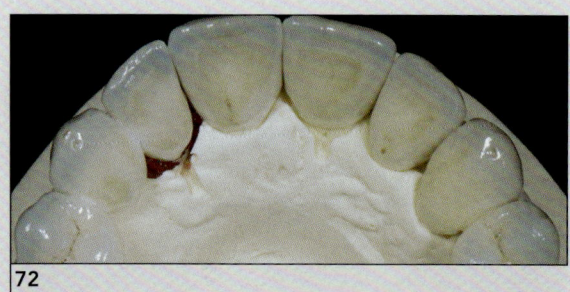

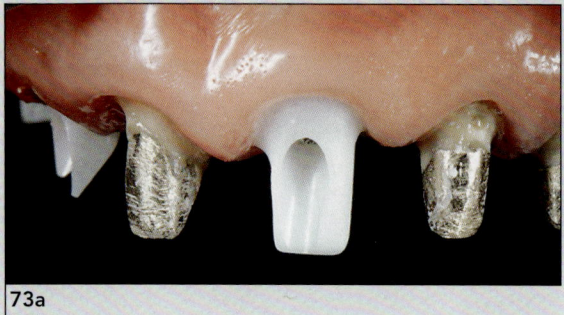

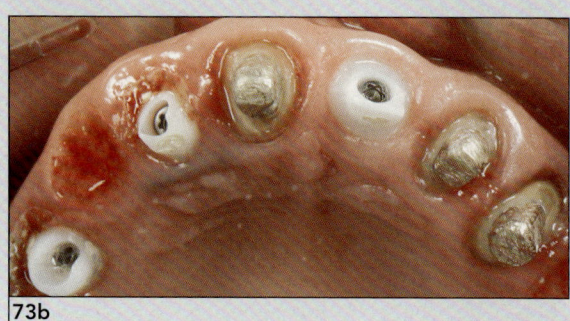

Fig 72 Occlusal view of the finished all-ceramic restorations.

Figs 73a and 73b Prior to placement of the definitive superstructure, excellent peri-implant soft tissue conditions and a natural emergence profile were observed.

are important because they provide a natural-looking depth effect, especially in the incisal area. Transparent materials should receive minimal firing to protect the character of the opalescence. If fired too often, their effects will diminish.

The zirconium restoration was then placed onto the abutments. The occlusal surfaces followed an international color-code occlusal compass concept. In the natural waxup technique, each functional direction is registered with a specific color. The German technician Dieter Schulz[8] came up with the idea of using colors to tranfer the individual directions to the respective tooth segments. In this case, the restoration exhibited proper cusp-fossa contacts along with sufficient space to allow excursive movements (Fig 72).

The preparation margin of the all-ceramic abutments was located slightly subgingivally. Before insertion of the definitive restoration, the peri-implant soft tissue situation was again evaluated. The individualized abutments were fixed on the implants. The ideally formed soft tissue architecture and implant emergence profile angle show the importance of a step-wise treatment plan (Figs 73a and 73b).[9] The screw cavity should then be covered with gutta-percha or self-curing acrylic resin.

The gingiva at the two pontics was reshaped concavely to achieve a natural-looking pontic design. Once the gingiva healed, the pseudopapillae and egg-shaped site for the ovate pontic were recognizable. Thanks to the newly developed gingival architecture, the pontic resembled a natural tooth.

At this stage, the patient was invited to the laboratory for shape correction, glazing, and finishing (Fig 74). The authors prefer to evaluate the patient's restoration in an unglazed bisque bake. Long contact surfaces were fabricated to prevent open interdental spaces. Any additional shaping and contouring can be done at this time to ensure the support of the gingiva. The ovate pontics can be fine-tuned directly in the patient's mouth. The crown margin should be designed to mirror that of a natural tooth (Fig 75). Any final characterization necessary to match the adjacent teeth should be performed at this stage as well.

A biologically natural tension will arise within a restoration when the width-to-length ratio of the teeth is in harmony. Studies have shown that the width of central incisors is approximately 80% of their optimum length.[3] In this case, the soft tissue reacted positively to the restoration, and tissue regeneration was observed. The margin of the crown

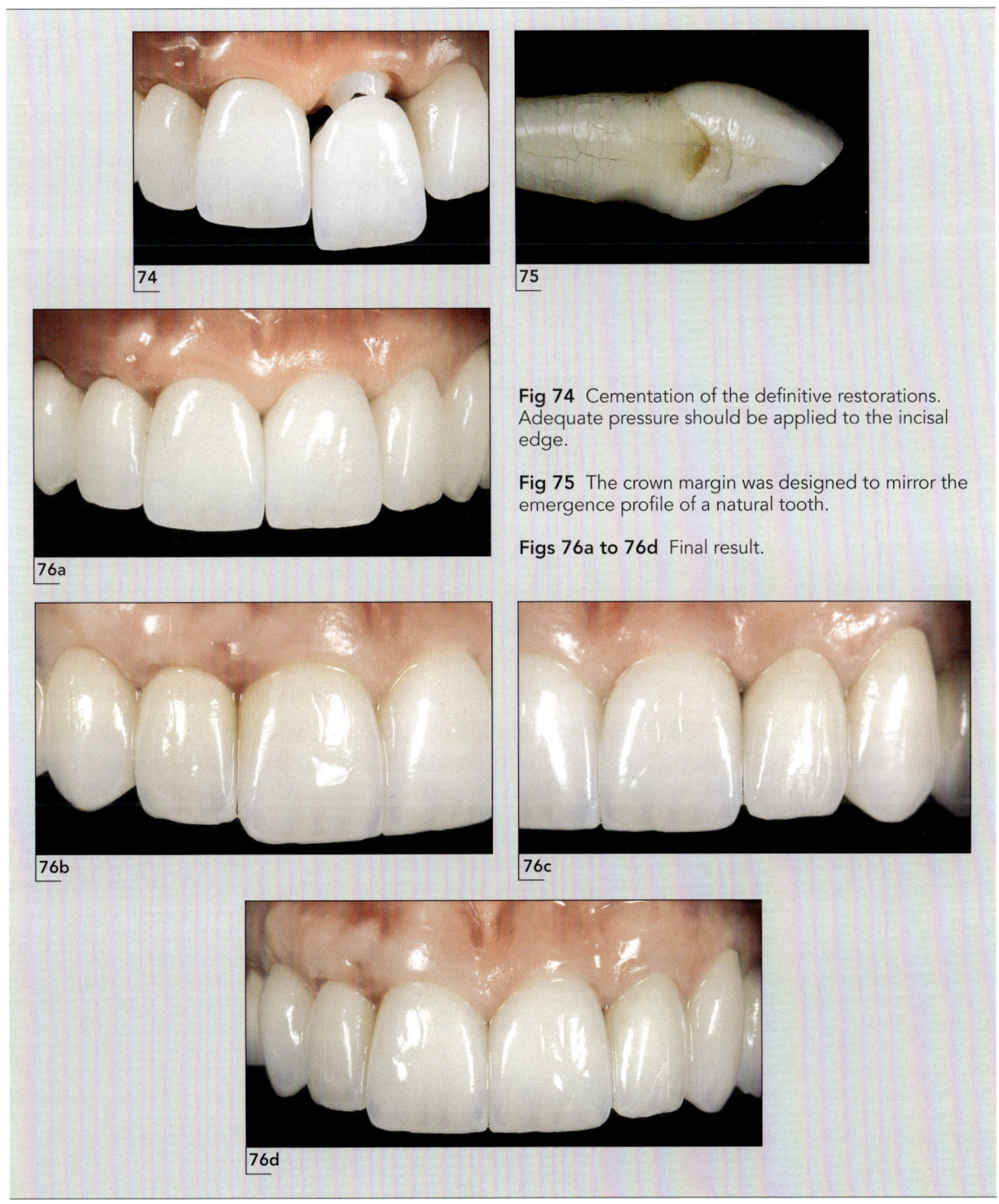

Fig 74 Cementation of the definitive restorations. Adequate pressure should be applied to the incisal edge.

Fig 75 The crown margin was designed to mirror the emergence profile of a natural tooth.

Figs 76a to 76d Final result.

should be no more than 0.5 to 1.0 mm subgingivally to allow for removal of any excess cement.

The final result is shown in Figs 76a to 76d. The gingival tissue was healthy, and optimal gingival support was evident. The success of this restoration was the combined result of perfect periodontal pre-treatment and appropriate technical execution. Due to the sizable change in shape, the patient's oral appearance was radically improved compared to the initial situation. It was impossible to distinguish the implants and ovate pontics from natural teeth—exactly what the treatment aimed to achieve.

CONCLUSIONS

This article demonstrated the advantages of zirconium dioxide using three complicated patient cases. Zirconium dioxide is biocompatible and can be easily integrated into the periodontal and gingival structures. Futher, its stability has been proven as a base for ceramic veneering materials.

Mother Nature is extremely complex, and it takes flexibility and virtuosity from the treatment team to produce a successful restoration. Solid treatment planning, a healthy dental and periodontal baseline situation, functional occlusion, and harmonious integration of the restoration in the patient's mouth are fundamental issues for a succesful treatment outcome.

ACKNOWLEDGMENT

The authors thank Dr Eric Van Dooren, Antwerp, Belgium, for his collaboration on the presented cases.

REFERENCES

1. Rompen E, Van Dooren E, Touati B. Soft tissue stability at the facial aspect of gingival converging abutments in the esthetic zone: A pilot clinical study. J Prosthet Dent 2007;97(suppl):S119–S125.

2. Tarnow D, Magner AW, Fletcher P. The effect of the distance from the contact point to the crest of bone on the presence or absence of the interproximal dental papillae. J Periodontol 1992;63:995–1004.

3. Fradeani M. Esthetic Rehabilitation in Fixed Prosthodontics: Esthetic Analysis: A Systematic Approach to Prosthodontic Treatment. Chicago: Quintessence, 2004.

4. Magne P, Belser U. Bonded Porcelain Restorations in the Anterior Dentition: A Biomimetic Approach. Chicago: Quintessence, 2002.

5. Rutten L, Rutten P. The fabrication of full ceramic abutments. In: Crown—Bridge and Implants. The Art of Harmony. Fuchstal, Germany: Teamwork Media, 2006:141–196.

6. Rutten L, Rutten P. The ovate pontic technique. In: Crown—Bridge and Implants. The Art of Harmony. Fuchstal, Germany: Teamwork Media, 2006:234–296.

7. Van Dooren E. Connective tissue grafts for the treatment of discolored roots and amalgam tattoos. Pract Proc Aesthet Dent 2000;12:461–465.

8. Schulz D. NAT—Die Naturgemässe Aufwachstechnik. Fuchstal, Germany: Teamwork Media, 2003.

9. Tarnow D, Elian N, Fletcher P, et al. Vertical distance from the crest of bone to the height of the interproximal papillae between adjacent implants. J Periodontol 2003;74:1785–1788.

PREFABRICATED ZIRCONIA ABUTMENTS: SURGICAL AND RESTORATIVE ADVANTAGES, HANDLING CONSIDERATIONS, AND CLINICAL OUTCOMES

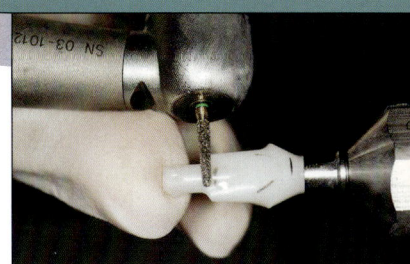

Sonia S. Leziy, DDS, Dipl Perio[1]
Brahm A. Miller, DDS, Dipl Pros[1]

Implant placement in the esthetic zone presents unique challenges that must be identified and considered to ensure treatment success. The dental literature clearly shows that an ideal gingival architecture supported by a physiologic ridge is essential to develop a pleasing framework around the definitive restoration.[1] Prior disease activity, traumatic injury, and extrac-

tions without ridge preservation result in bone loss in the area of treatment and can adversely impact the esthetic outcome. Bone loss can be reduced and ideal esthetics can be more predictably achieved through comprehesive treatment planning and ridge augmentation precedures. With high implant survival rates, clinicians are increasingly focused on subtle refinements to the treatment outcome. Fine-tuning to improve the esthetic result includes the following key factors:

1. *Correct three-dimensional implant placement.* There is extensive literature related to the impact of implant position on esthetics as assessed by gingival tissue levels. Current reviews suggest that even if implants are correctly positioned

[1]Associate Clinical Professor, University of British Columbia, British Columbia, Canada; Private practice, North Vancouver, British Columbia, Canada.

Correspondence to: Dr Sonia Leziy, 401-221 West Esplanade, North Vancouver, British Columbia, Canada V7M 3J3. E-mail: sonia@imperio.ca

three-dimensionally, facial tissue recession of up to 1 mm is still common and can be expected in the first year following implant restoration because of postsurgical bone remodeling.[2] Extensive bone remodeling and adverse and obvious changes in gingival tissue level are expected when implants are incorrectly positioned; unfortunately, this problem is still all too frequent and reflects treatment errors that cannot be predictably corrected.

2. *Treatment of the residual horizontal defect.* If an implant is ideally positioned in a socket, this typically creates a residual horizontal defect between the extraction socket wall and the implant body. Several studies support the concept of spontaneous defect fill without the addition of bone grafting products.[3,4] However, this does not prevent facial bone resorption, which leads to unfavorable facial tissue level changes. With this in mind, filling the residual horizontal defect, regardless of its size, is now recognized as a key step in preventing facial tissue recession. A prospective study by Chen et al[5] reported that placement of a bone grafting product (Bio-Oss bovine bone mineral, Osteohealth, Shirley, NY) in the residual horizontal defect significantly reduced facial tissue recession. They also noted a correlation between facial positioning of implants and buccal recession. Placement of an implant in an unfavorable facial orientation resulted in thinning of the facial bone and an increased likelihood of facial bone loss and corresponding recession of the facial tissues.

3. *Gingival biotype.* The periodontal literature clearly links the negative impact of a thin gingival biotype and gingival tissue stability around teeth. The evidence concerning the effect of a thin biotype on gingival health and stability around implants is weak at best.[6,7] Regardless, it is the authors' opinion that tissue quality is a critical issue that impacts gingival tissue stability and color esthetics. In an in vitro study, Jung et al[8] showed that thicker tissues hide or mask underlying abutments better than thin tissues. They did not comment on the potential impact of biotype enhancement on gingival stability. Chen et al's[5] findings suggest that the biotype had less impact on tissue stability than implant positioning.

4. *Minimizing crestal bone remodeling.* There is currently a developing interest in implant and/or abutment design changes that may minimize crestal bone remodeling. Implant manufacturers and clinicians are embracing concepts such as abutment undercontouring to thicken the connective tissue around an abutment and protect the underlying bone. Conceptually, this is akin to nonsurgical soft tissue augmentation. There is also interest in minimizing crestal bone remodeling by changing the position of or eliminating the implant-abutment microgap. The method that has attracted the most interest in reducing the impact of the implant-abutment junction on bone remodeling is platform switching. Platform switching involves moving the implant-abutment microgap medially and away from the bone crest toward the center of the implant.[9] This inward horizontal repositioning results in the preservation of crestal bone around the implant head. A recent in vitro study by Maeda et al[10] suggests that this medial movement of the abutment microgap could result in more abutment screw deformation because of the increased stress around the outside of the abutment and implant connection area. Another approach to alter the implant-abutment position is to move the microgap coronally away from the ridge crest with scallop-design implants.[11]

An interesting but less studied issue that potentially contributes to crestal bone remodeling is prosthetic component handling (dis- and reconnection). Based on their observations in an animal model study, Abrahamsson et al[12] suggested that repeated disruption of the epithelial and connective tissue attachment potentially contributes to crestal bone remodeling toward the first major thread. These subtle bone changes can negatively impact soft tissue stability, especially when multiple/adjacent implant placement is considered. In contrast, removal of a single healing abutment and replacement with a final abutment did not induce marginal bone loss.[13]

The potential benefits of zirconia abutments are clearly documented from an esthetic perspective. Zirconia positively impacts tissue health due to its superior biocompatibility and potential to position the cement line coronally and close to the gingival margin because of the white color of the material.[14-16] In contrast, titanium abutments in the esthetic zone generally force the clinician to place margins deeper under the gingiva to minimize the graying effect, thus increasing the risk of cement trapping. Furthermore, this leaves less biocompatible restoration material, such as porcelain or gold, in the subgingival area.

PREFABRICATED ZIRCONIA ABUTMENTS

This article describes and illustrates the use of prefabricated zirconia abutments (Procera Esthetic Abutment Selection Kit, Nobel Biocare, Göteborg, Sweden) with Nobel Biocare implants (NobelReplace or Brånemark implants). Other implant systems have similar abutments that can be modified by the clinician; however, those systems have a less complete "library" of abutment shapes and sizes. Prefabricated abutments can be used in many but not all cases. Several issues will affect whether the use of a prefabricated abutment is appropriate or whether the situation is best suited for a customized abutment, including:

1. *Correct three-dimensional implant positioning.* Use of any zirconia abutment, prefabricated or customized, requires precise three-dimensional implant placement to avoid excess reduction of the abutment in the subgingival area. For example, facially positioned implants require more substantial facial zirconia adjustments and may result in thinning to a point where the structural integrity of the abutment is compromised.

2. *Space availability between the implant and adjacent teeth.* Narrow spaces may necessitate significant reshaping of generic abutment profiles. From a practical perspective, this is time-consuming and may negatively impact the flexural strength of the zirconia abutment by thinning the areas around the abutment screw head.

3. *Degree of gingival scallop relative to the prefabricated margin/cement line profile.* "Average" gingival profiles lend themselves well to the use of stock forms, but flat or highly scalloped gingival architectures mandate that the margin and future cement line be specifically customized. As the library of choices grows, these various situations will be easier to handle. At this time, these cases are best managed through fabrication of customized abutments.

4. *Flat edentulous areas.* In sites where the gingival anatomy is ill-defined as a result of prior tooth loss and subsequent bone and soft tissue remodeling, provisionalization with screw-retained implant-level provisional res-torations may be preferable to the use of a definitive zirconia abutment and provisional restoration. Once tissue form is redeveloped, a customized final abutment is then fabricated and delivered along with the final crown. In this situation, a chairside-modified zirconia abutment with a crown delivered at a separate appointment offers few benefits to the patient and clinician in terms of time or cost.

5. *Impact of grinding/polishing of zirconia.* The impact of grinding or polishing procedures on the flexural strength of zirconia is controversial. Some literature suggests that the strength of zirconia is adversely affected by the various chairside procedures necessary to appropriately shape the abutments, while other authors propose that there is no impact on the structural integrity of the material.[17,18] Judicious management must be emphasized at this time, with specific attention paid to adequate cooling during grinding and to the types of burs and bur quality used for specific zirconia products.[19]

PROCEDURE REVIEW (Figs 1 to 11)

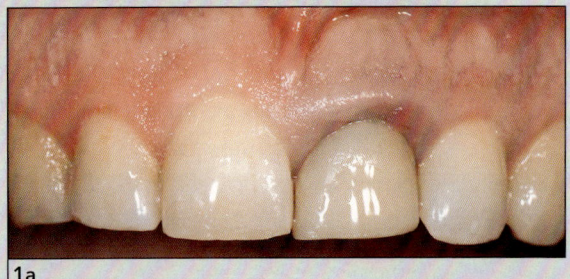

1a

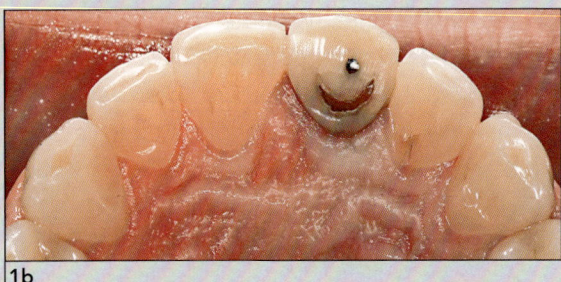

1b

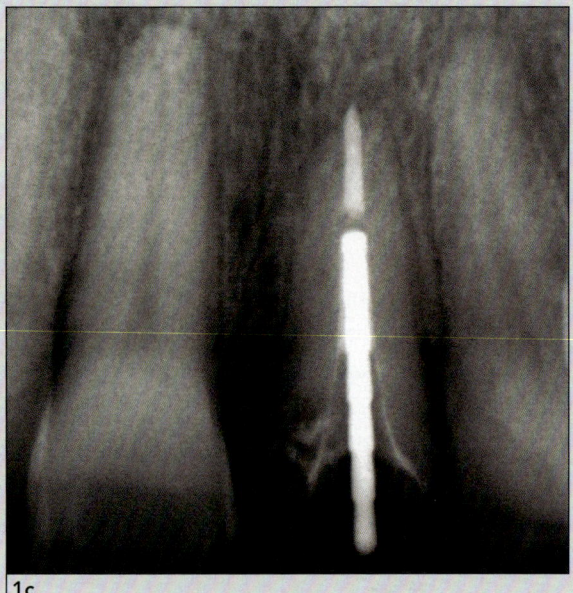

1c

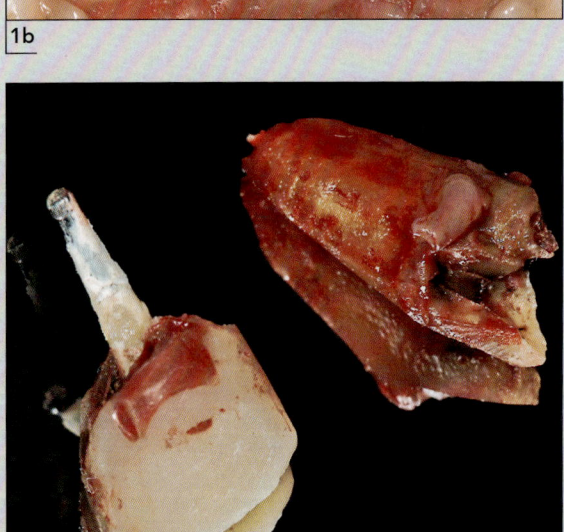

2a

Fig 1a Preoperative view showing slight gingival edema. Approximately 20% excess facial tissue was created by prior orthodontic extrusion.

Fig 1b Preoperative occlusal view.

Fig 1c Preoperative radiograph showing the crestal bone height after extrusion.

Fig 2a Extracted root and crown.

Figs 2b and 2c Atraumatic extraction minimizes the damage to bone and gingival tissues.

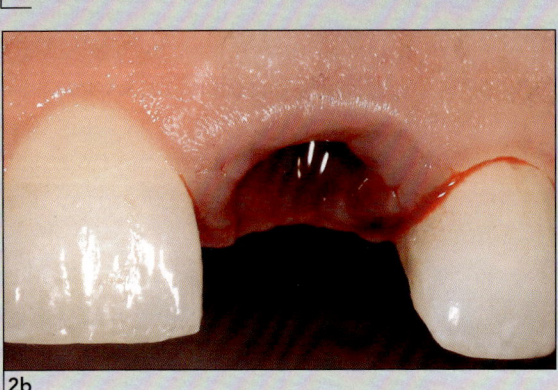

2b

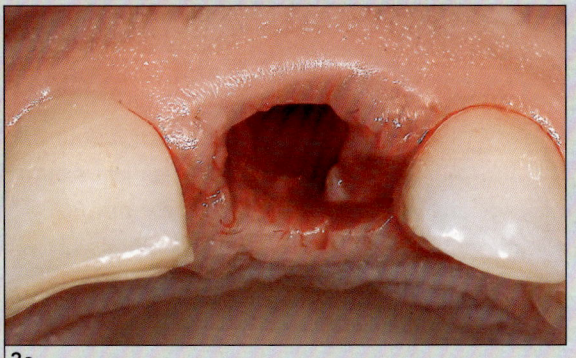

2c

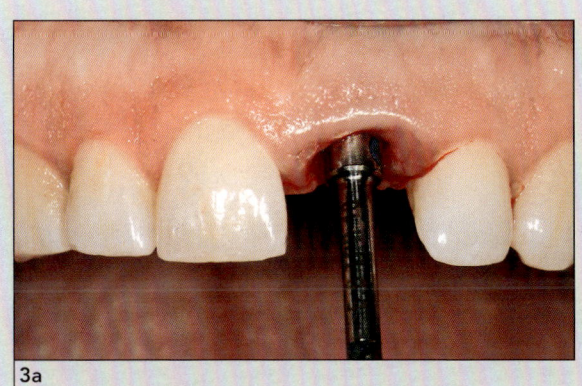
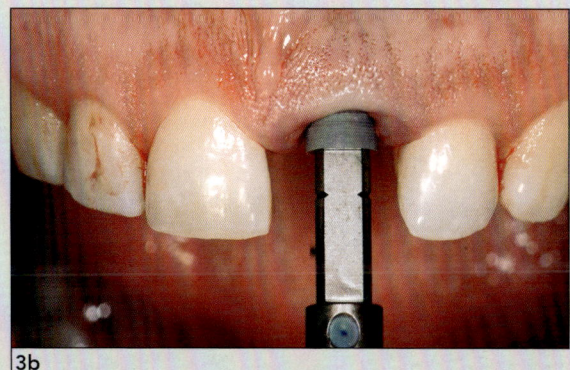

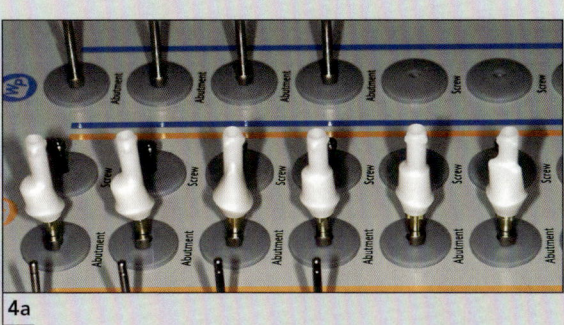
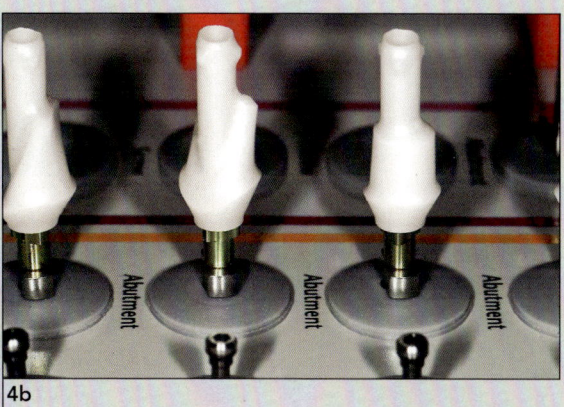

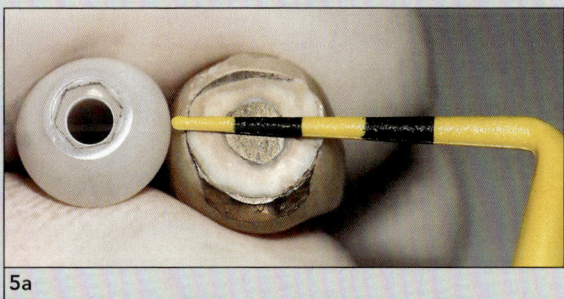
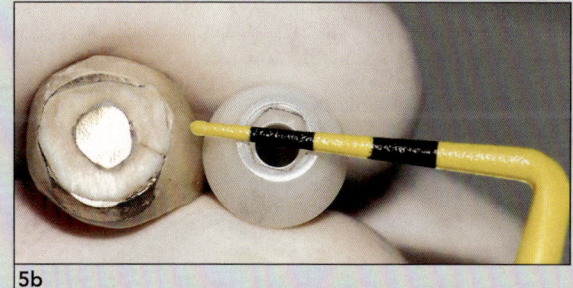

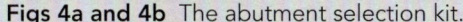
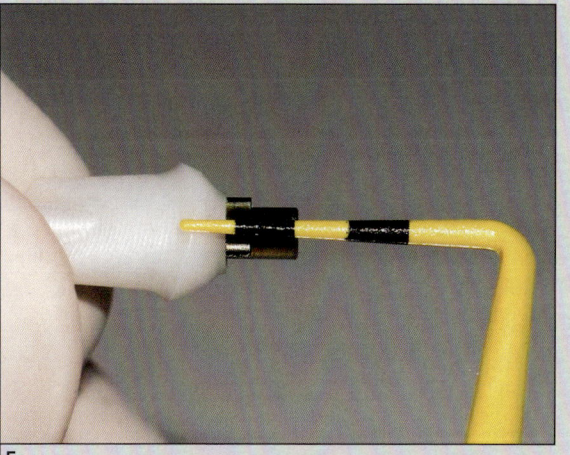

Fig 3a Extraction site with the implant drill in place to verify the drilling angle and stability of the prepared site.

Fig 3b Implant insertion. Adequate primary stability is essential (minimum 35 Ncm insertion torque). The implant should be inserted to a depth and angulation that will permit positioning of the abutment margin close to or minimally submerged (up to 1 mm) relative to the ideal or desired gingival tissue margin position.

Figs 4a and 4b The abutment selection kit.

Figs 5a to 5c Sectioning of an extracted incisor and comparative cross-sectional view with a zirconia abutment. This is useful when selecting the size and angle of the abutment and the appropriate margin height.

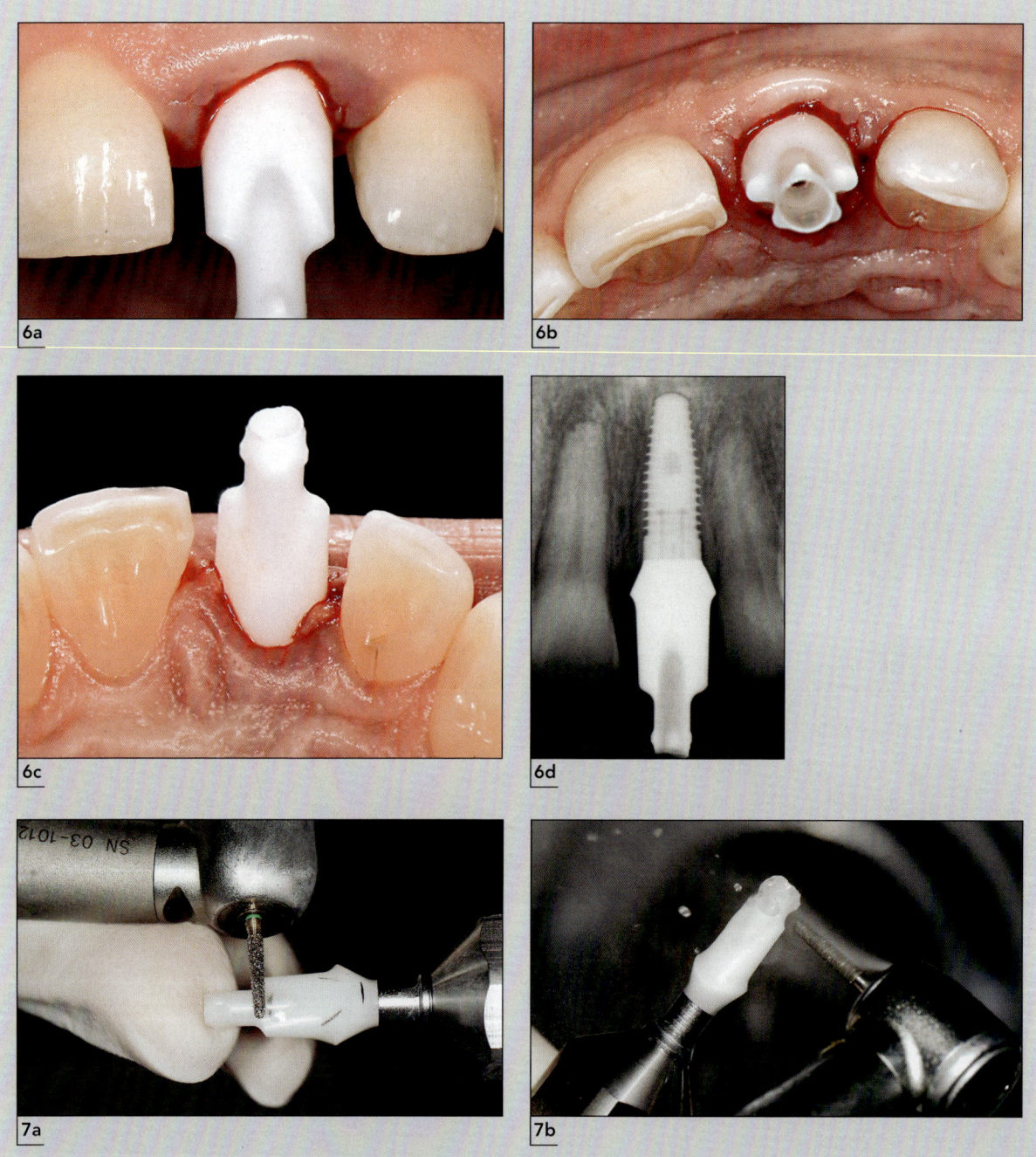

Figs 6a to 6d Correct three-dimensional positioning is the primary issue that must be considered to permit the use of zirconia abutments as previously discussed. *(a)* Ideal mesiodistal positioning of an implant between adjacent teeth. *(b)* Correct facial-palatal positioning may be the most significant cause of facial tissue recession. *(c)* Palatal view of the abutment prior to modification. *(d)* Radiograph showing the abutment margin height relative to the socket depth.

Fig 7a Modification of the abutment. Once an appropriate abutment has been selected, areas requiring modification are identified. The abutment is placed on a protection analog in a handle designed to facilitate extraoral modification.

Fig 7b The abutment is then modified as marked intraorally, using diamond burs with copious water-irrigation for cooling.

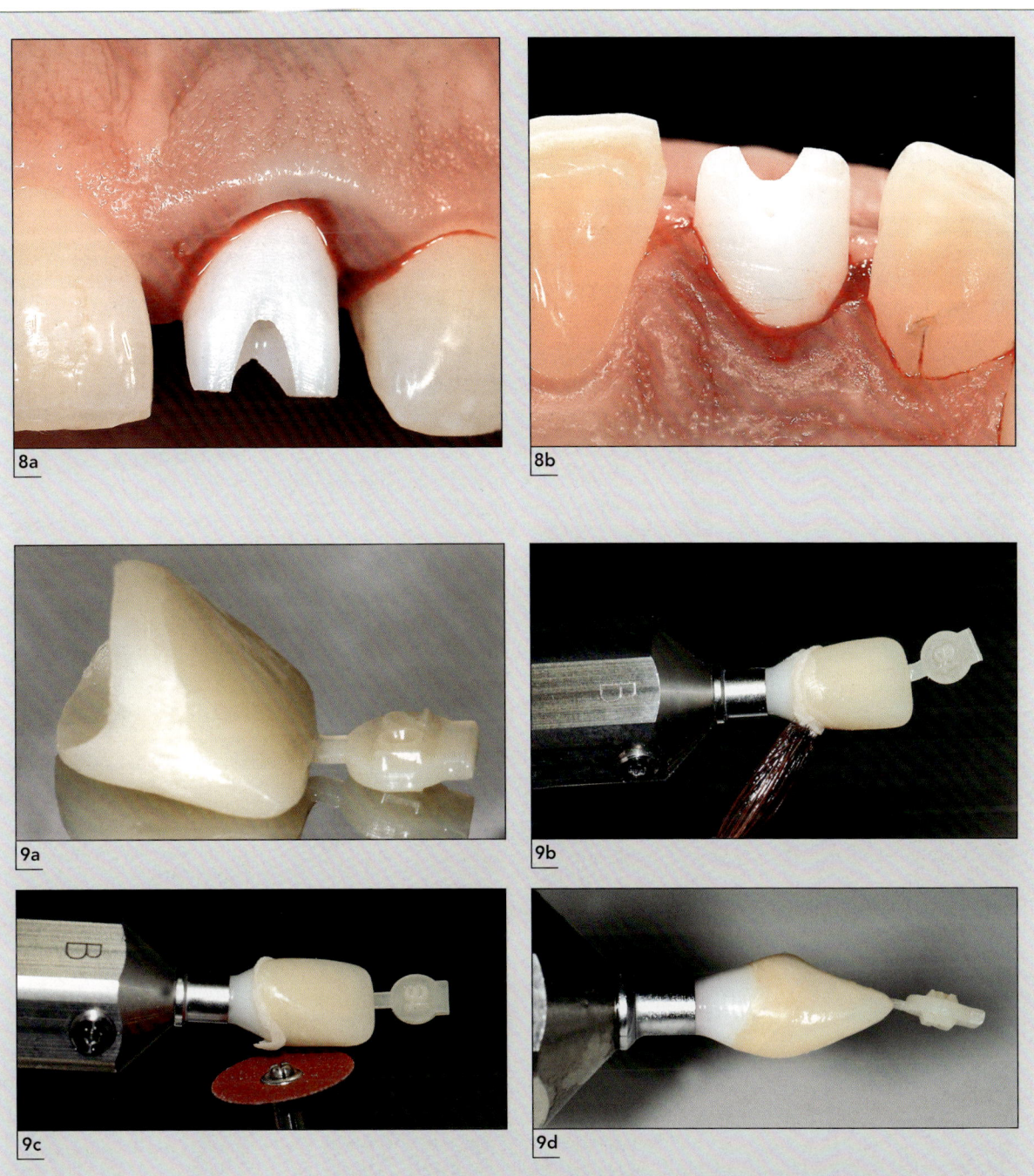

Figs 8a and 8b Abutment try-in following modification. The abutment is removed from the handle and analog and assessed intraorally. If needed, further modification can be carried out, ideally extraorally, although minor refinements can be performed intraorally. It is recommended to avoid embedding zirconia particles into the surgical site. The clear advantage of this abutment kit is the possibility for clean and precise crown margin modification extraorally on the handle/protection analog.

Figs 9a to 9d Fabrication of the provisional restoration following satisfactory abutment modification. Several techniques can be used, as previously discussed by Leziy and Miller.[20] Note the excellent crown margin adaptation to the abutment, which is possible because of its extraoral preparation. (a) Modified/trimmed prefabricated provisional shell. (b) Following intraoral indexing, the crown margin is refined extraorally on the abutment holder. (c) Finishing of the crown margin. (d) Typical crown margin finish quality.

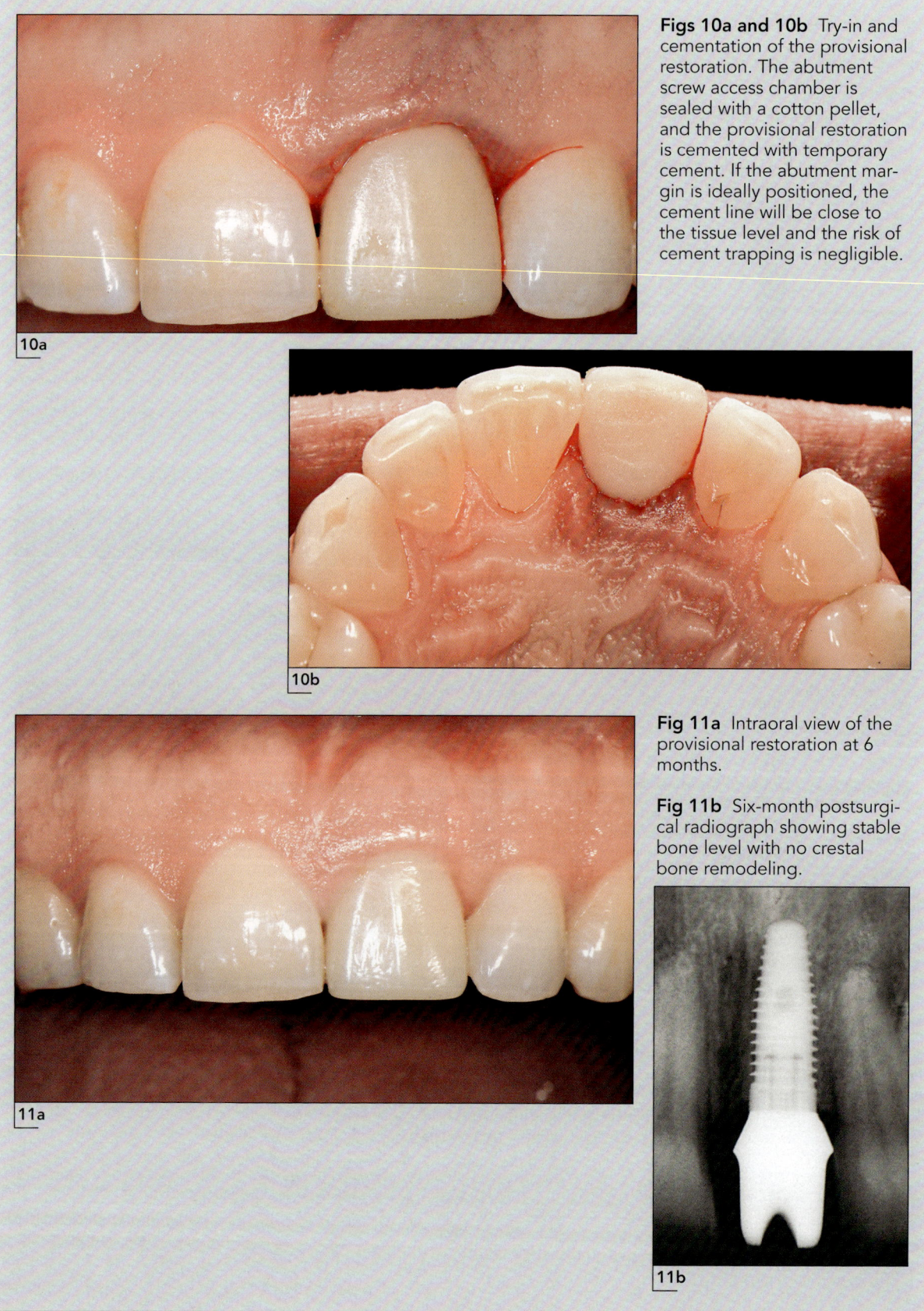

Figs 10a and 10b Try-in and cementation of the provisional restoration. The abutment screw access chamber is sealed with a cotton pellet, and the provisional restoration is cemented with temporary cement. If the abutment margin is ideally positioned, the cement line will be close to the tissue level and the risk of cement trapping is negligible.

Fig 11a Intraoral view of the provisional restoration at 6 months.

Fig 11b Six-month postsurgical radiograph showing stable bone level with no crestal bone remodeling.

DISCUSSION AND CONCLUSION

The authors' initial experience with this product has been very encouraging, in part because of its simplicity and easy introduction into clinical practice. The learning curve, for both the restoring dentist and the surgeon familiar with the concept of immediate implant restoration, is minimal. By taking into account the controversy over the impact of grinding/polishing on zirconia and using sound judgment when handling the material, no complications, such as abutment fracture or subsequent restoration failure, have been observed. Although this prefabricated abutment system was designed for chairside modification, ideally at the time of surgery, there is also an important potential role for the dental technician. In cases with appropriate gingival tissue profiles, these abutments could theoretically be used by technicians instead of waxing and scanning for the production of customized abutments. This may be advantageous in terms of time.

The authors' experience over the last 2 years using this prefabricated abutment system suggest that it could be used in approximately 80% of the cases assessed (premolar to premolar area in the maxillary dentition). The primary limitation, as long as implant placement was ideal, was in areas with limited mesiodistal space relative to the available abutment diameters. This problem was most commonly encountered in the lateral incisor site, where 3.5-mm narrow-platform implants are generally placed. Abutment diameters for narrow-platform implants range from 5.1 to 5.5 mm. These abutment diameters resulted in inadequate space for preservation or development of ideal papilla architecture, thus increasing the probability for blunting of the papilla. It is the authors' opinion that customized zirconia abutments are generally better suited for these situations. The second limitation encountered was in cases with highly scalloped gingival anatomy, since the degree of abutment margin scallop was generally deemed to be insufficient in these cases and resulted in deep margin positioning interproximally. This disadvantage relates primarily to the increased risk for cement trapping or challenging cement removal during both the provisional and definitive cementation protocol. Again, highly scalloped gingival anatomy appears to be better suited to customized abutments.

The most encouraging and compelling reason to consider the use of these prefabricated abutments, especially when they can be placed at the time of surgery, relates to the observation that crestal bone remodeling around the implant collar is predictably reduced. Whereas traditional implant placement and restoration protocols often result in crestal bone remodeling to the first major implant thread, a review of 36 consecutively treated cases involving placement of prefabricated zirconia abutments at the time of surgery has consistently resulted in no or minimal radiographic crestal bone remodeling. This leads to enhanced gingival tissue stability and diminishes the significance of the adjacent periodontium for maintaining papilla stability. The risk of progressive facial tissue recession resulting from repeated prosthetic dis- and reconnections may also be reduced.

REFERENCES

1. Buser D, Martin W, Belser UC. Optimizing esthetics for implant restorations in the anterior maxilla: Anatomic and surgical considerations. Int J Oral Maxillofac Implants 2004;19(suppl):43–61.

2. Cardaropoli G, Lekholm U, Wennstrom JL. Tissue alterations at implant-supported single-tooth replacements: A 1-year prospective clinical study. Clin Oral Implants Res 2006;17:165–171.

3. Paolantonio M, Dolci M, Scarano A, et al. Immediate implantation in fresh extraction sockets. A controlled clinical and histological study in man. J Periodontol 2001;72: 1560–1571.

4. Botticelli D, Berglundh T, Lindhe J. Hard tissue alterations following immediate implant placement in extraction sites. J Clin Periodontol 2004;31:820–828.

5. Chen ST, Darby IB, Reynolds EC. A prospective clinical study of non-submerged immediate implants: Clinical outcomes and esthetic results. Clin Oral Implants Res 2007;18:552–562.

6. Kan JY, Rungcharassaeng K, Umezu K, Kois JC. Dimensions of peri-implant mucosa: An evaluation of maxillary anterior single implants in humans. J Periodontol 2003;74:557–562.

7. Saadoun AP, Touati B. Soft tissue recession around implants: Is it still unavoidable? Part II. Pract Proced Aesthet Dent 2007;19:81–87.

8. Jung RE, Sailer I, Hammerle CH, Attin T, Schmidlin P. In vitro color changes of soft tissues caused by restorative materials. Int J Periodontics Restorative Dent 2007;27:251–257.

9. Lazzara RJ, Porter SS. Platform switching: A new concept in implant dentistry for controlling postrestorative crestal bone levels. Int J Periodontics Restorative Dent 2006;26:9–17.

10. Maeda Y, Miura J, Taki I, Sogo M. Biomechanical analysis on platform switching: Is there any biomechanical rationale? Clin Oral Implants Res 2007;18:581–584.

11. Leziy S, Miller B. Replacement of adjacent missing anterior teeth with scalloped implants: A case report. Pract Proced Aesthetic Dent 2005;17:331–338.

12. Abrahamsson I, Berglundh T, Lindhe J. The mucosal barrier after abutment dis/reconnection. An experimental study in dogs. J Clin Periodontol 1997;8:568–572.

13. Abrahamsson I, Berglundh T, Sekino S, Lindhe J. Tissue reactions to abutment shift: An experimental study in dogs. Clin Implant Dent Relat Res 2003;5:82–88.

14. Rimondini L, Cerroni L, Carrassi A, Torricelli P. Bacterial colonization of zirconia ceramic surfaces: An in vitro and in vivo study. Int J Oral Maxillofac Implants 2002;17:793–798.

15. Digidi M, Artese, L, Scarano A, Perrotti V, Gehrke P, Piattelli A. Inflammatory infiltrate, microvessel density, nitric oxide synthase expression, and proliferative activity in peri-implant soft tissues around titanium and zirconium oxide healing caps. J Periodontol 2003;77:73–80.

16. Scarano A, Piattelli M, Caputi S, Favero GA, Piattelli A. Bacterial adhesion on commercially pure titanium and zirconium oxide disks: An in vivo human study. J Periodontol 2004;75:292–296.

17. Zang Y, Lawn BR, Malament KA, Thompson VP, Rekow ED. Damage accumulation and fatigue life of particle-abraded ceramics. Int J Prosthodont 2006;19:151–157.

18. Papanagiotou HP, Morgano SM, Giordano RA, Pober R. In vitro evaluation of low-temperature aging effects and finishing procedures on the flexural strength and structural stability of Y-TZP dental ceramics. J Prosthet Dent 2006;96:154–164.

19. Park SW, Driscoll CF, Romberg EE, Siegel S, Thompson G. Ceramic implant abutments: Cutting efficiency and resultant surface finish by diamond rotary cutting instruments. J Prosthet Dent 2006;95:444–449.

20. Leziy SS, Miller BA. Developing ideal implant tissue architecture and pontic site form. Quintessence Dent Technol 2007;30:143–154.

SNOW WHITE AND TRANSPARENCE

Hiro Tokutomi, RDT
Cusp Dental Research
381 Pearl Street
Malden, MA 02148, USA
E-mail: info@cuspdental.com

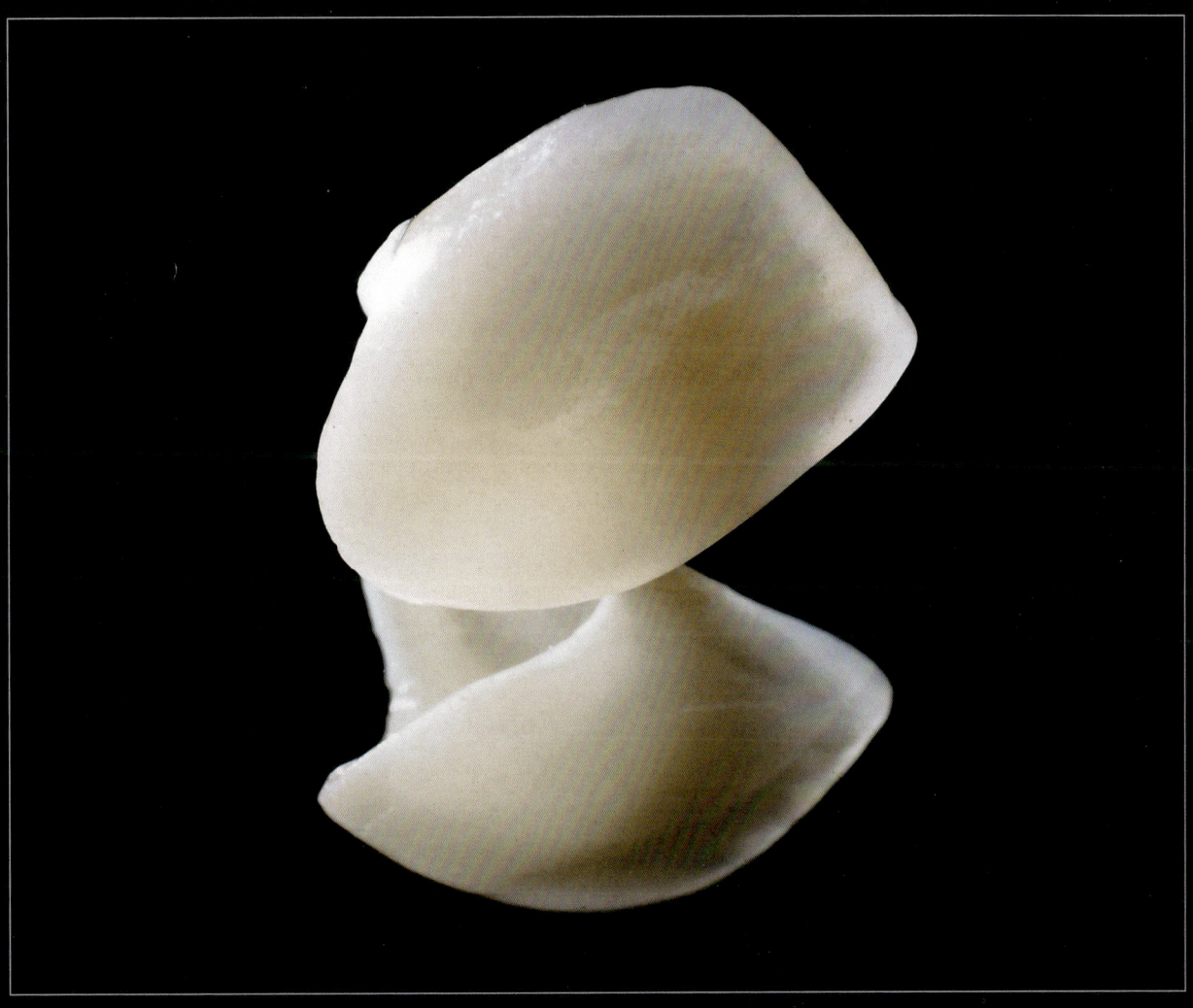

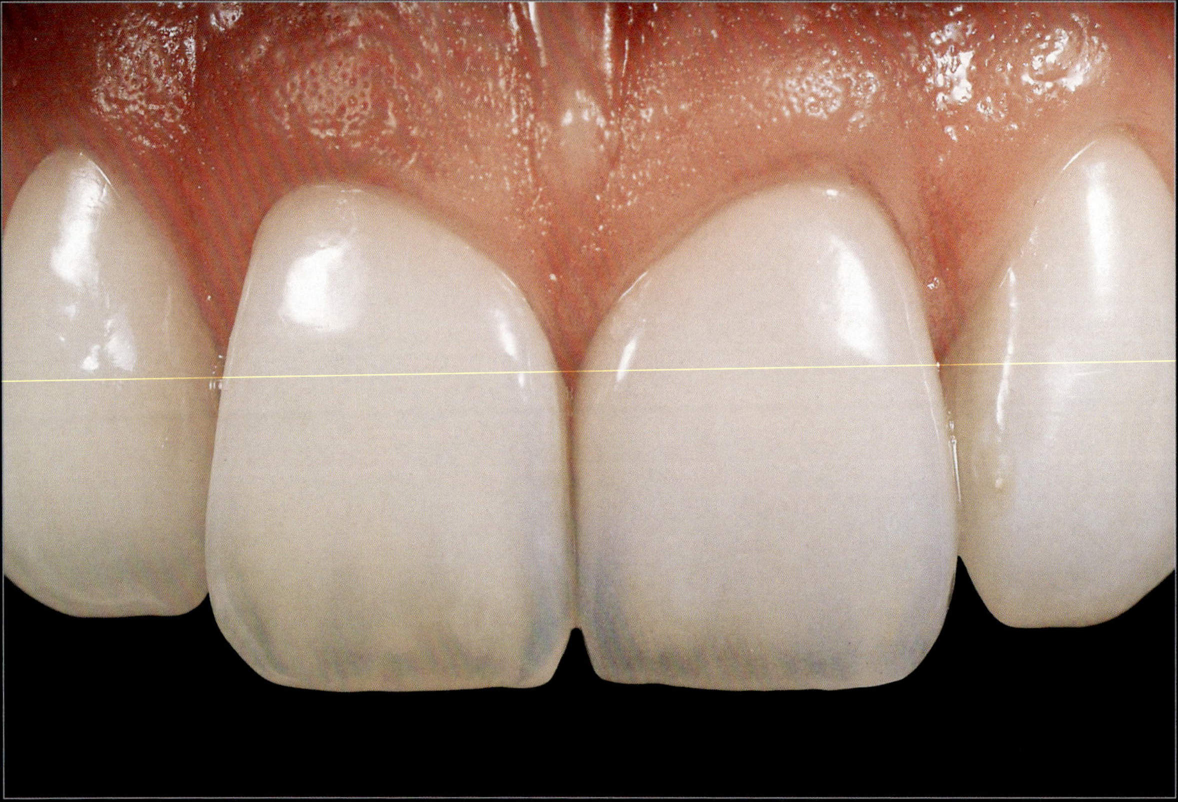

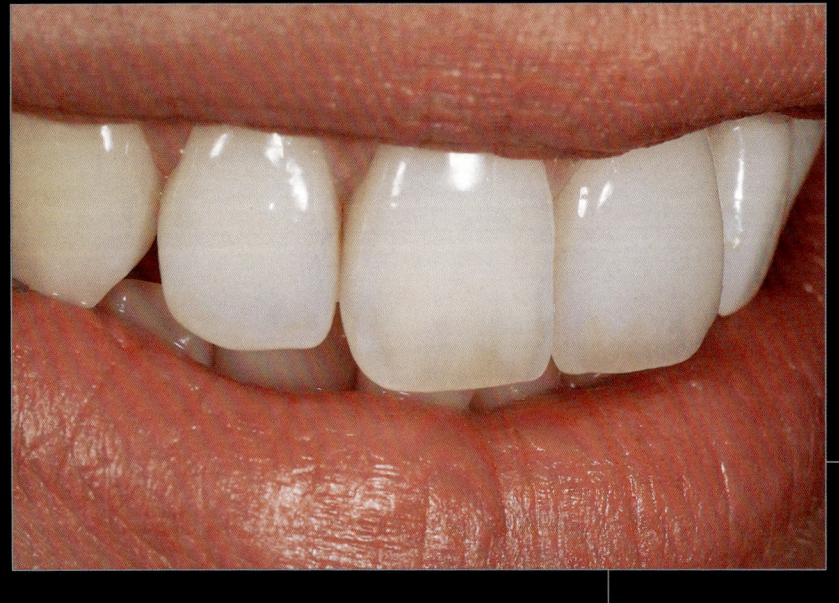

Case 1

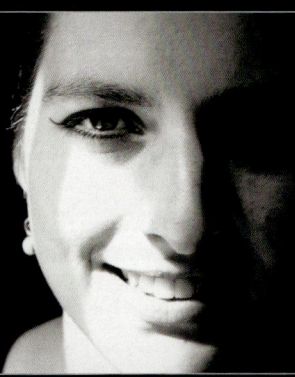

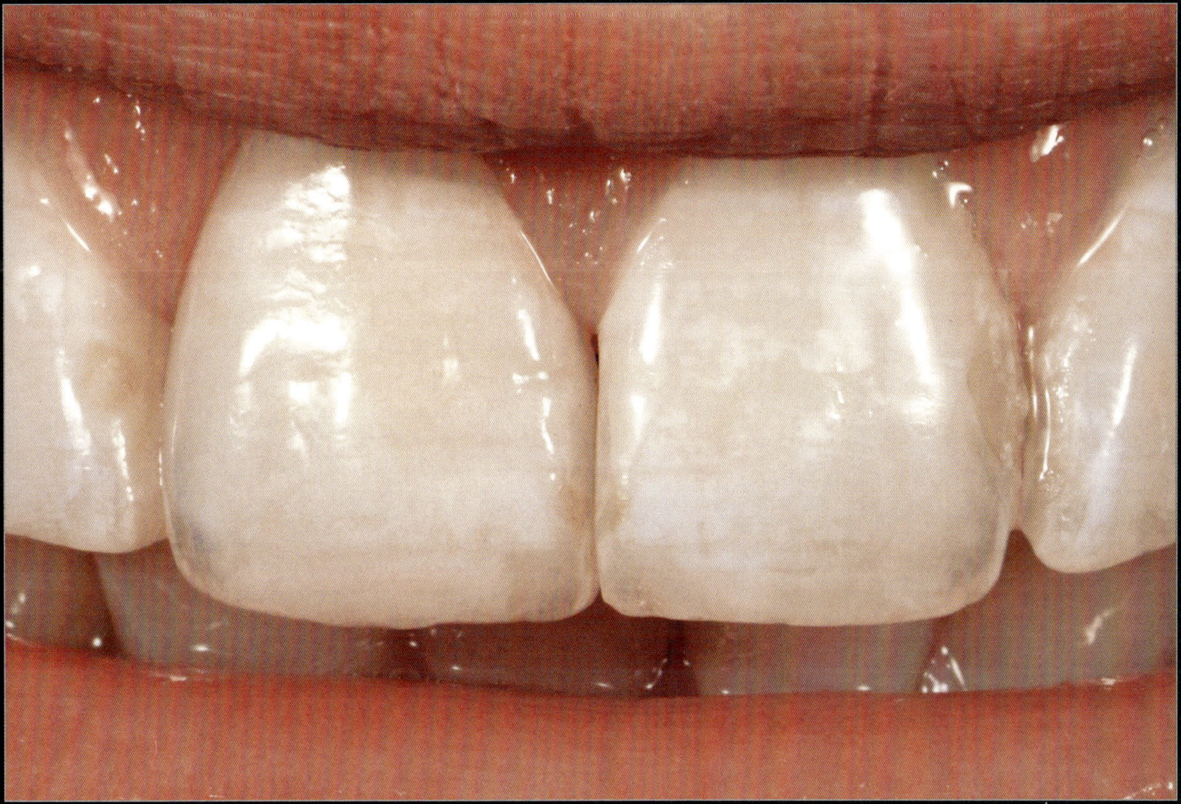

Case 2

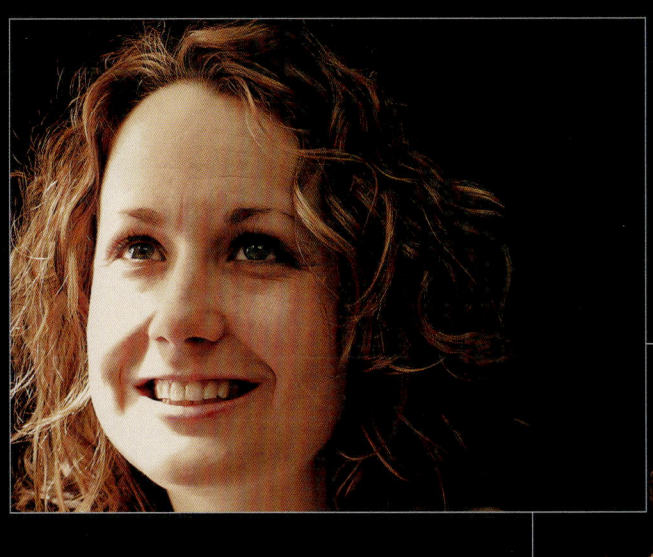

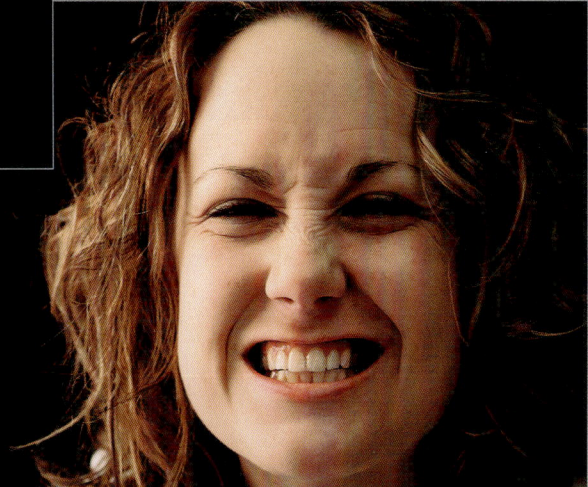

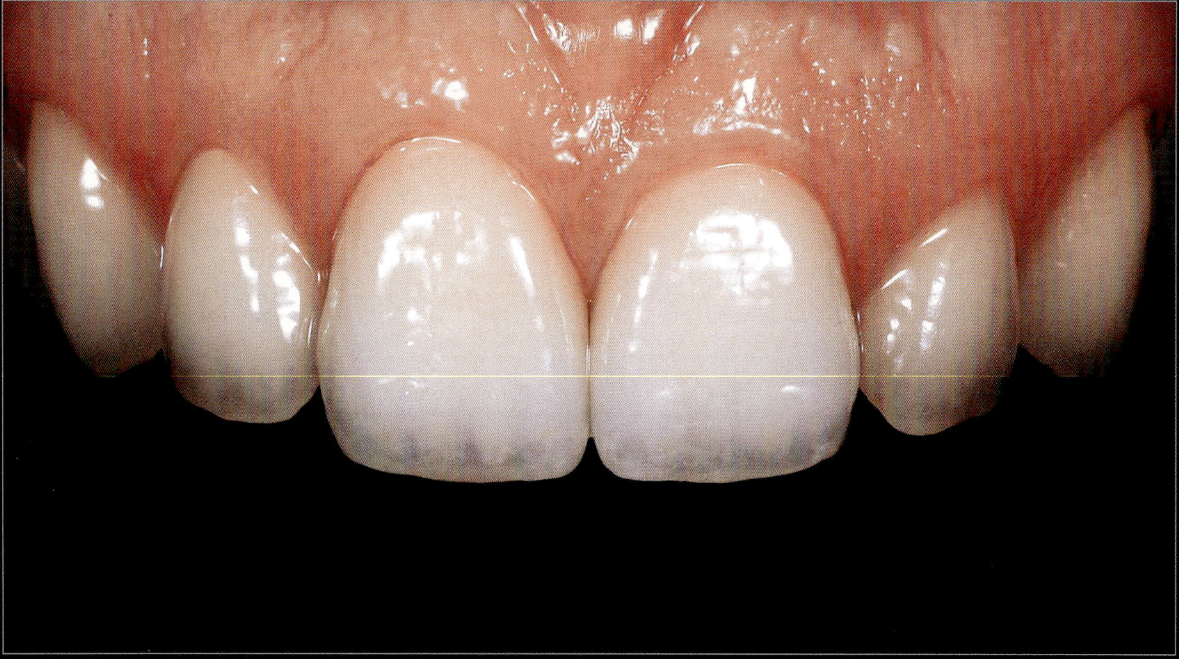

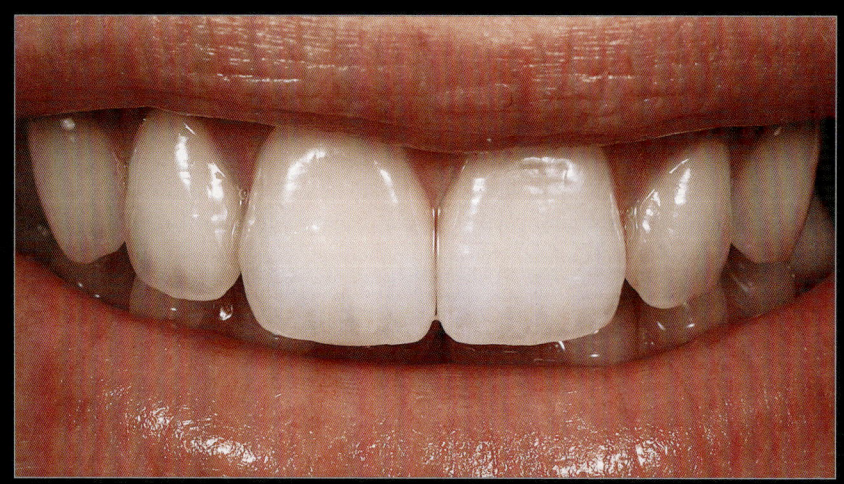

Case 3

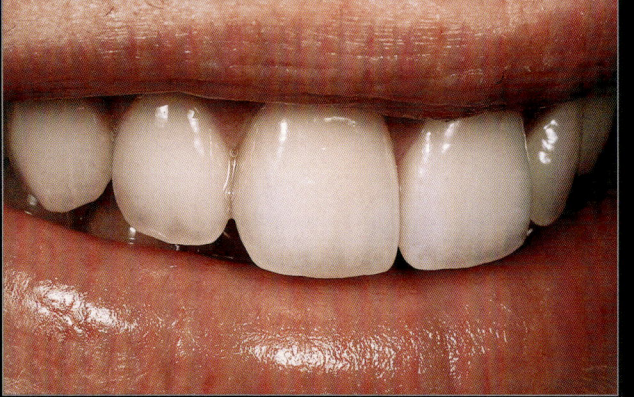
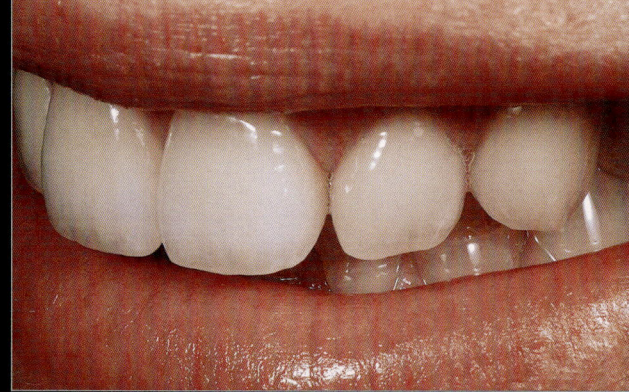

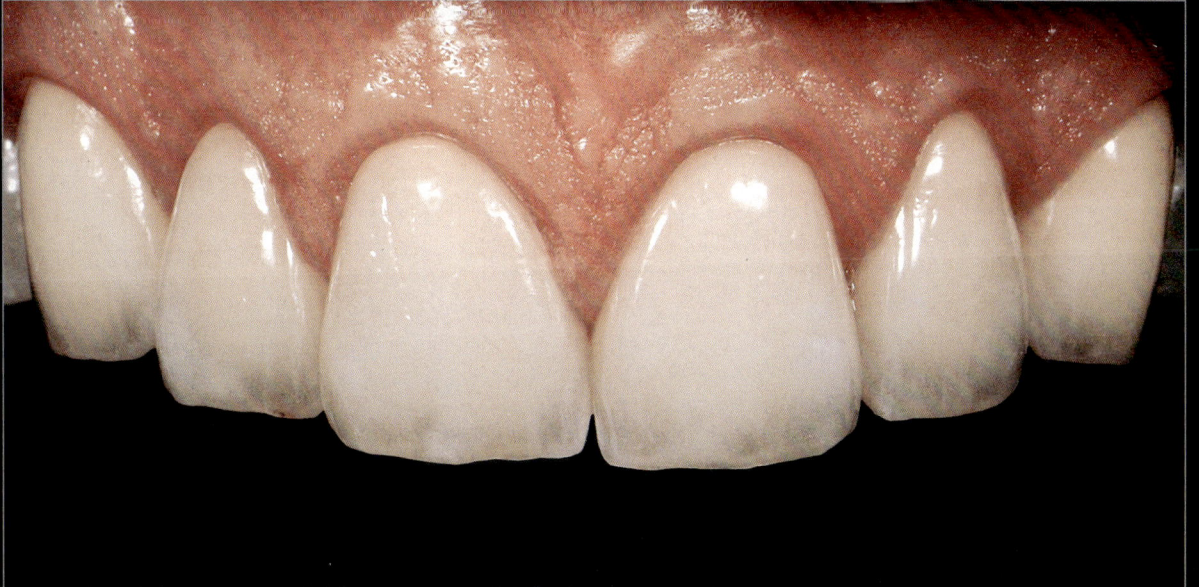

Case 4

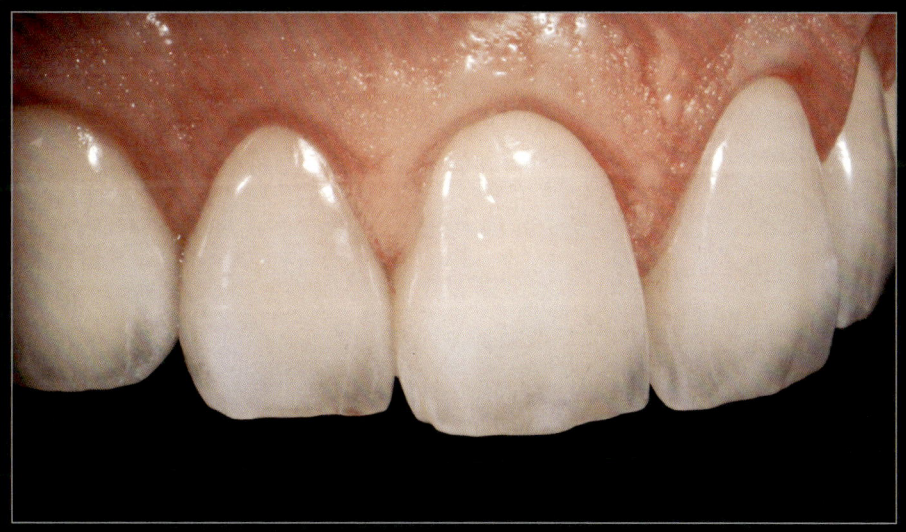

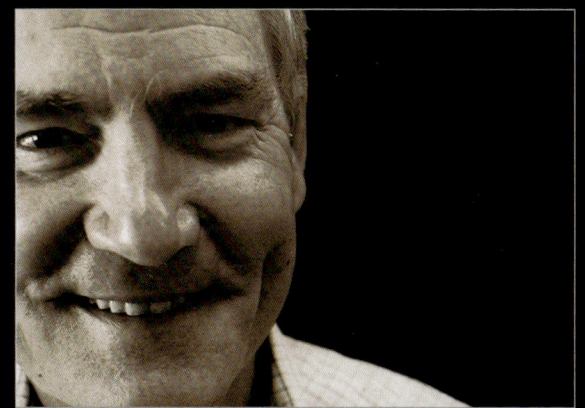

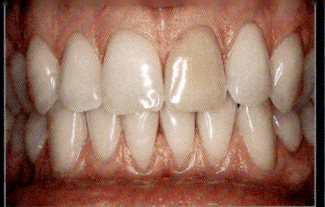

Fig 1 Pretreatment.

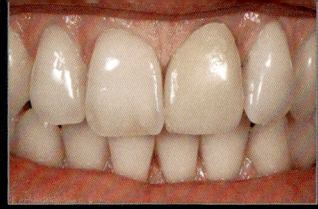

Fig 2 Provisional crown placed.

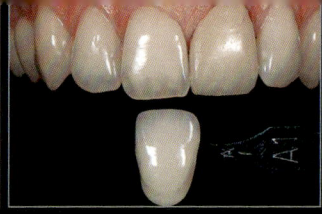

Fig 3 Basic shade is determined at the dentin layer.

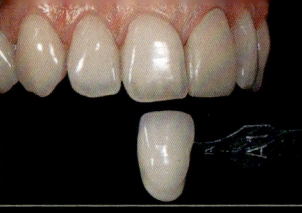

Fig 4 Color variations are best seen with a slight lateral shift of the dentition and shade tab.

CASE 1

Restoration: Maxillary left central incisor, Noritake Katana CZR crown.

Patient: 23-year-old female. Endodontic therapy, performed several years earlier, resulted in discoloration of the tooth.

Shade information: Shade taking was performed at the dental laboratory 3 days after the treatment, at about 1 pm. Conditions were ideal: Dry teeth were recovered from the chairside treatment, and natural light was used to record the tooth shade. Also, the ceramist took the shade under the same light setting as his work bench.

Key notes: Figures 3 and 4 show that the surface layers are translucent; the value is lower than A1 The use of a lower-value dentin powder is required along with the use of the same-value dentin powder as shown in an A1 shade tab. The value is controlled by the thickness of the translucent powder A bright translucency is achieved. It is important to create a blue wash translucency from the incisal edge to proximal area. The yellow mamelons are also important. It is best to minimize the orange characterization in the translucent area at the incisal edge.

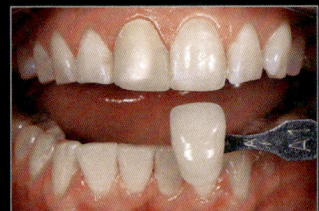

Fig 5 When the shade tab covers the dentition, it is difficult to analyze the shade differences.

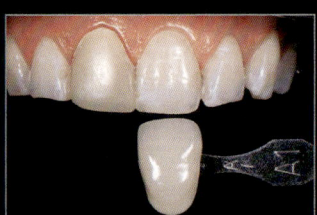

Fig 6 Edge-to-edge positioning of the shade tab to the tooth is suggested.

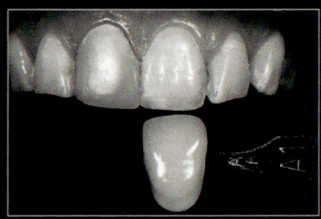

Fig 7 To better show differences in value, the photograph is adjusted to monotone, which eliminates the hue and chroma

CASE 2

Restoration: Maxillary right central incisor, Noritake CZR Press & CZR LF veneer.

Patient: 33-year-old female. She desired uniform-looking central incisors. Esthetics was paramount.

Shade information: Shade was taken at the dental laboratory with ideal natural light conditions. However, it was 1 hour after the chairside treatment, so

Key notes: For color determination, it was important to record the white calcifications on the surface and the translucency at the proximal areas. A color photograph was adjusted to monotone on a computer to verify the value of the dentin color (Fig 7). A higher value than the A1 shade tab was determined based on the information from the monotone photograph. NW 0.5 which is one shade brighter than A1, was used as the base color. Detailed characterizations had to be cre-

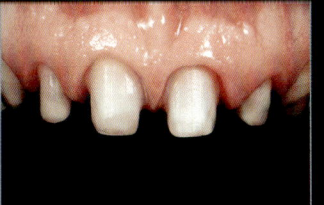

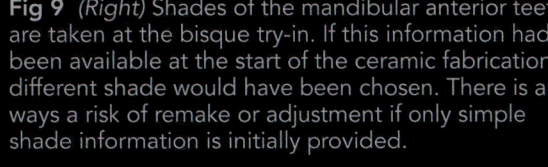

Fig 8 *(Left)* Multiple tooth preparations.

Fig 9 *(Right)* Shades of the mandibular anterior teeth are taken at the bisque try-in. If this information had been available at the start of the ceramic fabrication, a different shade would have been chosen. There is always a risk of remake or adjustment if only simple shade information is initially provided.

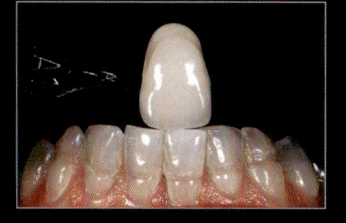

CASE 3

Restorations: Maxillary anterior teeth, Noritake Katana CZR crowns.
Patient: 43-year-old female.
Shade information: The only instructions provided by the clinician were that the central incisors should be brighter than shade A1. It was left to the ceramist to create the variations in color to achieve optimal results.

Key notes: The ceramist was required to arrange life-like characterizations along with the requested shade. Shade gradations were created from the central incisor to the canine. A blue wash translucency was used on the incisal edge of the central incisors. A snow-white modifier was used to create detailed white bands so that the crowns would not lose their color value.

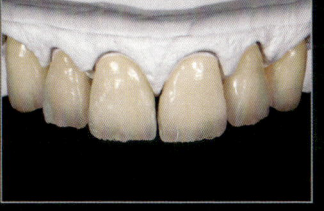

Fig 10 *(Left)* Strong characterization is expressed by using an internal stain technique.

Fig 11 *(Right)* The chroma appears strong, showing a dark appearance that is reflected in the teeth. Maintaining the color value is expressed in the mandibular teeth essence.

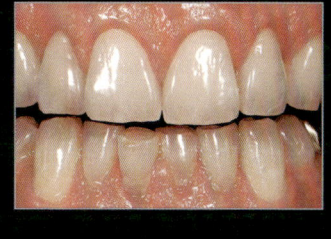

CASE 4

Restorations: Maxillary anterior teeth, Noritake Katana CZR crowns.
Patient: 50-year-old male.
Shade information: Several photographs with shade tabs were provided with instructions for an A3 base.

Key notes: Chroma usually needs to be increased for middle-aged men in order to express aging characteristics. All colors decrease the value. The same base color and hue as the shade tab should be used for the dentin powder to provide the strong characterization required in this case. In this way, the ceramist could control the value as well as color addition and color adjustment.

SNOW WHITE AND TRANSPARENCE

Translucency is key to the creation of natural tooth color. By managing the translucency, ceramists are able to create lifelike prostheses. If the vitality is lost by using materials of low color value or of an inappropriate volume, then the finished results will not be satisfactory.

White spots, white bands, or areas of calcification, along with the halo effect on the enamel, can enhance the lifelike characteristics of the restoration. With the use of a snow-white modifier, the color effect can be discreetly shifted to achieve the desired results. On the other hand, the inappropriate use of a snow-white modifier can destroy the natural appearance that has been created.

Based on the value chromatics, snow white reflects light completely, so its value is 100%, whereas glasslike transparency transmits and absorbs light completely, so its value is 0%. Transparency and snow white are two extreme values. They should not be used individually to express colors. Ceramists create various translucencies between transparent and snow-white values. They also create milk wash, which has a glasslike translucency along with a chroma and hue, to achieve a desired color. To the eye, the combination of the value, chroma, and hue make a difference. By using various translucencies, one can control color value, which is the key to obtaining a natural esthetic appearance. The use of the various translucent combinations, along with snow white, is essential in achieving our result.

A SMILE WITH BALANCE

Naoki Hayashi, RDT
Ultimate Styles Dental Laboratory
12 Mauchly Unit M
Irvine, CA 92618, USA
E-mail: nao@ultimate-dl.com

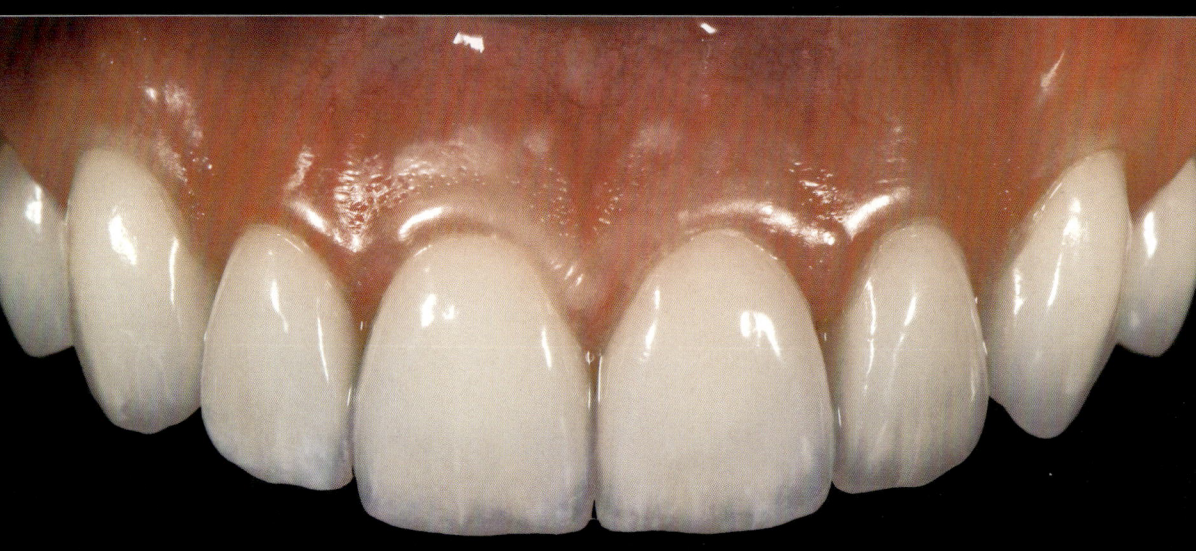

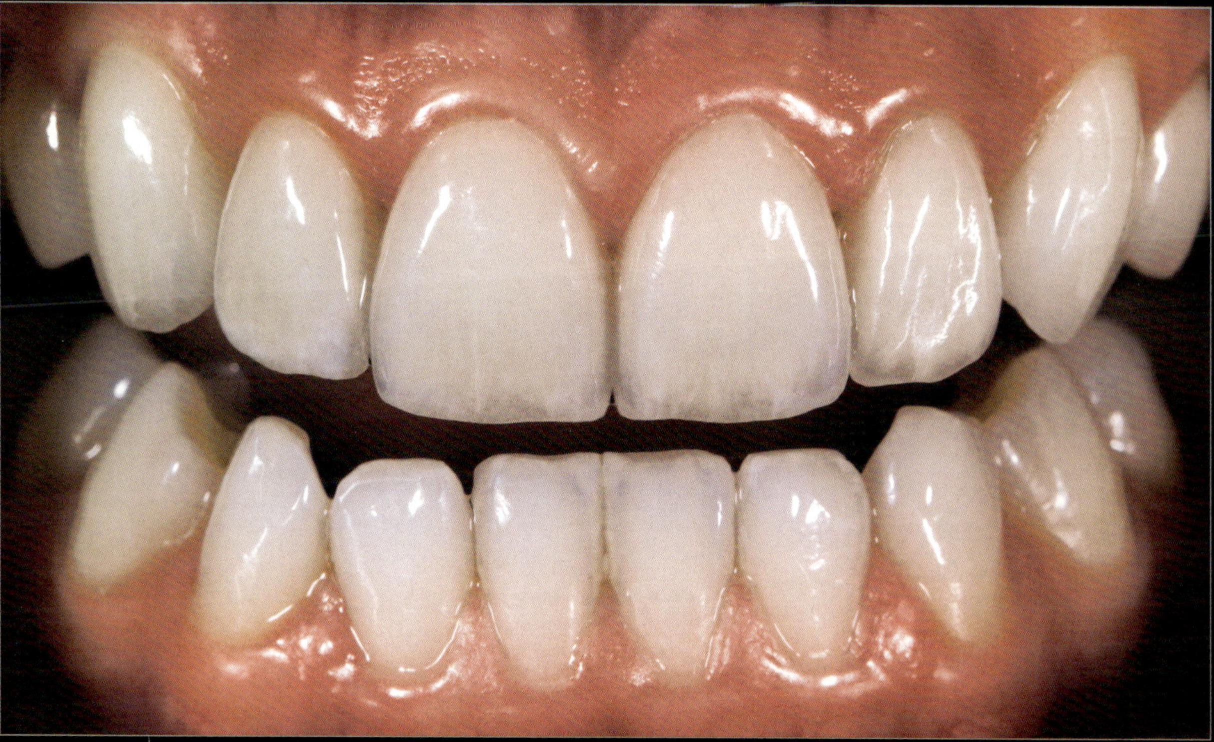

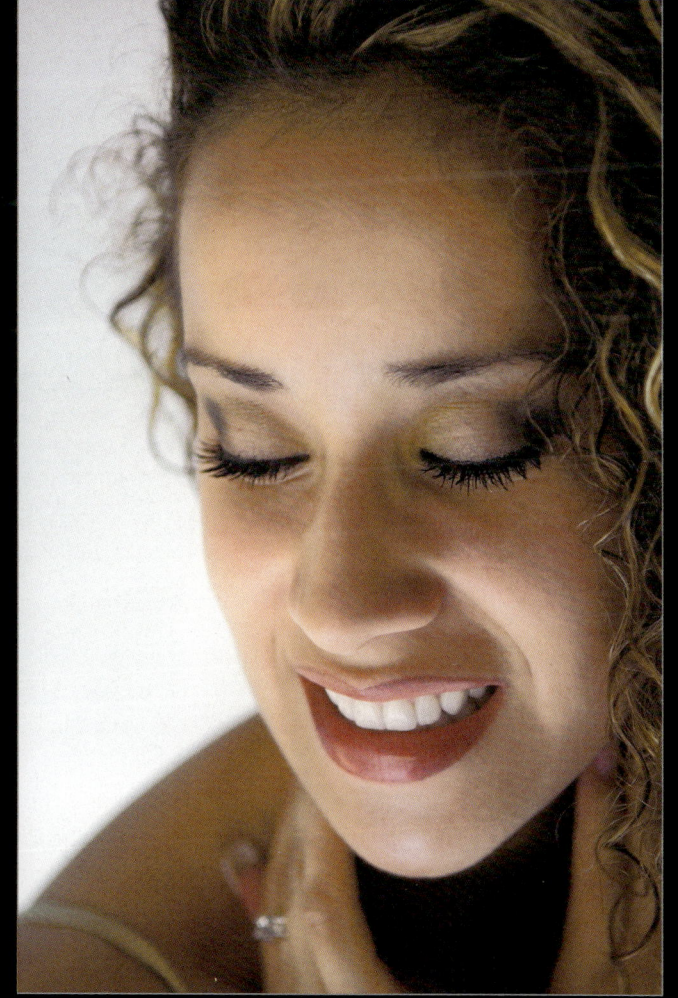

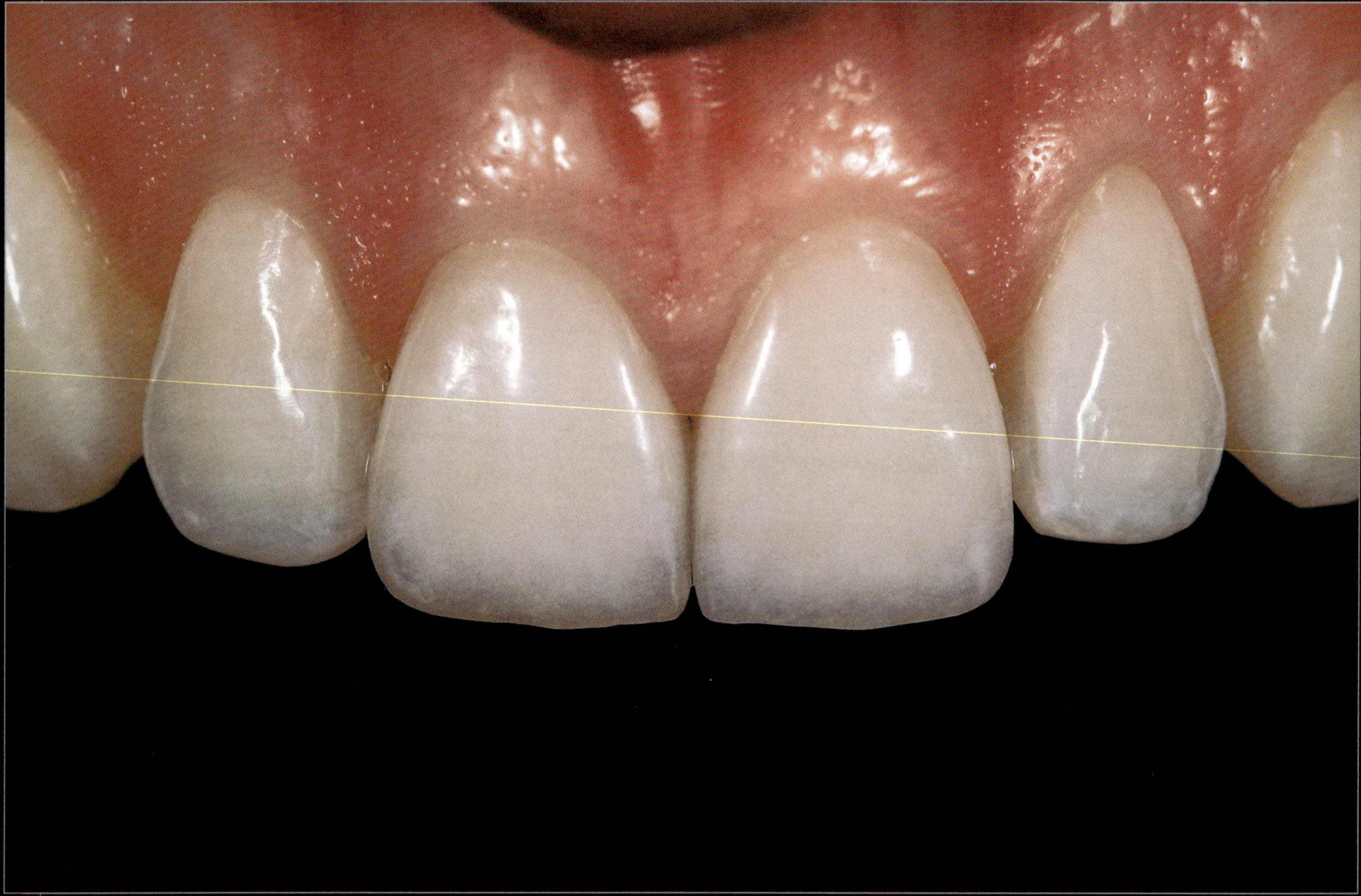

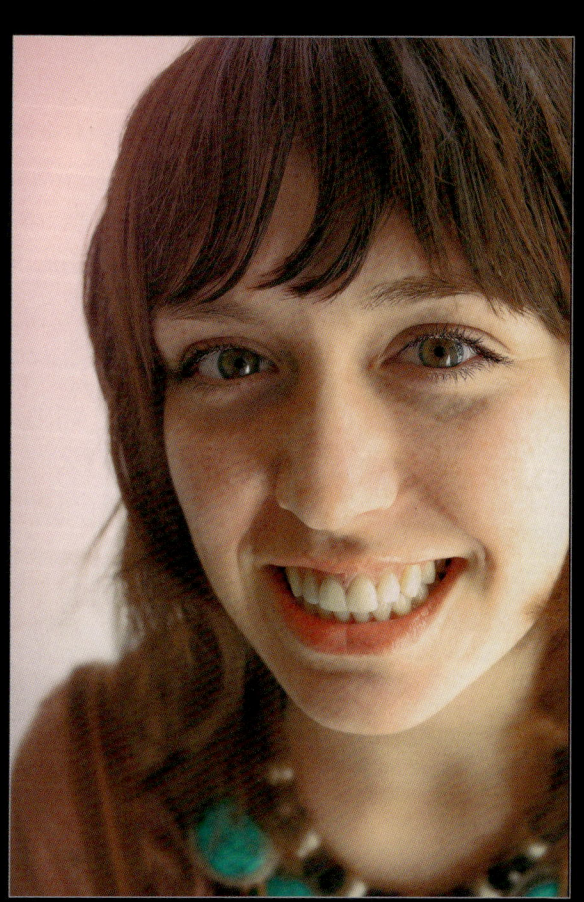

Case 2   Dentist: Dr Kurt R. Schneider

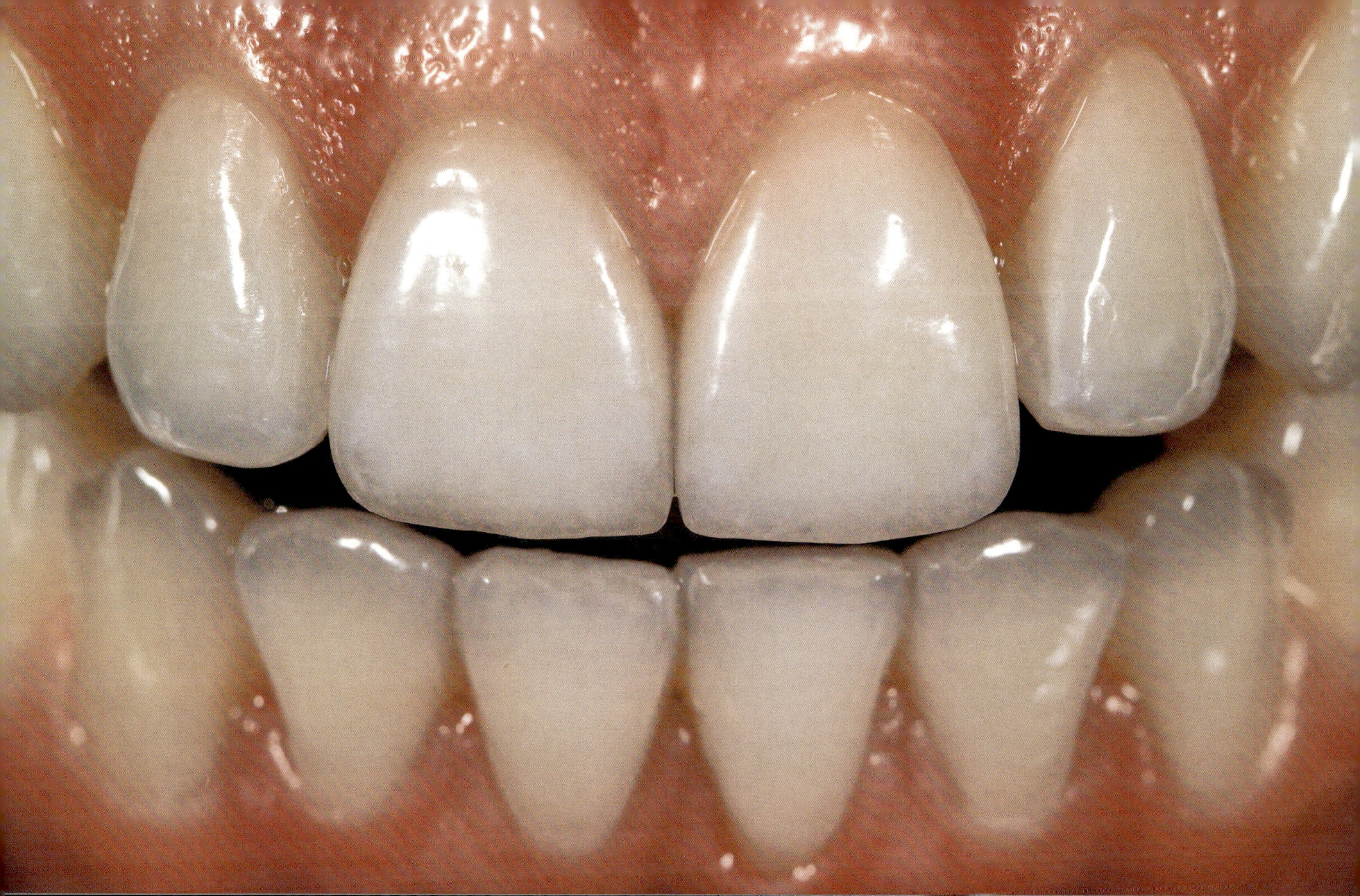
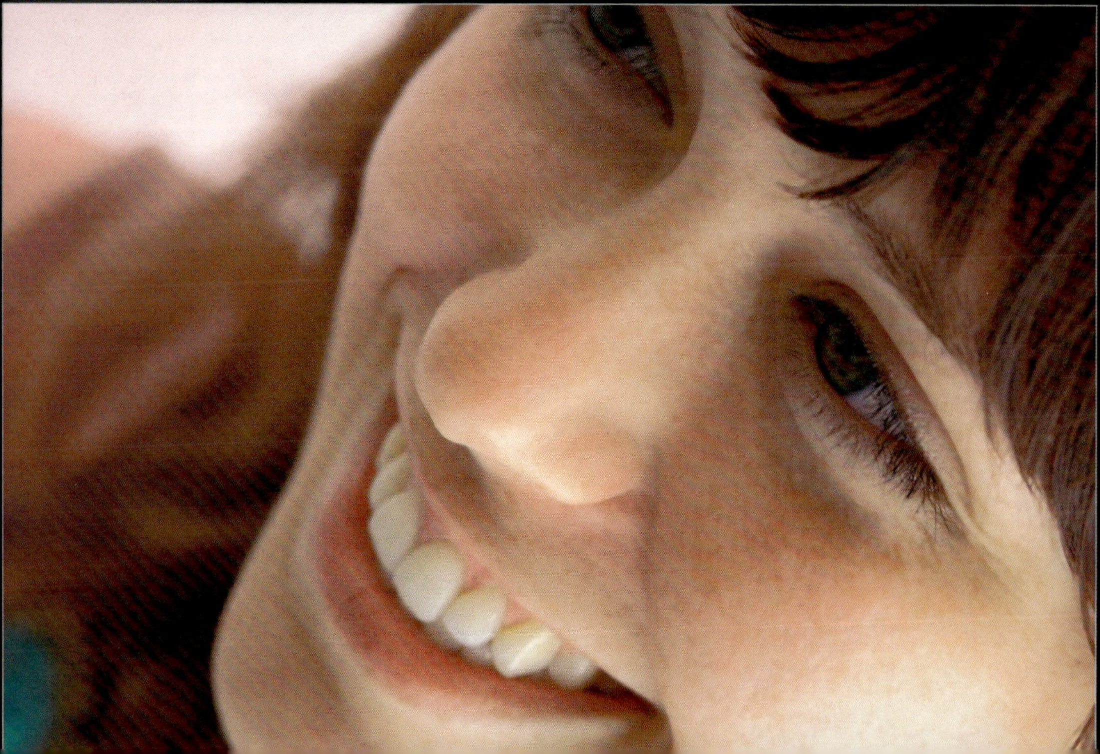

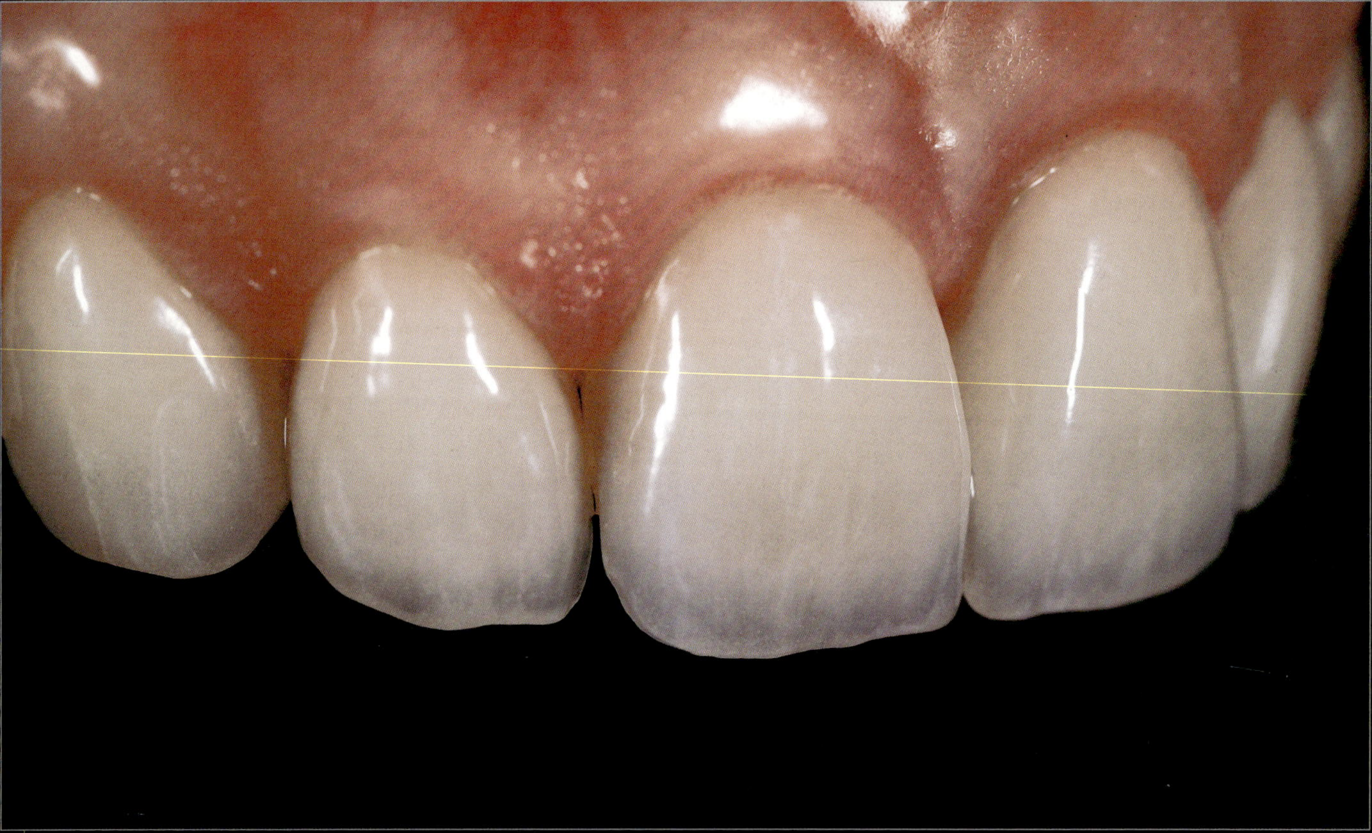

Case 3

Dentist: **Dr Chris C. Liu**

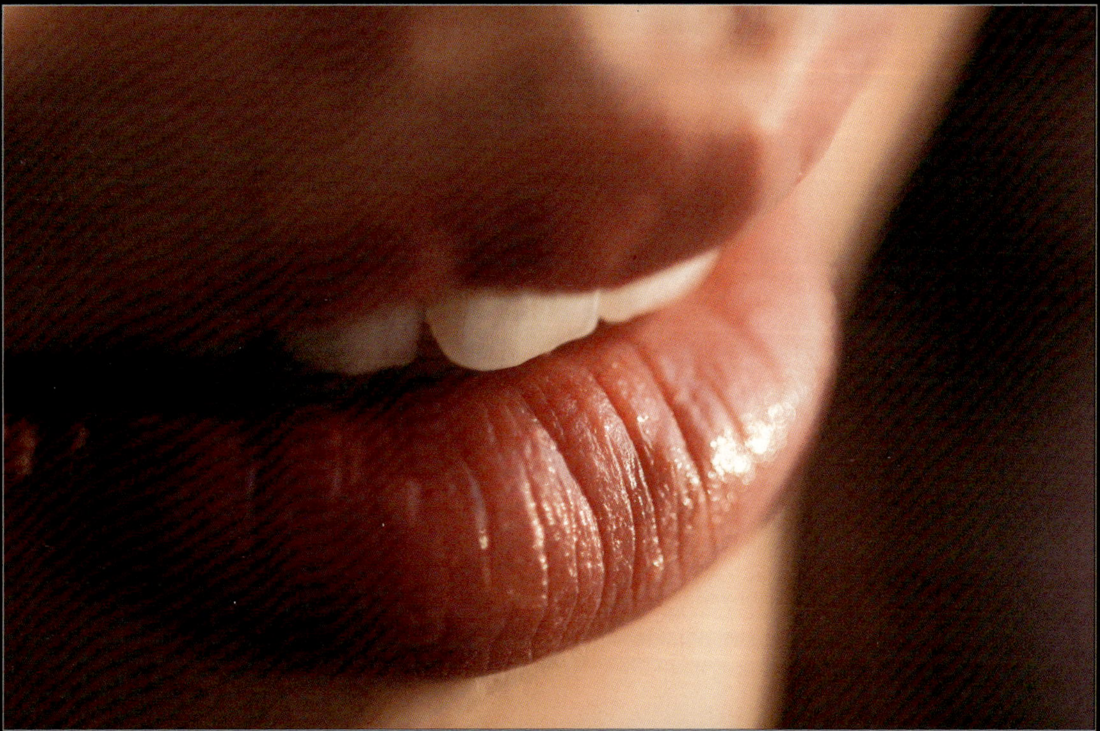

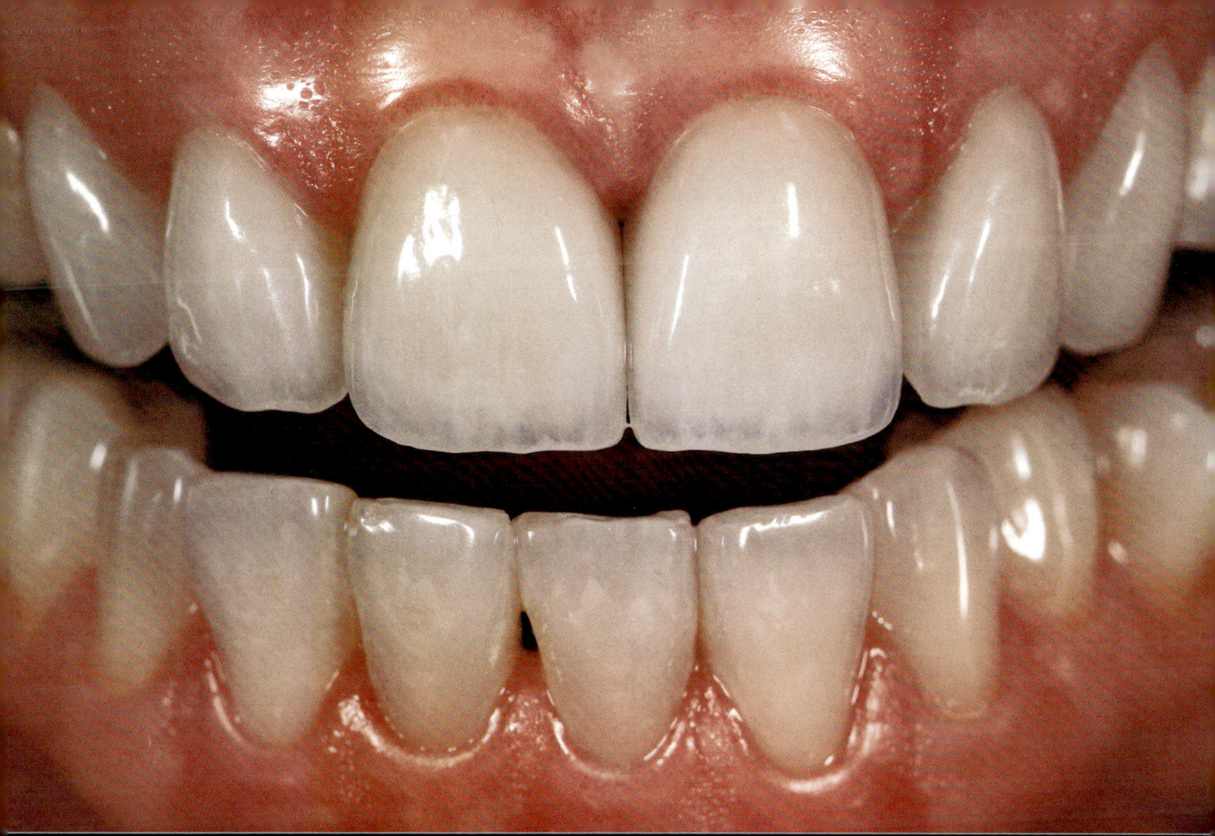

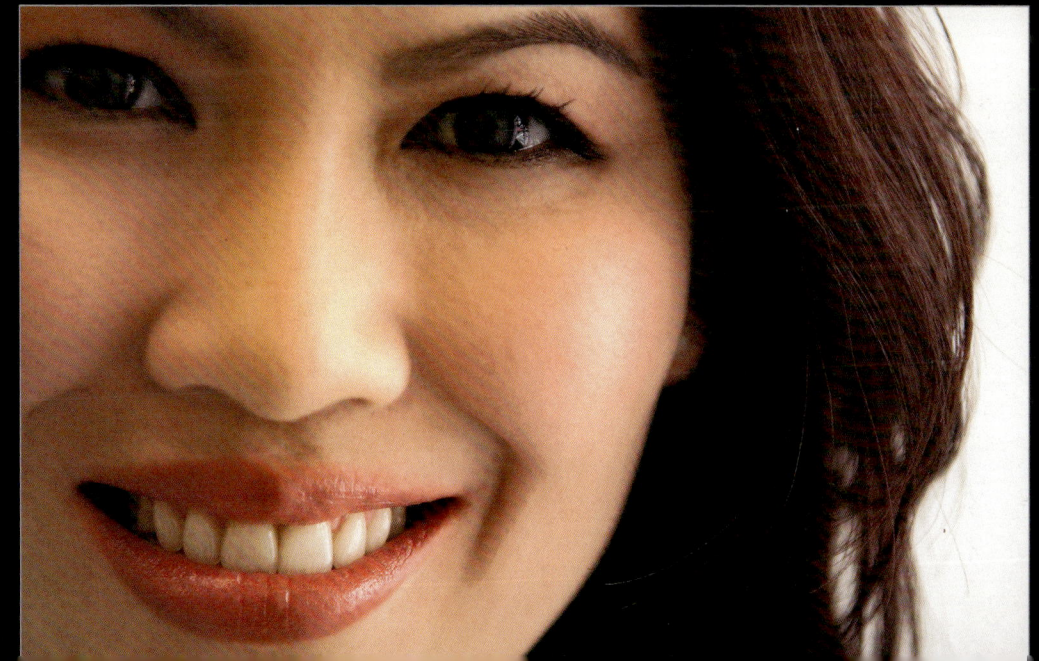

A SMILE WITH BALANCE

In esthetic restorative treatment of the anterior region, the appearance of a restoration is as important as its function. Evaluating the appearance is best done at a normal speaking distance from the patient. Remember that the evaluator's opinion is as important as the patient's esthetic preference, as it often can change the patient's perception.

Esthetic restorations should be in balance with various facial expressions. Ideal, well-balanced restorations are not distinguishable from the natural dentition. A naturally balanced restoration is such an important goal for each patient. Properly included irregularities sometimes add balance. Facial architecture, sex, and age, as well as skin, eye, and hair color, are other important determinant factors for well-balanced restorations.

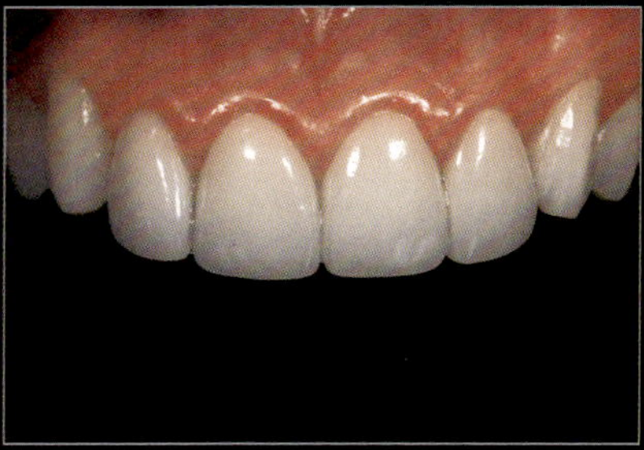

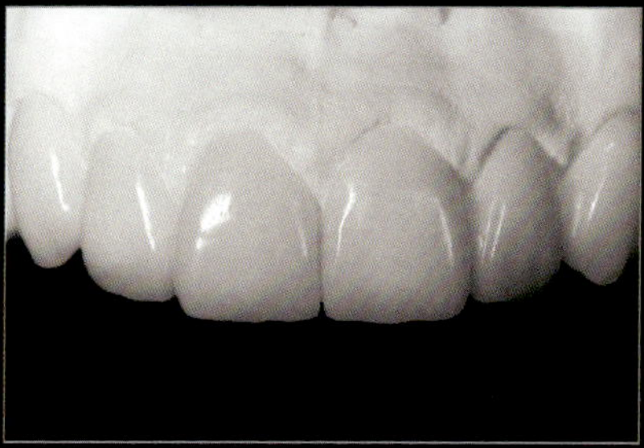

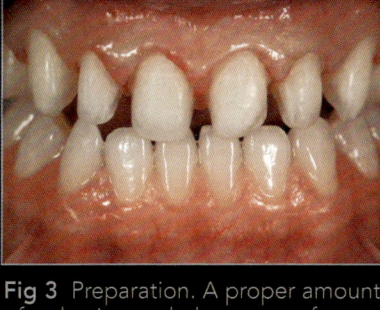

Fig 1 Preoperative view of patient's existing restorations.

Fig 2 Diagnostic waxup.

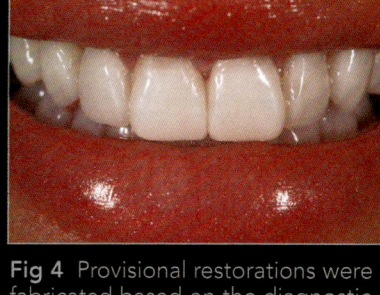

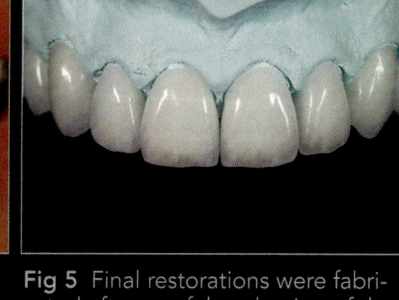

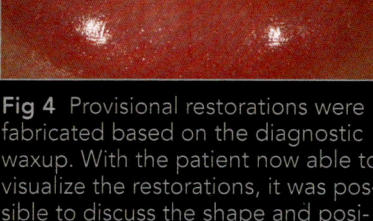

Fig 3 Preparation. A proper amount of reduction and placement of margin line was determined. Space between the mandibular central incisors was to be restored with composite resin.

Fig 4 Provisional restorations were fabricated based on the diagnostic waxup. With the patient now able to visualize the restorations, it was possible to discuss the shape and position of the final restorations in detail.

Fig 5 Final restorations were fabricated after careful evaluation of the provisionals with input from the patient. The line angle of the central incisors was made more prominent, and the lateral incisors were positioned more facially than the provisional restorations.

CASE 1

The treatment goal of this case was to improve the esthetics of existing restorations. Length, long axis of teeth, and incisal arch line were out of balance with the patient's face. The patient was also not happy with the unnaturally white shade of the restorations.

Since the patient's esthetic demand was so high, because her job involved being in front of people, a good amount of discussion took place among the dental ceramist, dentist, and patient to ensure a common goal. It was made clear that the final restoration would be properly balanced in color, shape, position, and function with the patient's face.

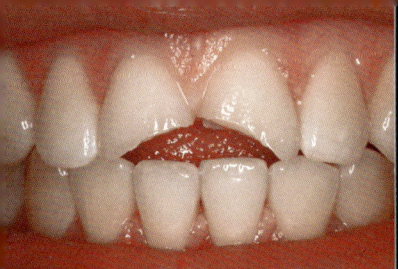

Fig 6 Preoperative fractured central incisors.

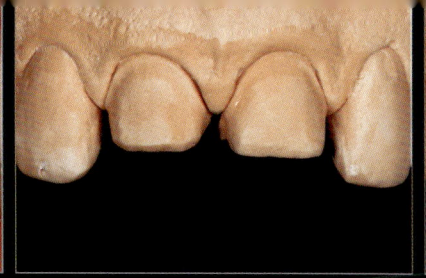

Fig 7 The master cast reproduced the abutments clearly and accurately. Porcelain laminate veneer restoration was indicated. The cervical margin was beveled since the shade of the abutment matched the intended shade of the restoration.

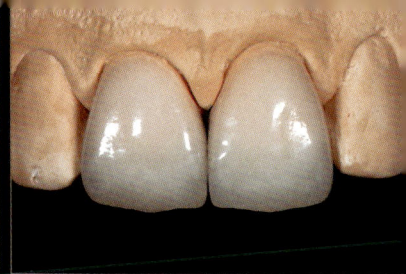

Fig 8 Completed restoration. All determinant factors were taken into consideration. The restorations were tried in the mouth for final evaluation.

CASE 2

This patient's maxillary central incisors were fractured at the incisal third in an accident. The patient wanted these teeth restored exactly the way they appeared previously. It was determined upon review of photographs from before the accident that the patient's original teeth were a little too long. After careful discussion with the patient, it was decided to shorten the central incisors according to the patient's facial architecture and smile line. Alignment of the restorations was also changed to balance them with the flared lateral incisors.

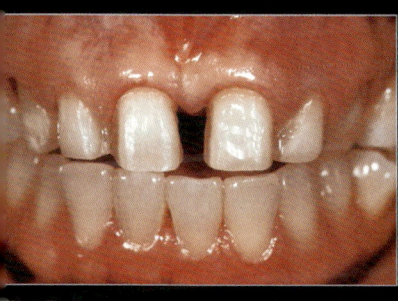

Fig 9 Preparation. Space between the maxillary central incisors was 4.5 mm. Restorations would be designed to balance the six anterior teeth in addition to filling the space.

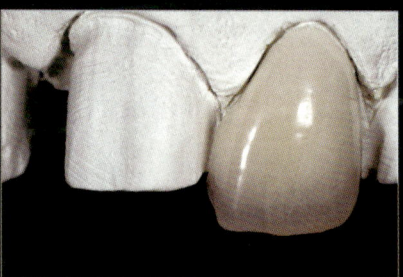

Fig 10 At the central incisors, the distance from the mesial line angle of the abutment to that of the restoration was 2 mm, so a mesial shift of the distal line angle by 2 mm was necessary to maintain the tooth width. The same modification was required for the other restorations. The mesial line angle of the lateral incisors therefore needed to be overlapped by the central incisors, but the restoration managed to conceal this overlap.

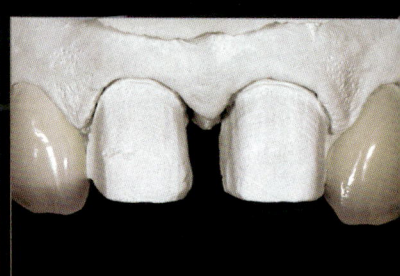

Fig 11 Margin placement of lateral incisor veneers at the mesial aspect. The width of the central incisors can be well-controlled by this manipulation.

CASE 3

Goals of this case were to improve color and shape and then close the diastema between the central incisors. Six anterior teeth were included in the restoration to be balanced with the facial architecture

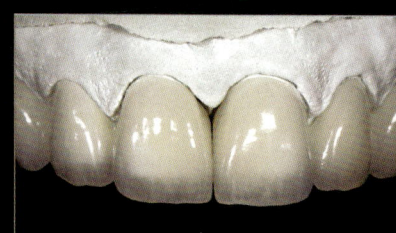

Fig 12 Completed restorations.

THRILLED BY SINGLES

Samuel C. Lee, CDT, MDC
Art Oral USA
13210 Estrella Avenue #1
Gardena, CA 90248, USA
E-mail: artoral@hotmail.com

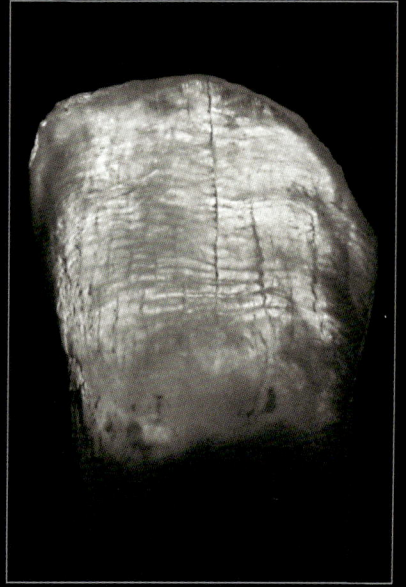 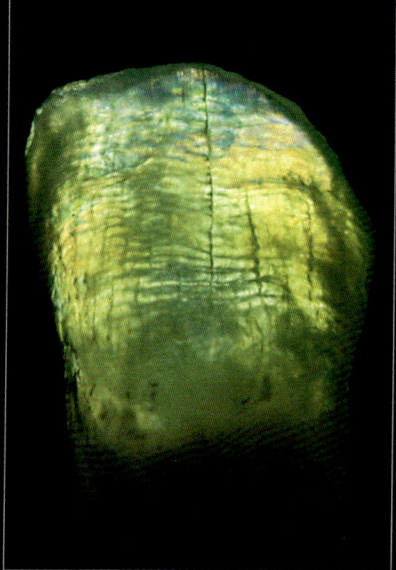 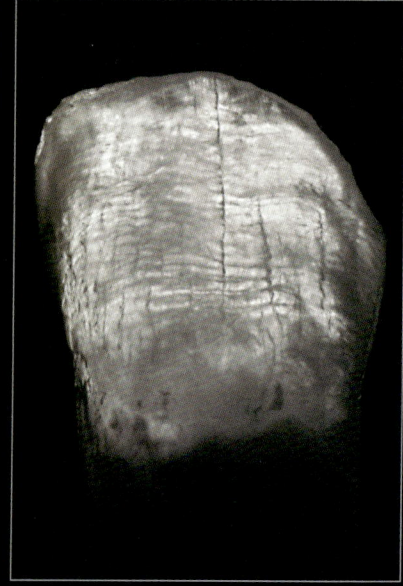

My treatment philosophy is to focus not only on restorations, but also on the patient's emotions. The emotion of excellence is not something we give the patient—it is something that is developed together through understanding. It takes commitment, dedication, and understanding of everyone involved throughout the entire process.

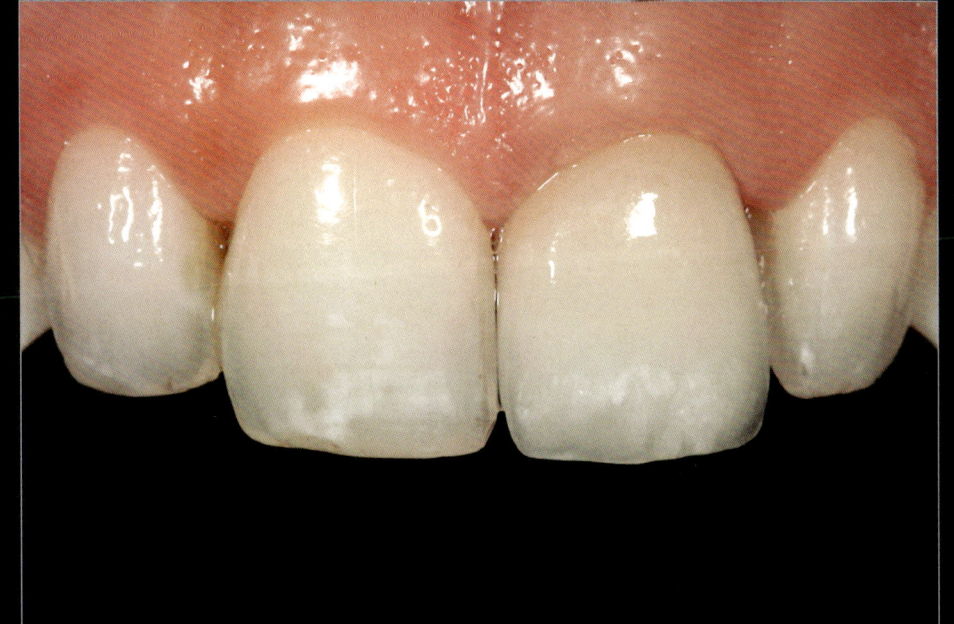

Case 1

All-ceramic restoration, maxillary left central incisor

Dentist: **Brian P. LeSage, DDS**, Beverly Hills, California

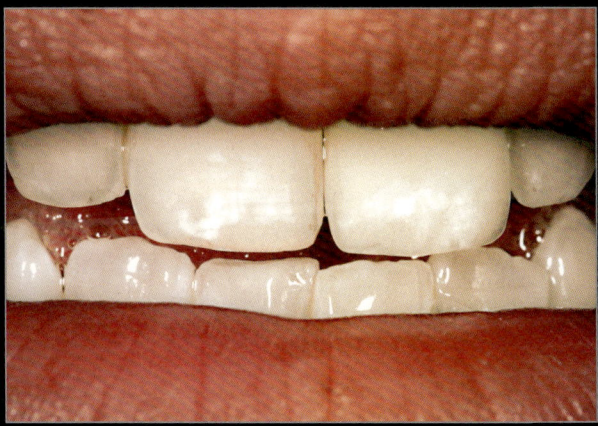

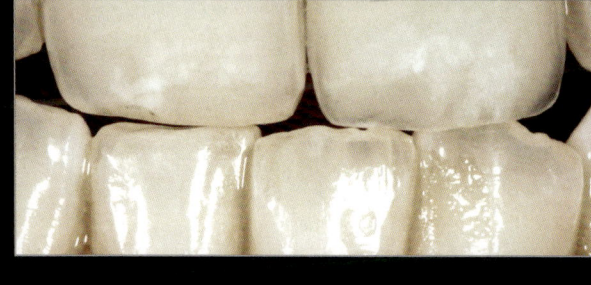

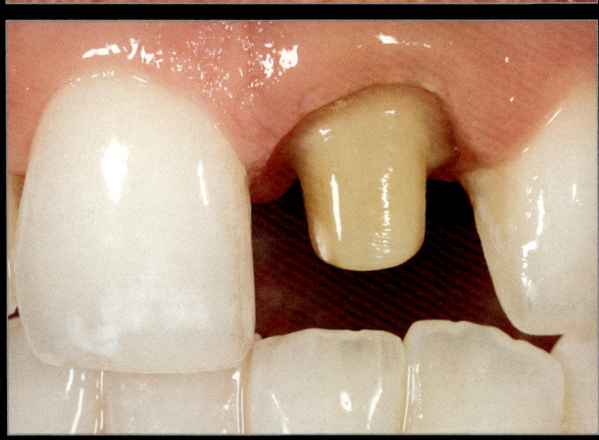

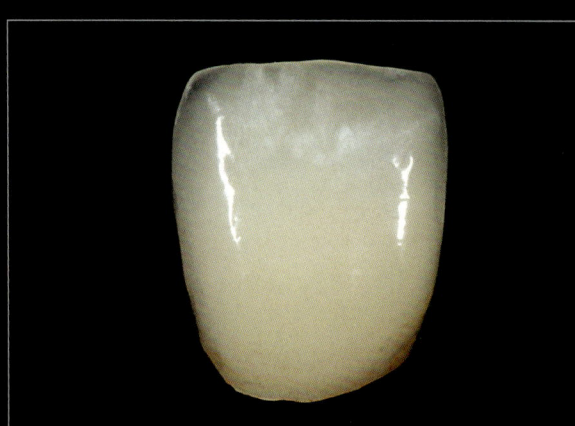

Pressable Technique (Vintage LF, Shofu)—Tooth bleaching.
Create the mottling-effect appearance and incisal translucency with the layering technique.

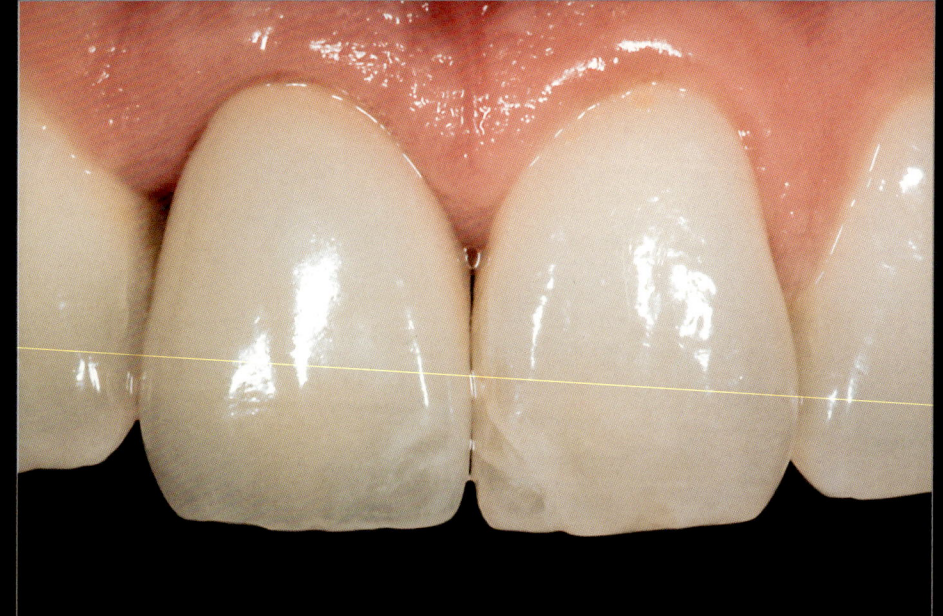

Case 2 — Metal-ceramic restoration, maxillary right central incisor

Dentist: **Kenneth D. Ochi, DDS**, Redondo Beach, California

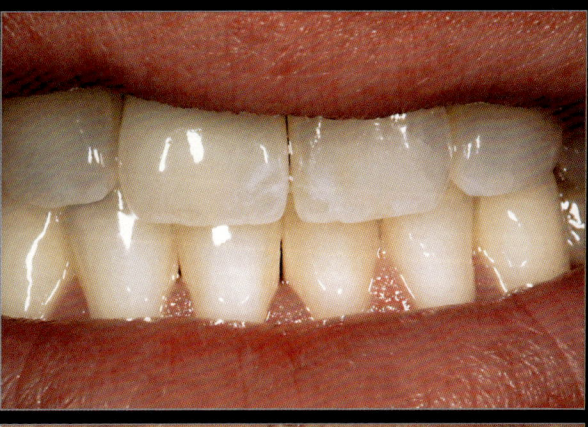

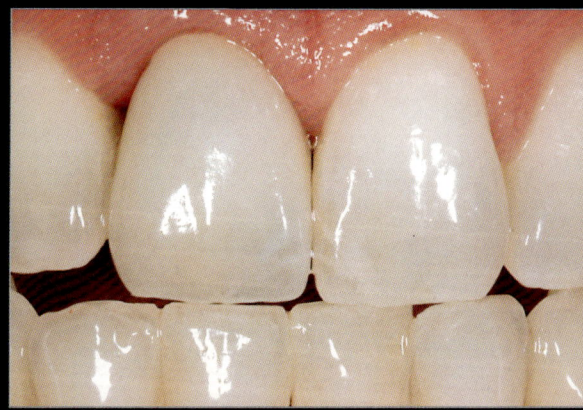

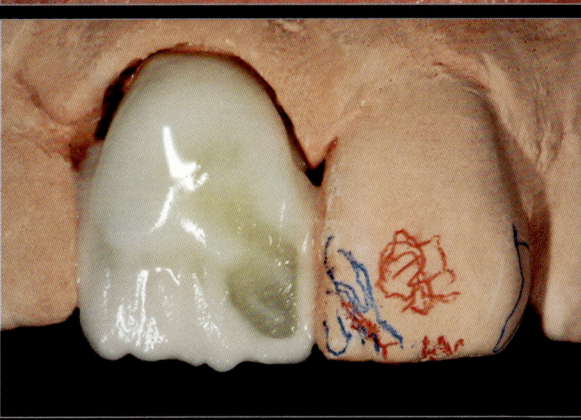

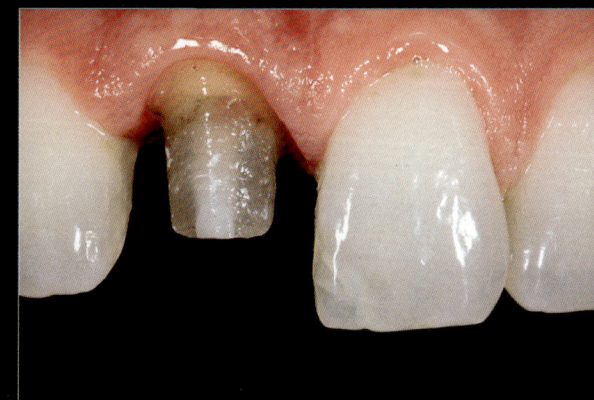

Porcelain fused to gold with porcelain margin technique (Vintage Halo, Shofu)—Unstable and discol-ored (gray/black) substructure.
Need to have strong substructure to completely mask the deep staining.

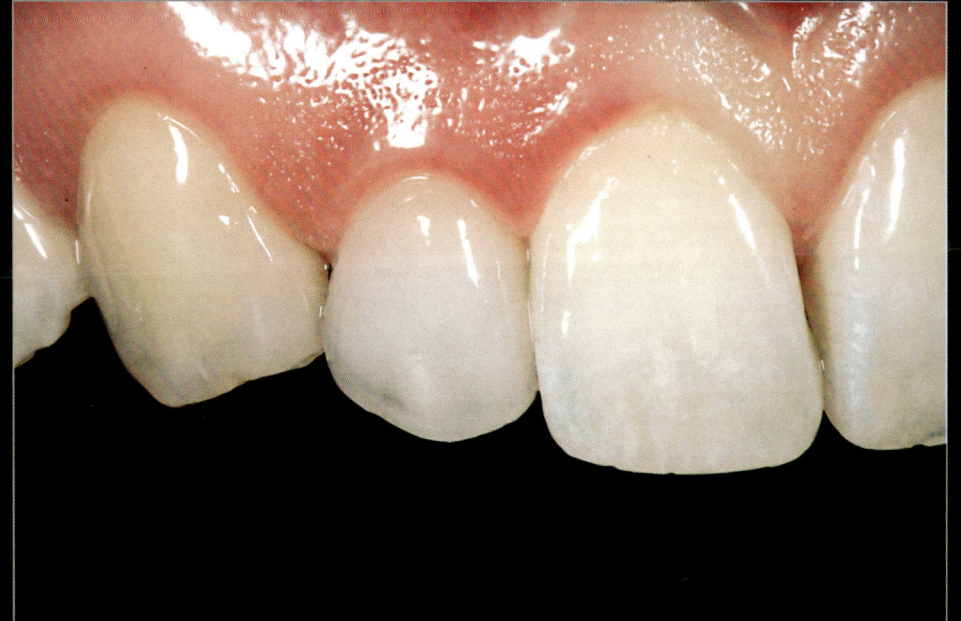

Case 3   Porcelain laminate veneers, maxillary right lateral incisor and canine
Dentist: **Hiroyuki Hatano, DDS, PhD,** UCLA School of Dentistry

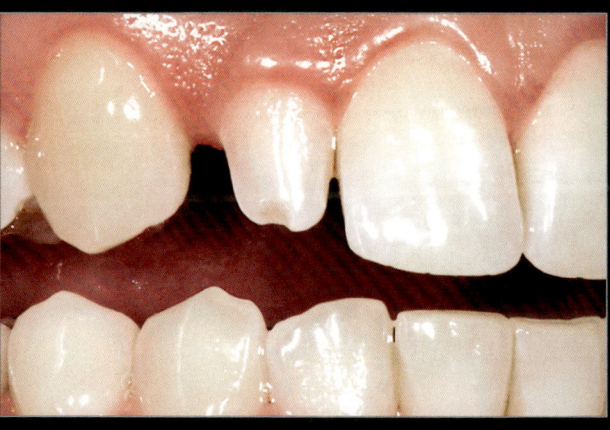

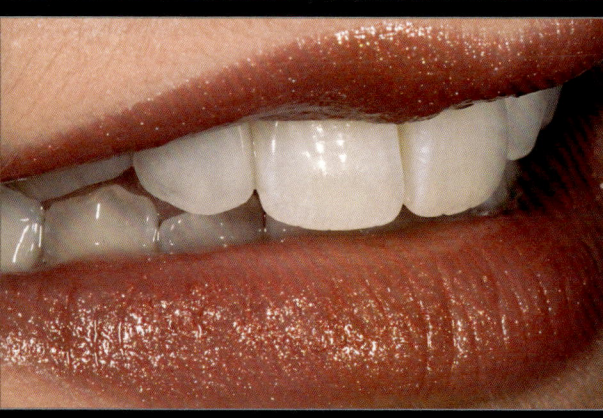

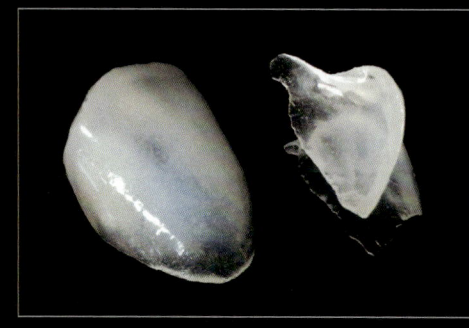

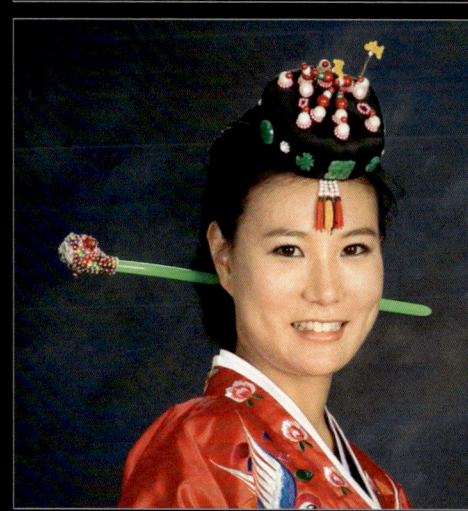

Refractory Model Technique (Vintage Halo)—Pegged lateral.
Create proper shape and close the diastema without teeth preparation. Use the contact lens effect tech-

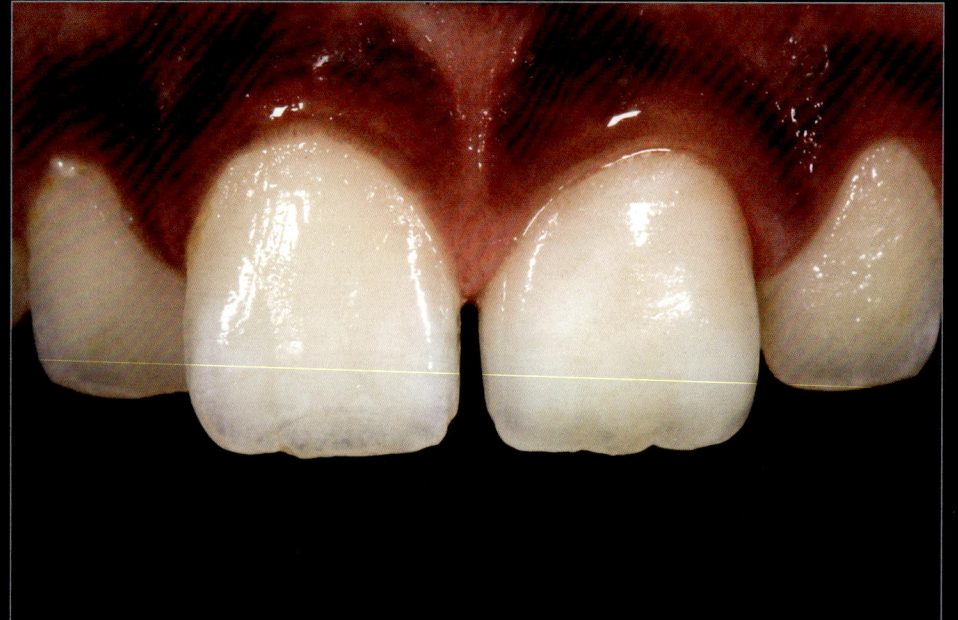

Porcelain jacket crown, maxillary left central incisor

Dentist: **Sunen G. Pandya, DDS**, Lawndale, California

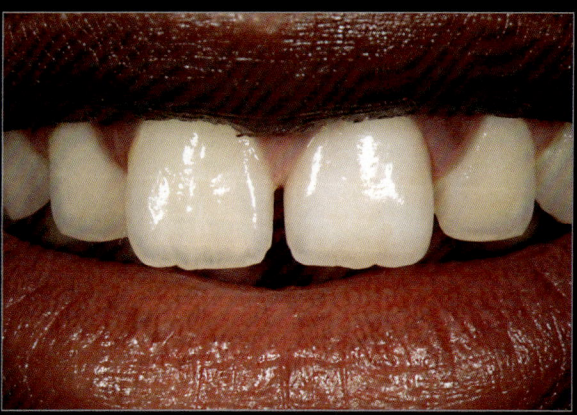
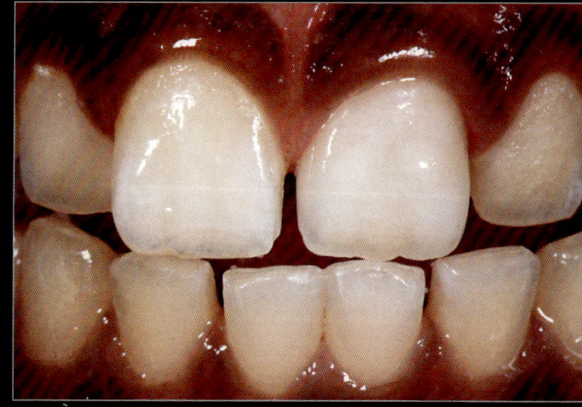
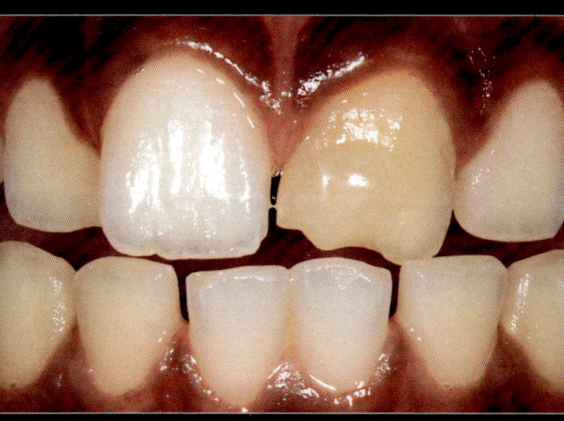
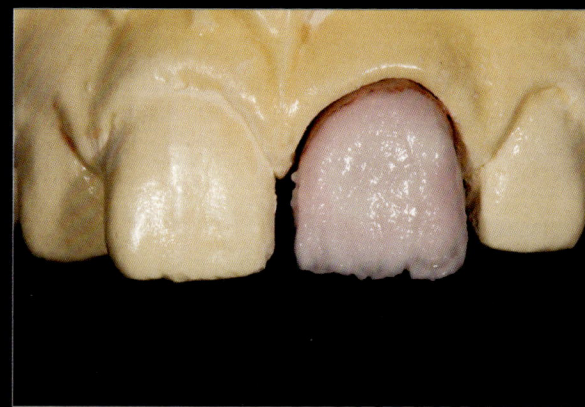

Refractory Model Technique (Vintage Halo)—Severely discolored tooth.
Create proper shape and shade within limited space by applying the multilayering technique.

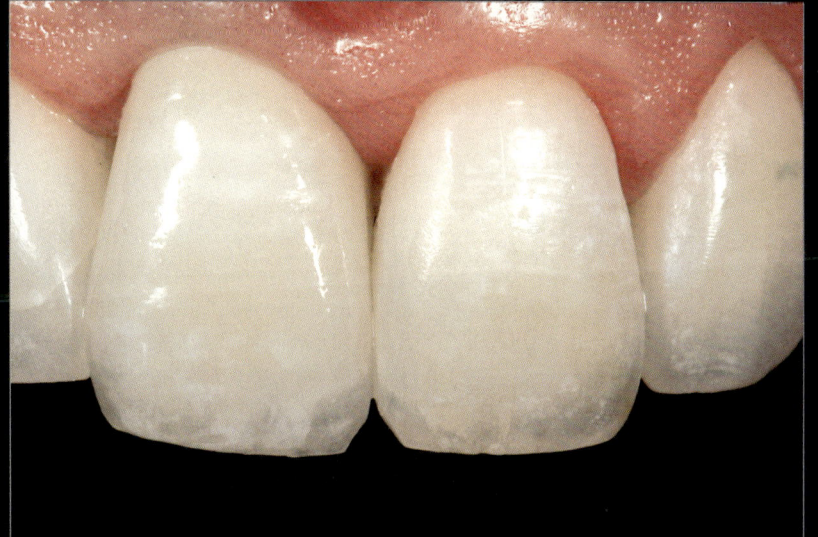

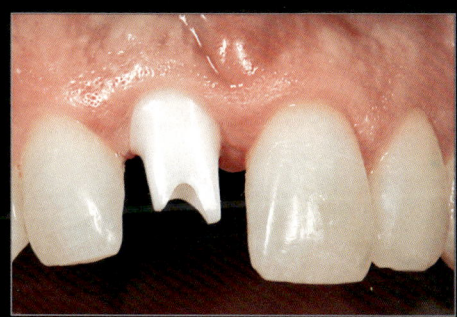

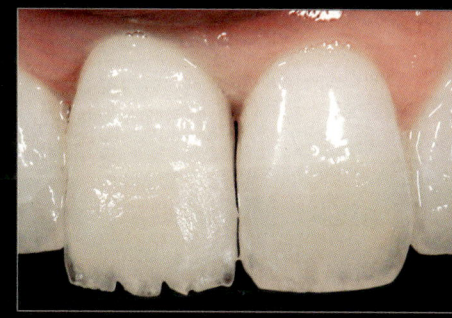

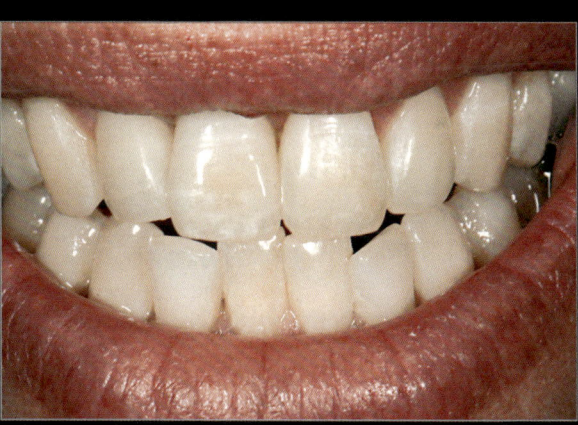

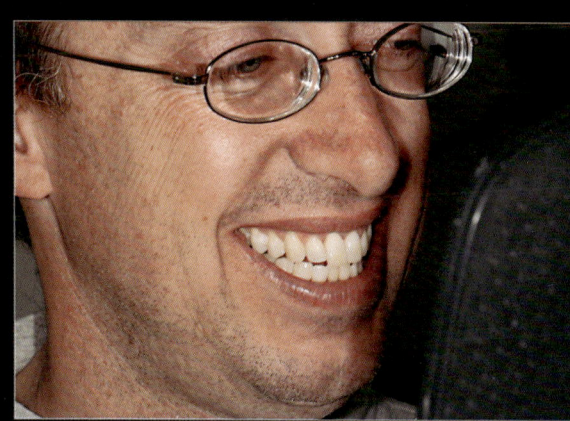

Zirconia All-Ceramic (Vintage ZR, Shofu)—Zirconia implant abutment.
Esthetic anterior implant with zirconia layering material.

smileDESIGN

A Guide for Clinican, Ceramist, and Patient

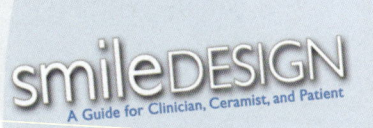

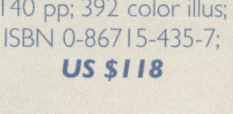

140 pp; 392 color illus;
ISBN 0-86715-435-7;
US $118

By Gerard J. Chiche and Hitoshi Aoshima

The patient's satisfaction with the outcome of esthetic treatment depends, in large measure, on the clinician's ability to understand the patient's desires and in turn to communicate effectively with the dental ceramist. Facilitation of this three-way communication is the purpose of this new clinical atlas that documents many years of collaborative work between a world-renowned clinician and educator and a master dental ceramist. This beautiful, full-color book presents patient objectives, treatment plans and outcomes, shade selection, and other elements of the smile design (ie, arrangement, brightness, character, and incisal effects) in a spare and straightforward style. For the patient, the book serves as a visual guide to various restorative treatment options and to methods for previewing the esthetic outcome of treatment; for the clinician, it is a communication guide to demonstrate the possible therapeutic approaches and to arrive at an understanding of the patient's preferences; and for the ceramist, it is a visual base for fully comprehending the desired smile composition, tooth shape, and nuances of shading. An indispensable adjunct to the practitioner's esthetic treatment armamentarium.

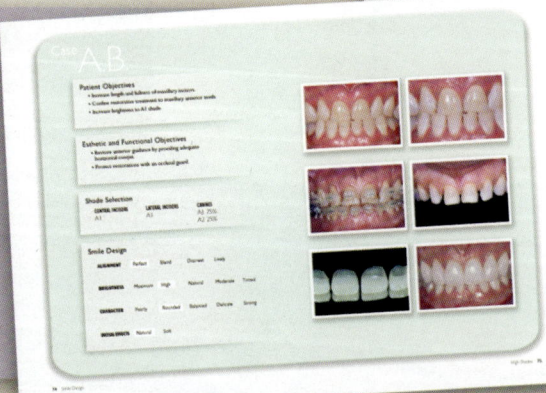

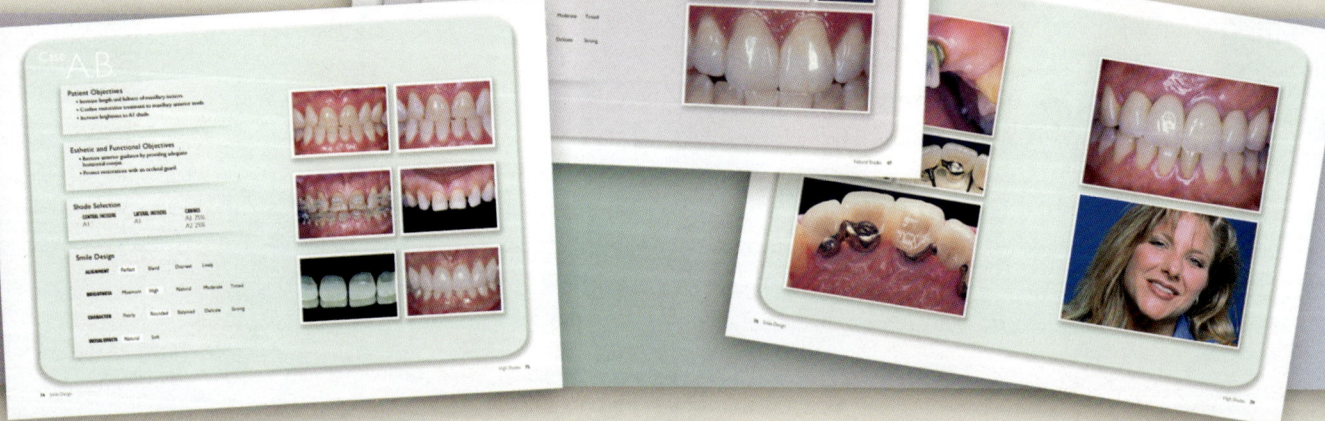

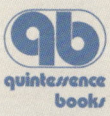

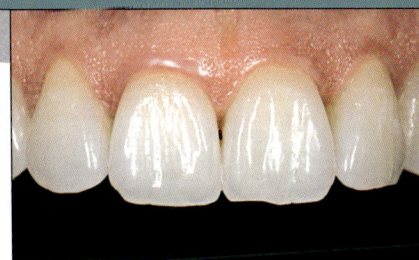

DOCUMENTATION VERSUS ARTISTIC PHOTOGRAPHY

James Fondriest, DDS[1]

The use of photography in dentistry is increasing rapidly due to the convenience and utility of digital images. Digital images are available instantly and are useful for diverse purposes. Even images captured with a film camera can be easily digitized with a scanner.

There are many ways to use digital images in dentistry. The ultimate use of an image determines how it is best composed. Every image conveys information, but not all images provide the same amount of diagnostic data. Clinicians need to learn to choreograph their photographs to increase value for each purpose.

The stylistic agenda of most images is generally either documentary or artistic. Documentation photography is dedicated to showing what is actually there. It provides an accurate rendering with no misrepresentations; there is a need to be true to your subject and tell the whole story. Artistic photography shows what is appealing or interesting; it focuses on what is attractive and has no responsibility to present the entire circumstance.

Artistic photography is used for educating, creative expression, and marketing.

DOCUMENTATION PHOTOGRAPHY

Visual clinical examinations with charted notes, however thorough, do not provide a lasting detailed description of the display of the dentition as framed by the face and lips. It is helpful to have documentation images that clinicians can review long after the patient has left the examination room. Having photos in addition to other work-up information allows for better evaluation of clinical circumstances and will generate more informed efforts in diagnosis, treatment planning, interdisciplinary communication, laboratory communication and development, self-improvement, and dental education.

Clinicians should learn to tell as much of the patient's circumstance with as few images as possible, just as we do radiographically with a full-mouth series. Before each diagnostic photograph is snapped, the photographer must determine what information is to be conveyed and how best to display it in the image. Figures 1 to 15 show how to best choreograph images to maximize documentation value.

[1]Private practice, Lake Forest, Illinois.

Correspondence to: Dr James Fondriest, 560 Oakwood Avenue, Suite 200, Lake Forest, IL, 60045, USA. E-mail: jimfondriest@cs.com

Portraits (1:10 to 1:15 magnification factor)

Documentation portraits illustrate facial shape, symmetry, facial proportions, and display of the dentition beneath the drape of the lips (Figs 1 to 6).

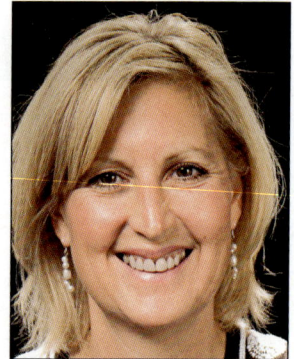

Fig 1 High artistic value, low documentation value. Nikon D200, Nikkor 28–70 mm zoom lens, ISO 100, F4.5, 1/250 sec, strobe lighting.

Figure 1 is a preoperative portrait that introduces the personality of this patient (artistic goal). However, this image has limited diagnostic/documentation value because it was exposed slightly from the side of the patient and the subject's head is subtly tilted. Oftentimes, people—especially females—pose with a slight head tilt, which softens their look. Even a minor angulation does not allow for proper assessment of facial symmetries, and how the dentition appears relative to the facial midline (axially or horizontally).

Facial symmetry is best evaluated by drawing a line on a photograph down the middle of the subject's face (see Fig 2). Two points of reference can be used to orient this line: the bridge of the nose and the center of cupid's bow at the bottom of the philtrum.[1] Ideally, the occlusal plane will be perpendicular to the midline. Have your patient hold her head straight to the camera with the facial midline perpendicular to the floor. Some practitioners compare the occlusal plane with the interpupillary line, but rarely are a person's eyes exactly level with each other.

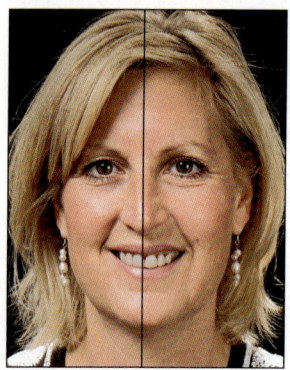

Fig 2 Medium artistic value, low documentation value. Nikon D200, Nikkor 28–70 mm zoom lens, ISO 100, f/4.5, 1/250 sec, strobe lighting.

The preoperative portrait in Fig 2 has documentation features that Fig 1 does not have. The image appears to have been exposed directly in front of the patient. If the individual's face were perfectly symmetrical, we would see exactly the same amount of cheek and temple on both sides of the face. It is important that hair be pulled behind the ears for an unobstructed view of the cheeks and temples. If the temples are exposed, any deviation to the right or left becomes visible. Figure 2 shows some asymmetry of the head, face, lips, and gingival display; horizontal midline discrepancies; and axial inclinations of the teeth. However, this photograph has been taken from too high an angle. When the image is taken from slightly above (high forehead/hairline), the occlusal plane can appear U-shaped and even minor occlusal plane cants become difficult to see. If the occlusal plane is flat, we want it to appear as such when photographed. In this photograph, the incisal edges are in contact with the lower lip, making it difficult to visualize the occlusal plane. Ideally, the mouth should be opened wider to expose the occlusal plane.

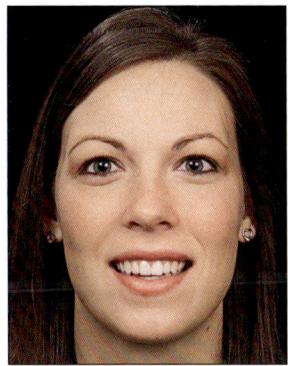

Fig 3 Low artistic value, medium documentation value. Nikon D200, Nikkor 28–70 mm zoom lens, ISO 100, f/3.2, 1/160 sec, strobe lighting.

It would appear that Fig 3 is a good documentation image that represents the reality of this patient's full preoperative smile. Actually it does not tell the entire story. Many people learn to smile with the correct tooth display or to show their good side while being photographed. This patient smiles with some restraint to show a relatively small amount of gingiva.

The maximum forced smile in Fig 4 gives a true representation of gingival display of this patient's smile. Often, the photographer has to catch the patient off guard to capture the true height of the smile (highest limit of lip mobility). Here the teeth are resting on the lower lip, thereby obscuring the incisal edges and occlusal plane.

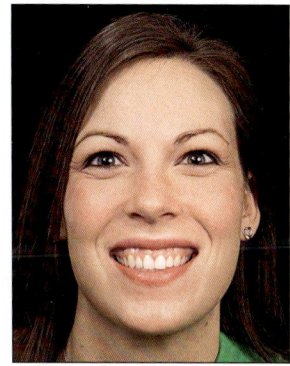

Fig 4 Low artistic value, medium-high documentation value. Nikon D200, Nikkor 28–70 mm zoom lens, ISO 100, f/4.0, 1/160 sec, strobe lighting.

Figure 5 is an intraoperative photograph (midtreatment documentation of provisionals) taken at the proper vertical and horizontal vectors. The same amount of cheek and temple on each side of the face is visible, and the height of the camera is at the same level as the occlusal plane. The mouth is open wide enough to display the occlusal plane. Ask the patient to open his mouth halfway and then smile while leaving his mouth open to prevent the incisal edges of the maxillary teeth from resting on the lower lip. It is often helpful for the photographer to model the pose for the patient.

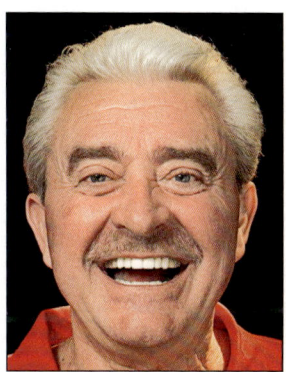

Fig 5 Low-medium artistic value, high documentation value. Nikon D70s, Nikkor 28–70 mm zoom lens, ISO 200, f/8.0, 1/80 sec, strobe lighting.

The profile portrait has diagnostic value. Common soft tissue profile documentation goals are to evaluate mandibular angle, facial plane, midface convexity, Ricketts' E-plane or Steiner's S-plane, nasolabial angle, and mentolabial angle.[2] Variations from norms can suggest orthodontic, orthognathic, plastic surgery, and restorative dental treatment. Orthodontists commonly orient the head so that the Frankfort plane is parallel to the horizon or a natural head posture.[2–7] Because the Frankfort plane is determined radiographically and the comfortable rest position is too variable and arbitrary, clinicians should consider using visible soft tissue landmarks to create consistency with their images. Try using the mid-ala of the nose to the mid-tragus of the ear (ala-tragus line), shown in Fig 6, or the Camper's plane.

To take a profile portrait, have the patient face the camera at a 90-degree angle. The patient should be relaxed and not smile. Make sure hair is pulled back to expose the ear. The camera height should be between the nose and mouth and centered in the face. The ala-tragus line should be parallel to the floor.

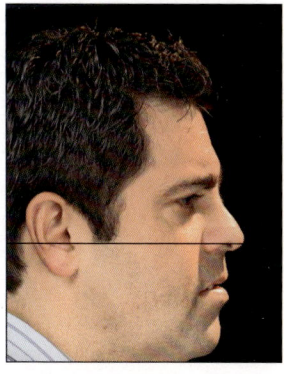

Fig 6 Low artistic value, high documentation value. Nikon D200, Nikkor 28–70 mm zoom lens, ISO 100, f/4.5, 1/160 sec, strobe lighting.

Extraoral Close-ups (1:2 to 1:3 magnification factor)

Gingival display and incisal edge position are parameters often taken into account while planning restorative dentistry. Although portraits render this information, the extraoral close-ups (commissure-to-commissure shots), as in Figs 7 to 10, show this better.

The postoperative lips-at-rest pose in Fig 7 and forced-smile pose in Fig 8 show lip mobility and the dentogingival display beneath the lips. (It helps to ask the patient to mouth breathe when this photograph is being taken.) This pair of images has significant influence on placement of incisal edge position in the final restorations.[8-10]

Do not orient the camera to the interpupillary line, intercommisure line, or the occlusal plane, as these are often canted. The horizontal plane of the camera should remain perpendicular to the facial midline. If the images are shared with the interdisciplinary team, draw an orientation line over the images, as in Fig 8, to confirm orientation.

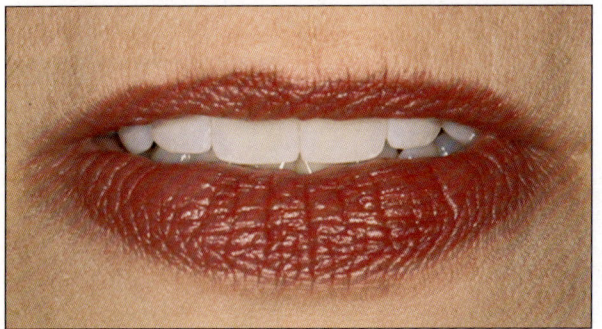

Fig 7 Low artistic value, high documentation value. Nikon N2000 35mm, Nikkor 105 mm macro lens, f/22, 1/100 sec, Nikon SB-29 flash.

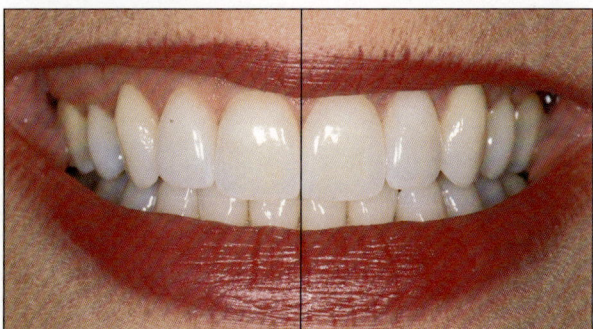

Fig 8 Medium artistic value, high documentation value. Nikon N2000 35mm, Nikkor 105 mm macro lens, f/22, 1/100 sec, Nikon SB-29 flash.

Extraoral lateral images such as those shown in Figs 9 and 10 are also taken as a pair. These preoperative forced-smile shots centered on the lateral incisor allow documentation of tooth and gingival display from the side view. These photos are taken at the height of the occlusal plane or the midbuccal of the lateral incisors, with the camera oriented so it is parallel to the horizon and perpendicular to the facial midline.

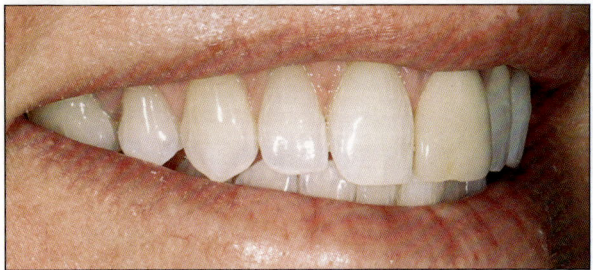

Fig 9 Medium-high artistic value, high documentation value. Canon 5D, Canon 100 mm macro lens, ISO 100, f/32, 1/125 sec, Canon MT-24EX Twin Lite Macro Flash.

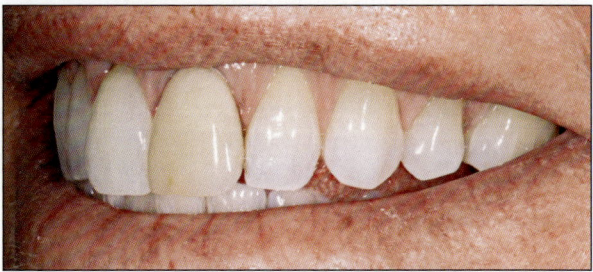

Fig 10 Medium-high artistic value, high documentation value. Canon 5D, Canon 100 mm macro lens, ISO 100, f/32, 1/125 sec, Canon MT-24EX Twin Lite Macro Flash.

Intraoral Close-ups (1:2 to 1:3 magnification factor)

Intraoral close-ups such as in Figs 11 and 12 document the full dentition as it appears, unrestricted by the lips. Images such as those shown in Figs 13 to 15 are especially good for communicating with laboratory partners. Shade information is improved by such choreography of your images.[11–12]

Figures 11 and 12 are intraoral close-ups also usually taken as a pair. Figure 11 shows the overbite relationship of the incisors. In Fig 12, the teeth are fully retracted and discluded and the incisors are 2 to 3 mm apart so a clinician can assess the occlusal plane. Take these images with the camera perpendicular to the facial midline. This allows discovery of occlusal plane cants. If restorative dentistry is to be completed, Fig 12 allows selection of landmarks when planning the eventual occlusal plane. Allowing for the subtle curves of Wilson and Spee, the occlusal plane normally is fairly flat. Taking the image from above would give the incorrect impression that the occlusal plane is U-shaped.

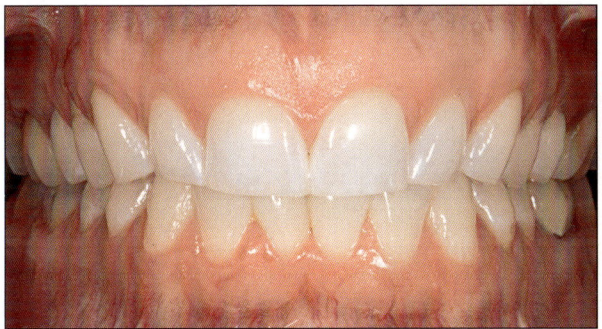

Fig 11 Low artistic value, high documentation value. Canon 5D, Canon 100 mm macro lens, ISO 100, f/28, 1/125 sec, Canon MT-24EX Twin Lite Macro Flash.

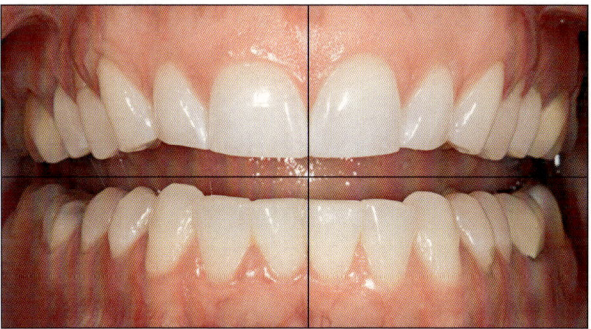

Fig 12 Low artistic value, high documentation value. Canon 5D, Canon 100 mm macro lens, ISO 100, f/28, 1/125 sec, Canon MT-24EX Twin Lite Macro Flash.

When documenting translucency as in Fig 13, use a black background, minimize reflections (which render the surface opaque) by vectoring your shot from above at 60 degrees, and underexpose the image.

When documenting silhouette and surface morphology (Fig 14), use a black background, maximize reflections by vectoring your shot perpendicular to the surface you are documenting, and clean and dry the teeth.

When documenting the chroma and hue as in Fig 15, use a neutral gray background, minimize reflections by vectoring your shots from above at 60 degrees to limit reflections, keep the shade tabs parallel to the teeth and equidistant from the camera, and underexpose your image.

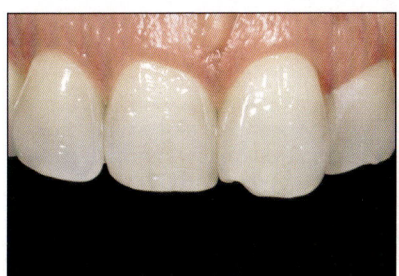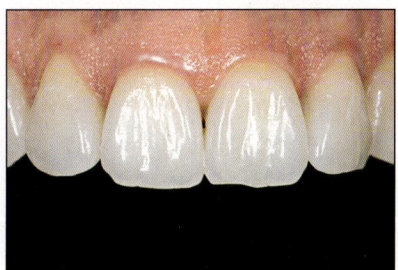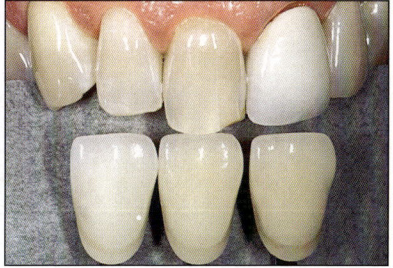

Figs 13 to 15 Medium artistic value, high documentation value. Nikon N2000 35 mm, Nikkor 105 mm macro lens, f/28, 1/100 sec, Nikon SB-29 flash.

Artistic images that are universally pleasing are extraoral, not re-tracted. Portrait or commissure-to-commissure photos are best.

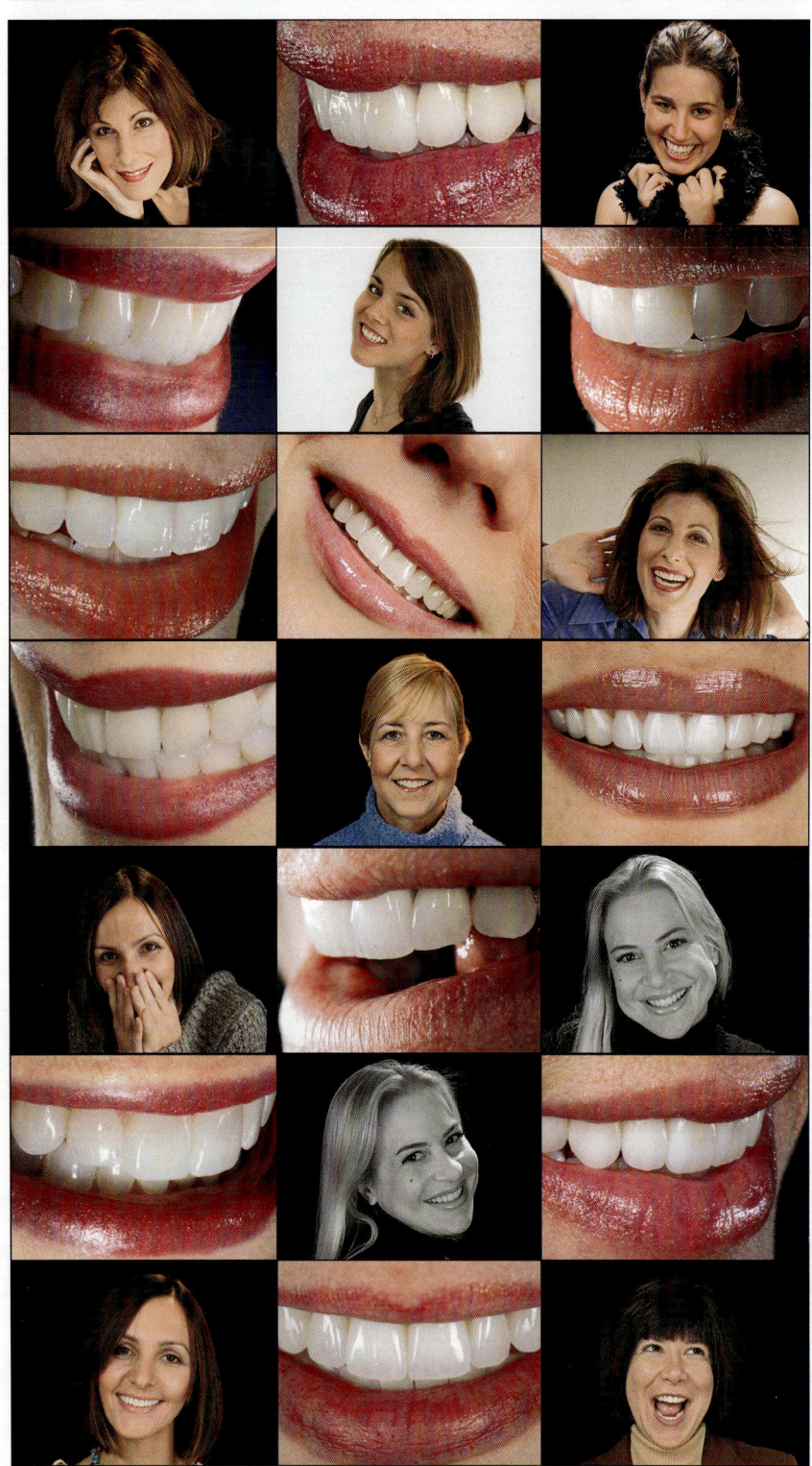

Portraits: High artistic value, low-medium documentation value. Nikon D200, Nikkor 28–70 mm zoom lens, f/4.5, 1/250 sec, strobe lighting.

Postoperative close-ups: High artistic value, low-medium documentation value. Canon 5D, Canon 100 mm macro lens, ISO 100, f/12-28, 1/100 sec, Canon MT-24EX Twin Lite Macro Flash.

ARTISTIC PHOTOGRAPHY

Artistic portraits of a patient introduce and portray personality, emotional status, sophistication, and mannerisms. Images of happy patients, smiles, and beautiful dentistry can display many artistic qualities and be influential to the viewer. The best artistic images elicit an emotional and/or intellectual response. Rather than having to be responsible, logical, and accurate, artistic photography allows the photographer the latitude to capture the viewer's imagination. Unlike the documentation shots, there are few rules as to camera angle or exposure level.

In dental education, a case report with photographic documentation of each step helps the audience see how procedures are performed and garner a better depth of knowledge of what can be done in particular clinical circumstances. When artistic images are included, the emotional and intellectual response they create can hold the audience's attention better and be more motivational.

Ansel Adams used his camera to share the breathtaking and tremendous beauty of our nation's national parks. Quality artistic photography can also show the beauty that nature has created in the mouth and what talented ceramists can produce in porcelain.

CONCLUSION

By properly staging your photograph and keeping your audience in mind, the resulting image will have captured the information necessary for its intended use. An image to be used for treatment planning or communication purposes can be improved when taken with specific angulations, focus points, and exposures while providing good illumination, retraction, isolation, and/or aspiration. If a photographer intends to use an image to show a successful treatment, the various steps of a procedure, or what a specific type of restoration looks like, any image that is pleasing to the eyes will do.

Always consider who your audience is. Whereas dentists will appreciate retracted intraoral images of detailed dental procedures, most nondentists prefer extraoral images and portraits. Because different audiences won't always find the same images esthetically pleasing, it is important to choose views common to the intended viewer.

REFERENCES

1. Yaremchuk M. Atlas of Facial Implants. Philadelphia: Saunders, 2007.

2. Jacobson A, Jacobson RL (eds). Radiographic Cephalometry: From Basics to 3-D Imaging ed.2. Chicago: Quintessence, 2006.

3. Ricketts RM. Divine proportion in facial esthetics. Clin Plast Surg 1982; 9:401–422.

4. Solow B, Siersbaek-Nielsen S. Cervical and craniocervical posture as predictors of craniofacial growth. Am J Orthod Dentofacial Orthop 1992;101:449–458.

5. Warren DW, Spalding PM. Dentofacial morphology and breathing: A century of controversy. In: Melsen B (ed). Current Controversies in Orthodontics. Chicago: Quintessence, 1991:45–76.

6. Showfety KJ, Vig PS, Matteson SR. A simple method for taking natural-head-position cephalograms. Am J Orthod 1983;83:495–500.

7. Profit WR, Fields HW Jr. Contemporary Orthodontics, ed 2. St Louis: Mosby, 1992:164–165.

8. Spear FM, Kokich VG, Mathews DP. Interdisciplinary management of anterior dental esthetics. J Am Dent Assoc 2006;137:160–169.

9. Hulsey CM. An esthetic evaluation of lip-teeth relationships present in the smile. Am J Orthod 1970;57: 132–144.

10. Chiche GJ, Kokich VG, Carrdill R. Diagnosis and Treatment Planning of Esthetic Problems. In: Chiche GJ, Pinault A (eds). Esthetics of Anterior Fixed Prosthodontics. Chicago: Quintessence, 1994:33–51.

11. Fondriest JF. Shade matching: The science and strategies. Int J Periodontics Restorative Dent 2003;23:467–479.

12. Fondriest JF. Shade matching a single maxillary central incisor. Quintessence Dent Technol 2005;28:215–225.

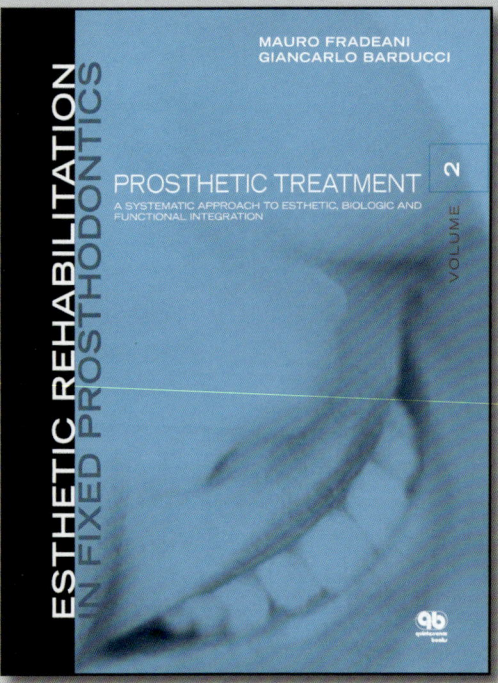

VOLUME 2

PROSTHETIC TREATMENT
A Systematic Approach to Esthetic, Biologic, and Functional Integration

Mauro Fradeani and Giancarlo Barducci

This much-anticipated book presents the procedural phases required to achieve optimal results in the esthetic rehabilitation of patients in need of fixed prostheses. Communication between the clinician and the technician, which is essential to the esthetic, biologic, and functional integration of the prosthetic rehabilitation, is highlighted through a step-by-step presentation of all clinical and laboratory procedures. Chapters demonstrate methods to obtain accurate facebow recordings, impression materials and techniques, fabrication of provisional restorations, and incorporation of interdisciplinary therapies for ideal comfort and esthetics. All of this information is transferred to the final restorations, which should provide patients with long-term prosthetic solutions exhibiting appropriate fit, form, and function. Hundreds of full-color clinical photographs and detailed illustrations accompany each treatment phase and situation described. This beautiful book picks up where Volume 1 ended and delivers its message with equal clarity and precision.

600 pp; 2,500 illus (mostly color); ISBN 978-1-85097-171-9; US $320

Contents

- Communication with the Laboratory for the Diagnostic Waxing
- The Fabrication and the Esthetic-Functional Integration of the Provisional
- Biologic Integration of the Provisional and Final Preparations
- From the Provisional to the Definitive Prosthesis: Impressions and Data Transfer
- Constructing and Finalizing the Prosthetic Rehabilitation

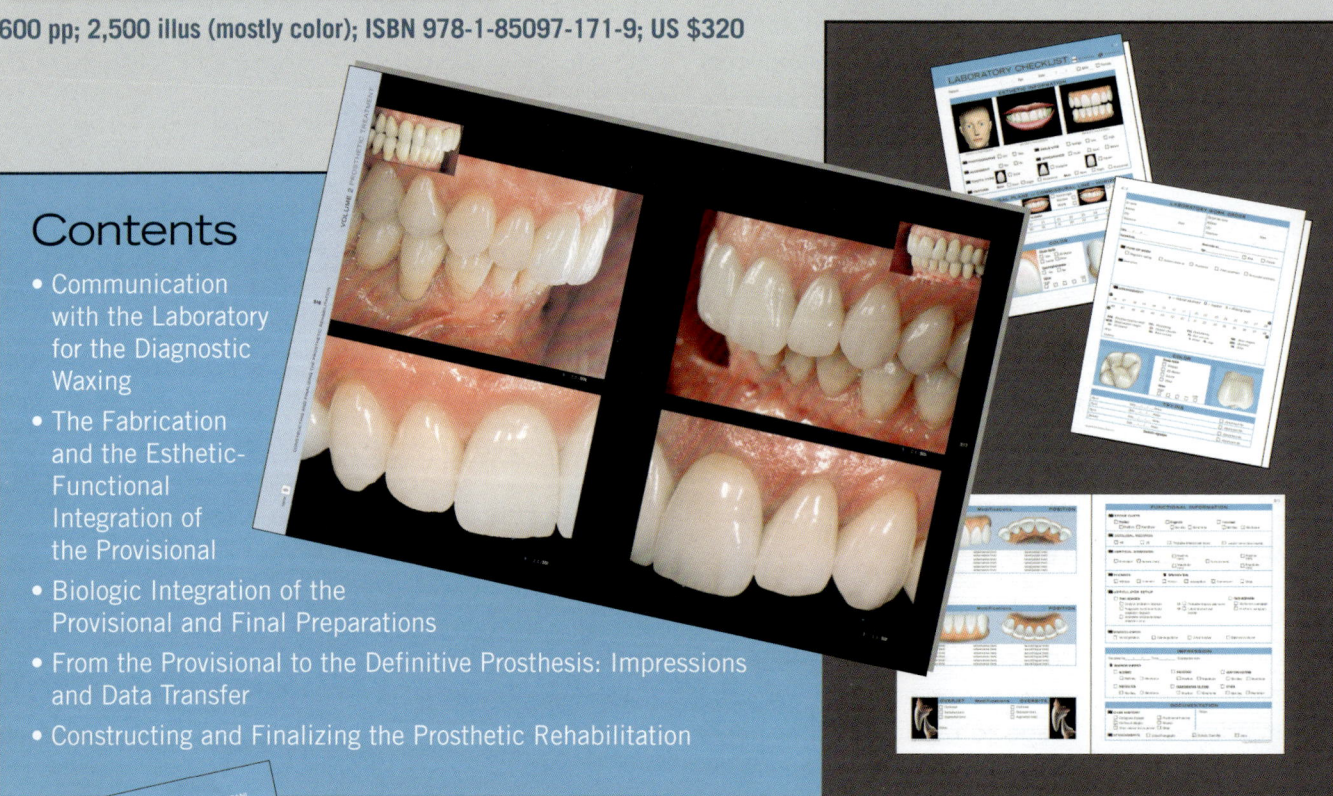

VOLUME 1—**Esthetic Analysis:**
A Systematic Approach to Prosthetic Treatment
Mauro Fradeani

352 pp; 1,136 illus (mostly color); ISBN 978-1-85097-108-5; US $258

TO ORDER

CALL: (800) 621-0387 (toll free within US & Canada) • (630) 736-3600 (elsewhere)
FAX: (630) 736-3633 **E-MAIL:** service@quintbook.com **WEB:** www.quintpub.com
QUINTESSENCE PUBLISHING CO, INC, 4350 Chandler Drive, Hanover Park, IL 60133

THE FUNCTIONAL-ESTHETIC COMPLEX: CONSIDERATIONS BASED ON CLINICAL CASES

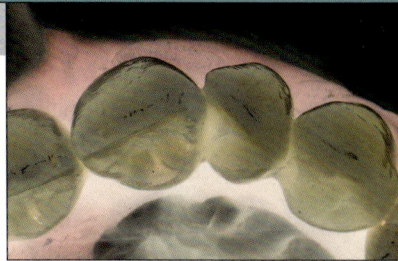

Stefan Schunke, MDT[1]

I s it at all possible to separate function from esthetics? These days, the trend seems to be to present oral rehabilitations that are highly complex and supported by various implants or that exhibit esthetics that would turn even Mother Nature green with envy. In this article, I would like to remind the reader of what we originally set out to do—to provide replacements for missing or damaged teeth. Ultimately, we fabricate our dental restorations—tooth replacements—to allow dentists to properly treat their patients. This article will present a number of topics related to the functional-esthetic complex. The question of tooth shade will not be discussed here, as it is too prone to subjective perception.

---

[1]Master Dental Technician, Fürth, Germany.

Correspondence to: Mr Stefan Schunke, Ate Reustrasse 170, 90765 Fürth, Germany. Fax: + 49 (0)911 7 0 37 52. E-mail: st.schunke@arcor.de

MATERIALS

The question of what materials to use can be a highly polarizing one. We may be shown ceramic crowns abrading natural tooth substance, citing the excessive hardness of ceramics, without ever mentioning the functional aspects of the case. Other authors show images of severely abraded teeth restored with gold inlays without exhibiting any adapted gold occlusal surfaces (Figs 1 and 2).

Whether a functional restoration should be executed in gold or whether using ceramics is preferable continues to be a subject of heated debate. Not infrequently, one hears that gold is the better of the two materials because it adapts more easily and exhibits superior abrasion behavior when compared to ceramics. But is that really the case? In my opinion, such a comparison is misleading. As far as I know, there has been no study on abrasion and gold occlusal surfaces. The abrasion behavior of ceramics, by contrast, has been sufficiently examined in the literature. (And of course we cannot compare the ceramics we have at our disposal

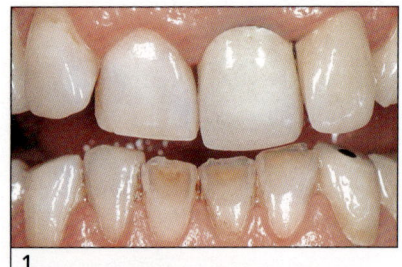

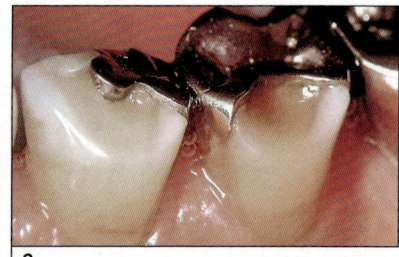

Figs 1 and 2 When comparing ceramics and gold, it is not just the material and its technology that counts. Functional aspects, especially of the more modern materials, also play a role.

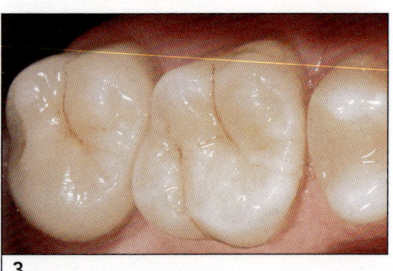

Fig 3 Today's materials permit esthetic and functional ceramic onlays using the adhesive technique. Dentist: A. Enssle.

Figs 4 to 6 Any material can be used to create the correct morphology.

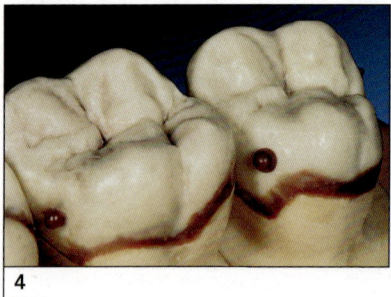

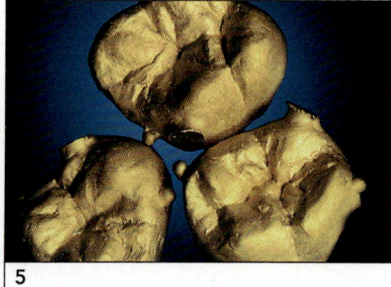

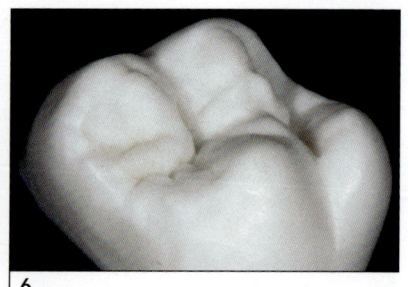

today with the materials we worked with in the 1960s and 1970s.)

So if gold, as has been claimed, is abrasive, it should exhibit a rough surface, but, contrarily, functional anomalies manifest themselves intra-orally as areas of high luster. Metals only exhibit high luster if they have been highly compressed, as in polishing, so high-luster areas simply consist of what would have to be considered cold-formed metal. That in turn means that a lot of tension will have been built in the metal, tension that will be relieved in the form of natural enamel cracks or chipping, depending on the shape of the crown. This is one of the reasons why onlays were promoted in the first place.

Preparation shapes, on the other hand, became ever more daring as dentists increasingly strove to respond to patients' demands for better esthetics.

The advent of adhesive techniques helped alleviate the ensuing problems (Fig 3).

Consider a natural mandibular first molar with a parafunction at the distolingual cusp. Now let us assume that this parafunction is very pronounced, causing the cusp to fracture. Let us further assume that we restore the tooth with a ceramic crown without changing the situation itself. What we get then is, of course, exactly the same situation as before, only in ceramics, and the ceramic cusp is ultimately bound to fracture, as well. Assuming we had restored the same situation with a gold crown, while there will be no fracture of that gold crown, the parafunction will persist but manifest itself elsewhere—in the periodontal tissues, the bone, the orofacial muscles, the temporomandibular joint, or even more remote parts of the body. Not a good prospect, either.

Figs 7 and 8 Ceramic inlays and a metal-ceramic crown. Dentist: A. Kreisl.

Figs 9 and 10 Ceramic inlay, ceramic onlay, and two all-ceramic molars. Dentist: A. Enssle.

Figs 11 to 13 Ceramic onlay and two all-ceramic molars. Dentist: A. Kreisl.

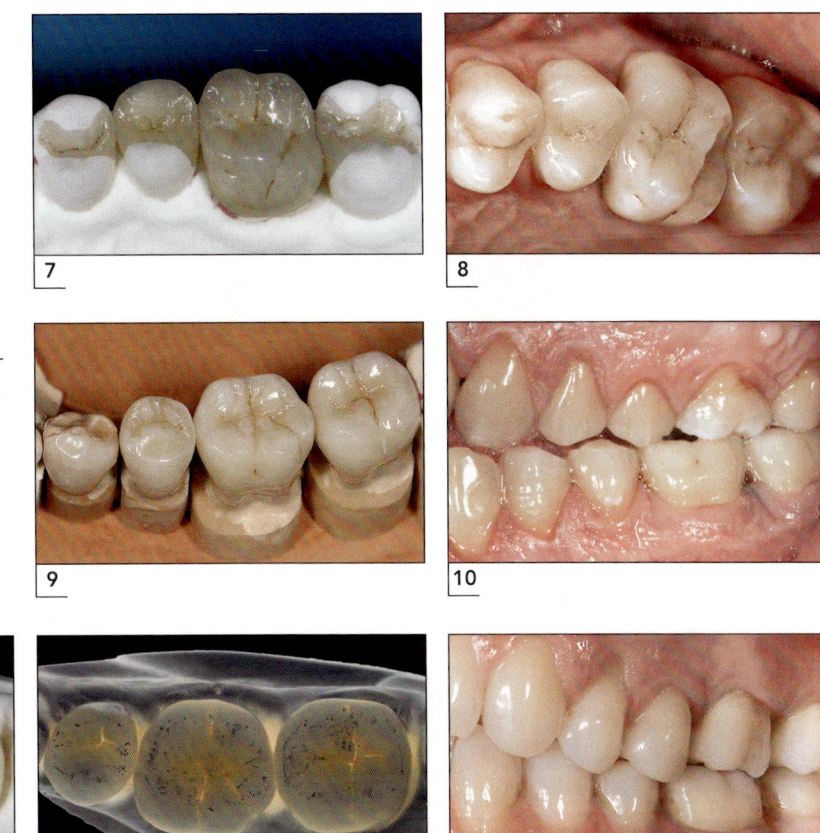

It is therefore imperative for us to have intimate knowledge of the esthetic, as well as functional, aspects of the anatomic and morphologic structures and to be able to imitate them. This is not only true of metal occlusal surfaces, but also, and especially, of ceramic occlusal surfaces (Figs 4 to 6).

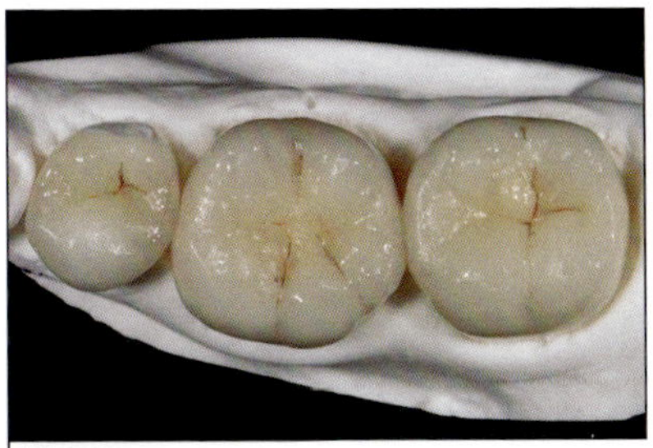

The question of what kind of ceramics is also answered in the literature, which likes to favor glass ceramics in this situation.[1-3] Glass ceramics exhibits the most favorable abrasion behavior. But due to the (in my opinion) esthetic disadvantages of pure glass ceramics, I currently prefer Inspiration (Heimerle + Meule, Pforzheim, Germany), a state-of-the-art two-phase leucite glass-ceramic material, for metal-ceramic restorations. The leucite is important for obtaining a beautiful esthetic result

that is convincing not only on the master cast but also intraorally. Personal observation over a period of approximately 4 years has shown me that this ceramic material is in fact abraded by natural antagonists (Figs 7 to 13).

There is no longer any reason to say no to ceramic occlusal surfaces, whether from the point of view of material technology and science or of adhesion technology. Technicians who are less comfortable with ceramics may utilize the more recent pressable ceramics to achieve their goals, although with some esthetic compromises. Given the enormous variety of materials on the market today, the number of challenges is rising exponentially. Alumina and zirconia ceramics are trendy materials that none of us can afford to ignore entirely.

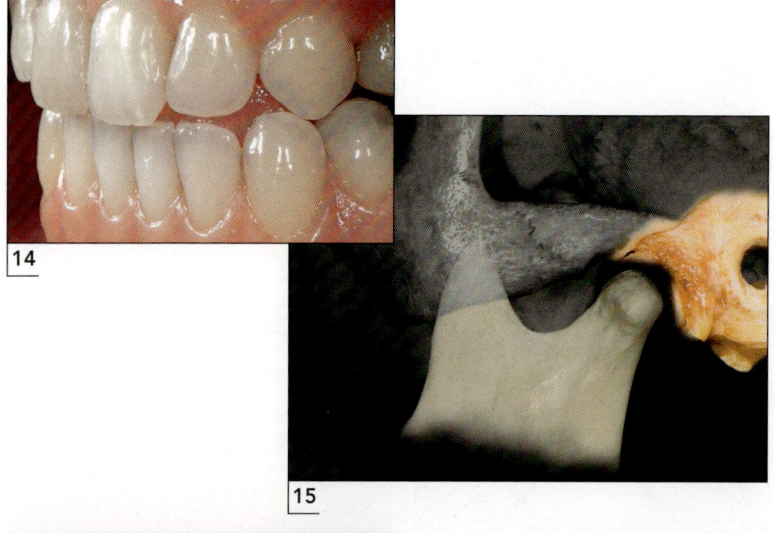

Figs 14 and 15 In Angle Class I situations, the temporomandibular joint is moved away from the sensitive dorsal bilaminar zone during lateral excursions due to the anatomic position of the teeth and jaws. The teeth automatically afford protection for the joint.

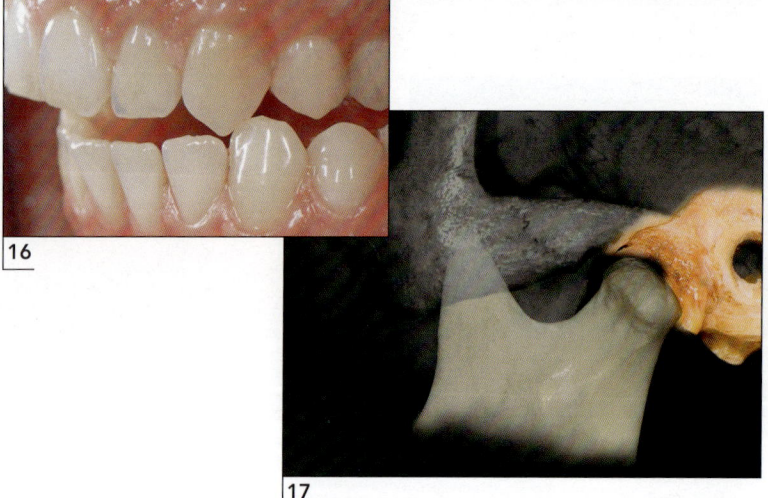

Figs 16 and 17 In Angle Class II, the temporomandibular joint is moved into the bilaminar zone during lateral excursions.

ANTERIOR/CANINE GUIDANCE

Many dental technicians, when discussing esthetics, will talk about beautiful anterior teeth, more beautiful than almost anything we ever see in nature. But while a beautiful appearance is one thing, function is another. Length-to-width ratios, gingival scalloping, and emergence profiles are the focus of attention, while the functional aspects of the anterior teeth are sometimes neglected. Let us therefore take a look at the definition and the effects of anterior/canine guidance.

In an Angle Class I situation, lateral movements are characterized as follows: The distal slope of the mandibular canine moves along the mesial slope of the maxillary canine. During the lateral movement, the temporomandibular joint is moved laterally and forward, away from the sensitive dorsal bilaminar zone. The teeth thus protect the temporomandibular joint during lateral excursions (Figs 14 and 15).

In an Angle Class II situation, by comparison, lateral movements are characterized as follows: It is the *mesial* slope of the mandibular canine that moves past the *distal* slope of the maxillary canine, based on the canine guidance that starts further distally. Consequently, the lateral movement guides the temporomandibular joint further into the dorsal cranial region, ie, into the sensitive bilaminar zone[4] (Figs 16 and 17).

Fig 18 In a distally oriented bite, the canine tip is positioned for functional reasons.

Figs 19 to 23 If the canine guidance is distalized, this will invariably result in a mandibular ledge between the canine and the first premolar.

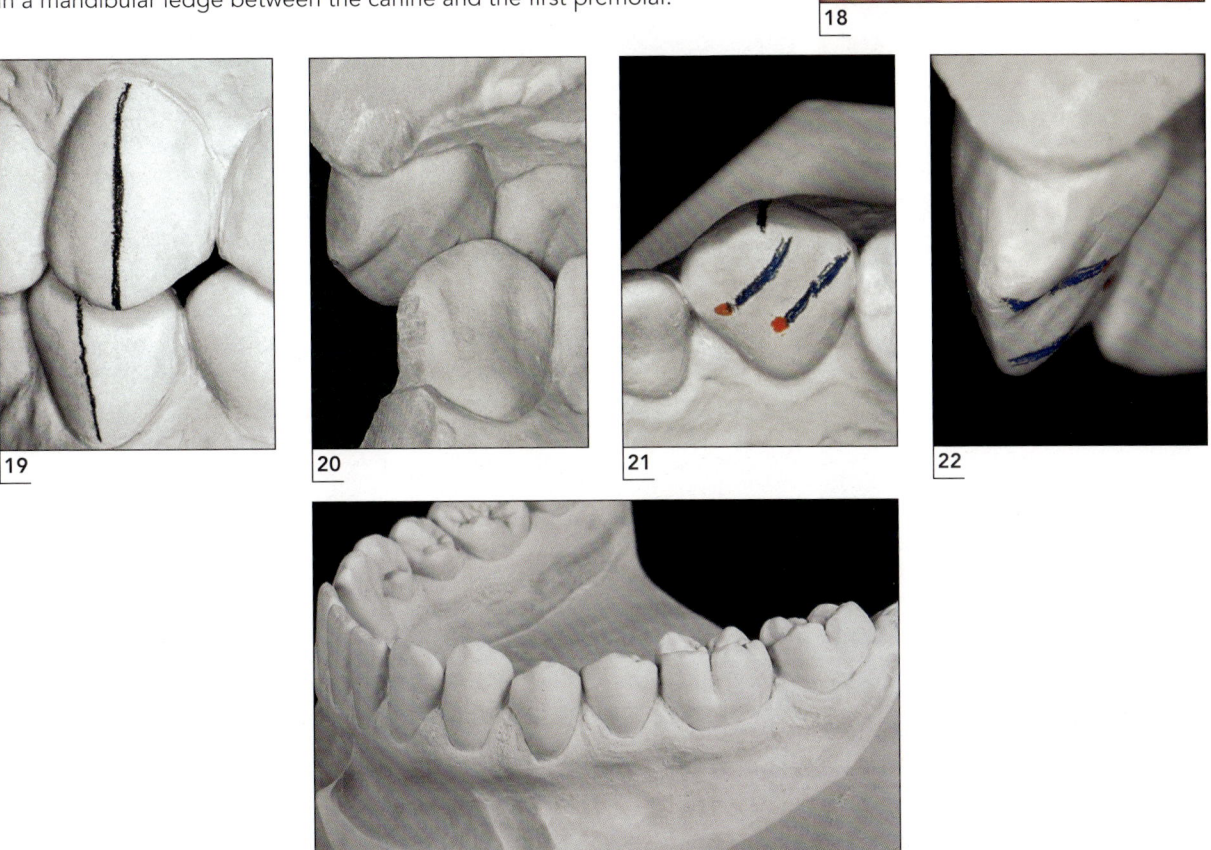

Various problems and options ensue. Esthetically speaking, the Class II situation mandates a different position of the canine tip, which, compared to Angle Class I, should be located further mesially. This mesialization of the maxillary canine tip in turn lengthens the distal slope. Therefore, if anterior teeth are designed following esthetic and functional principles, the overall result will be harmonious only if these details are taken into account (Fig 18).

Normally, then, canine guidance serves to protect the joint. If the canines cannot provide this protection, the posterior teeth will have to perform this task, as will be shown below.

Other functional considerations also ensue. In an Angle Class I situation, the mandibular canine is positioned to the mesial of the maxillary canine. Due to the conical shape of the maxillary canine, the canine guidance will be relatively steep and long. In an Angle Class II situation, the starting point (actually the ending point, since the movement is intrusive in nature) is located further distally and cranially. The starting point is located behind a cone, making the canine guidance shallower and shorter than in Angle Class I. This is why these dentitions typically feature a ledge between the mandibular canine and the mandibular first premolar (Figs 19 to 23).

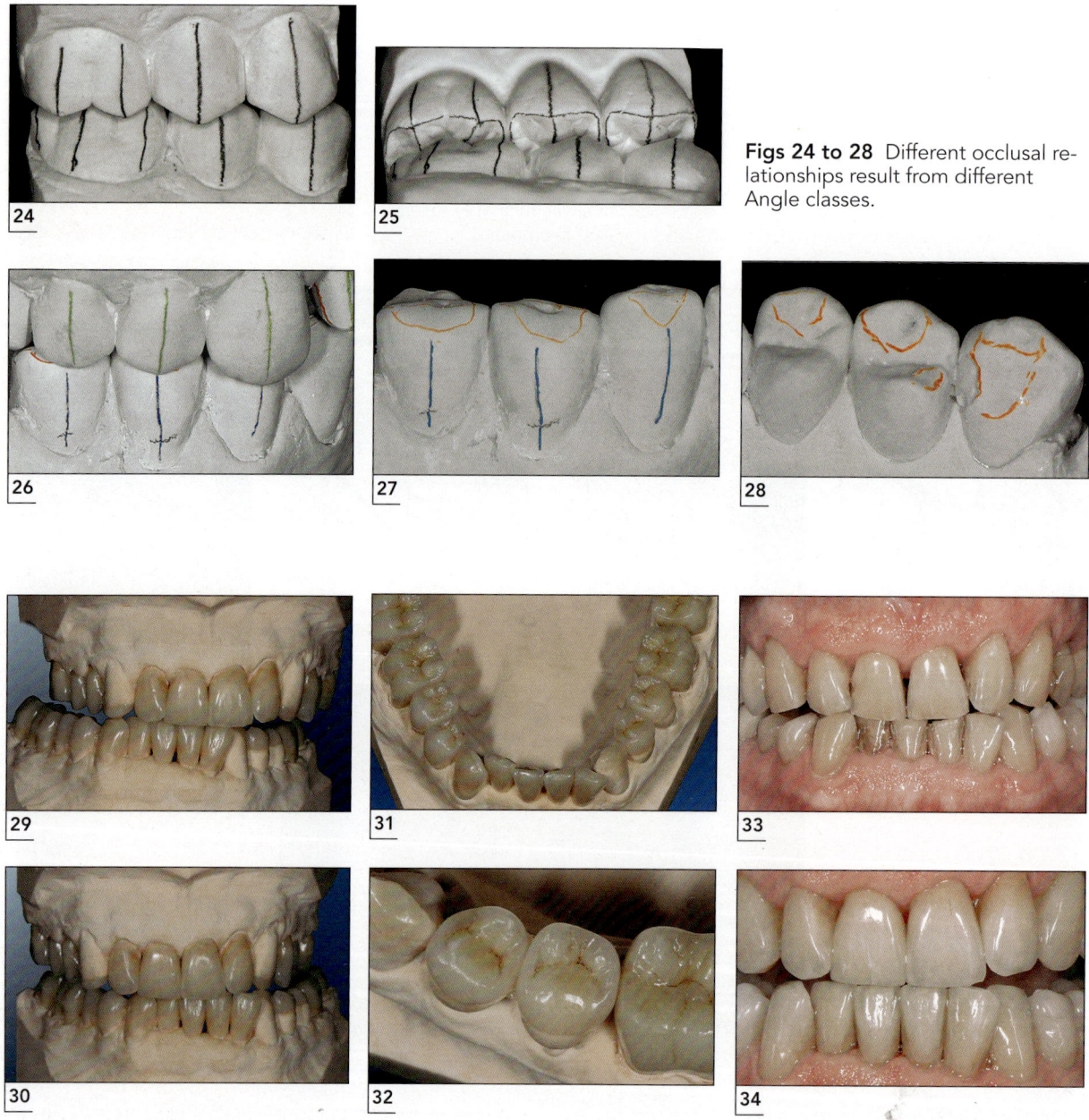

Figs 24 to 28 Different occlusal relationships result from different Angle classes.

Figs 29 to 34 Differences in canine guidance steepness and intercuspation based on the anatomy of the teeth and their positions in the jaw. Dentist: A. Kreisl.

The problem discussed also affects the posterior teeth. A healthy occlusion will typically show a cusp-fossa relationship or a cusp-ridge relationship, as is normally found in Angle Class I or in a distalized neutral occlusion. But in a distalized occlusion, depending on how pronounced the distalization, we may find a tooth-tooth relationship, permitting only "abrasion teeth" instead of a cusp-fossa relationship (Figs 24 to 28).

These characteristics vary between patients and should be examined on a case-by-case basis (Figs 29 to 34).

Figs 35 to 37 The immediate side shift requires sufficient space by providing "backpacks" in the correctly designed occlusal morphology.

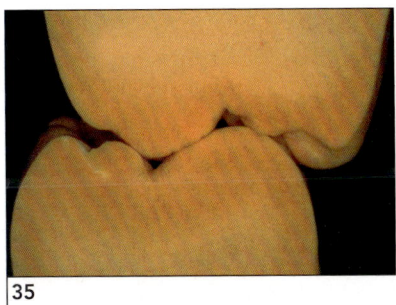

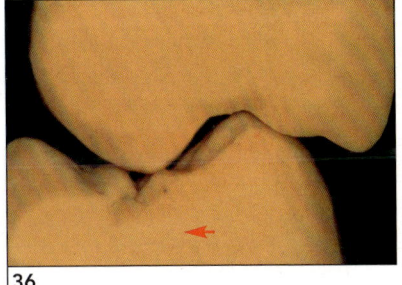

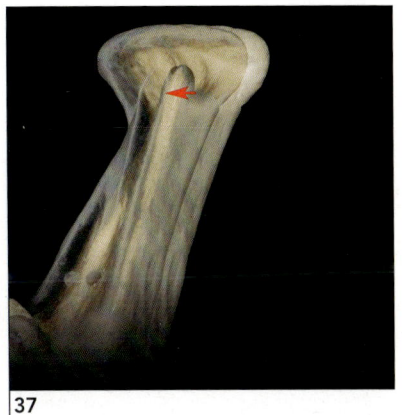

35

36

37

THE BIOMECHANICAL CONCEPT ACCORDING TO POLZ

Many and very different concepts of function are being propagated today. Dentists have the luxury of being able to concentrate on a single system to guide all their treatment efforts. Dental technicians, on the other hand, are faced with having to deal with different dentists favoring different concepts—or no concept. In any case, dentists expect the finished restoration to create no problems, whether at the time of insertion or later. This is where the biomechanical concept according to Master Dental Technician M. H. Polz comes into play.

A frequently discussed aspect is the number of contacts to provide. The literature clearly indicates an average of 3.9 contacts per tooth.[5,6] Too many occlusal stops restrict movement, especially in the molar region, which is strongly influenced by the temporomandibular joint. This is demonstrated below on the basis of two directed movements.

One of these movements is the immediate side shift. The question has been raised whether this movement exists at all, but it has been demonstrated in various publications.[7–10] Whether it is physiological or pathological in nature is a question that must be answered by scientific research. The following two options exist in clinical practice: Either the dentist believes that this movement should be disregarded because it does not exist or the dentist believes it to be pathological, taking the requisite precautions to avoid this movement.

But not infrequently, the dental technician will simply be confronted with the task and will have to resolve it somehow, without any additional information. The movement as such is defined as the temporomandibular joint first moving medially (inward) on the mediotrusive (nonworking) side during lateral excursions before performing the remainder of the usual mediotrusive movement. Imagining this movement and its effect on the temporomandibular joint and the molars in the frontal view illustrates the problem.

If the joint really performs this type of movement, the classical gnathological waxup scheme will soon reach its limits. Even the early gnathologists knew about this problem, and since they could not compensate for it in their waxup concept, they accommodated it with an elaborate articulation technique.[11,12]

So what do we do if we do not have the requisite information? M. H. Polz, being a keen observer of nature, was the first to describe the morphologic structures as resembling "backpacks."[13–15] Occlusal stops would be placed on these backpacks, creating space for the respective movements. For the immediate side shift, this would mean that the mandibular first molar has a prepended occlusal element (the backpack) on its middle (distobuccal) cusp. It is this backpack that is contacted by the mesiopalatal cusp of the maxillary first molar. This provides the necessary space for the excursion in the occlusal vicinity (Figs 35 to 37).

Another very important direction of movement is called *laterotrusion*. This term implies that the jaw

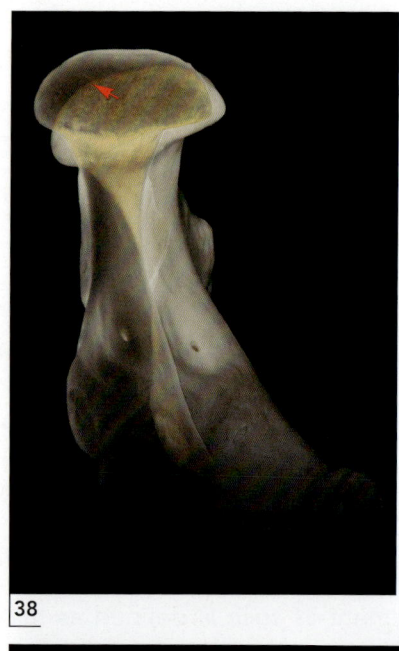

Figs 38 to 40 Laterotrusion can create facets that protect the temporo-mandibular joint from sliding further into the bilaminar zone.

Fig 41 The occlusal compass is an abstract pattern of movement that can be superimposed on a tooth or on any individual contact.

Figs 42 and 43 In the biomechanical concept, occlusal stops can be arranged nearly within a single plane. This means more rapid decoupling and easier occlusal adjustment.

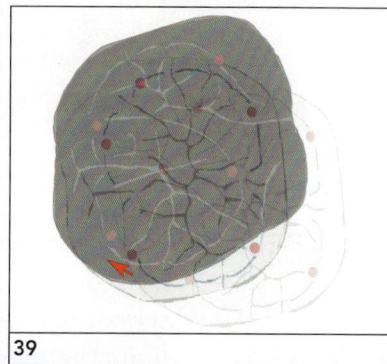

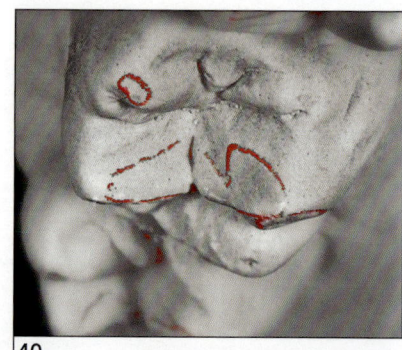

38

39

40

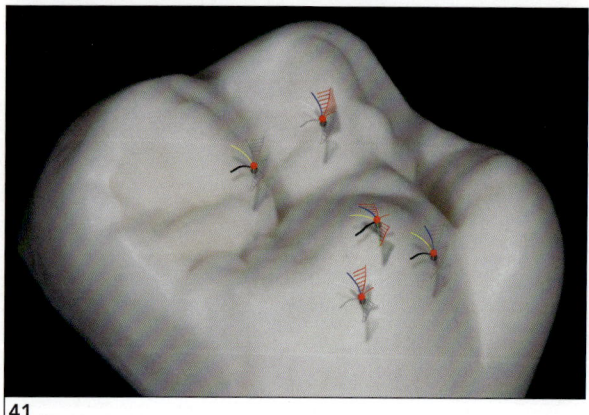

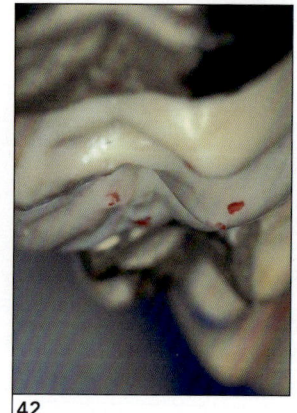

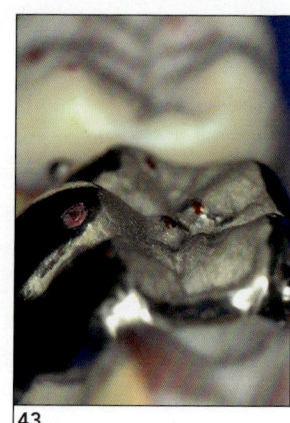

41

42

43

moves backward and upward during lateral excursions. In the horizontal plane, it can be seen that the distobuccal cusp of the mandibular first molar moves toward the distobuccal cusp of the maxillary first molar. Because this movement is three-dimensional and has a cranial aspect, wear facets are frequently the result—now often viewed as protective facets in the literature in that the cusp ensures that the temporomandibular joint does not slide even further into the dorsocranial region (Figs 38 to 40).[16–19]

In an Angle Class II situation, or in similarly structured anomalies, the posterior teeth thus serve to protect the temporomandibular joint. The "occlusal compass" is nothing but a representation of the movements in the form of an abstract bar code of the respective cusps on the occlusal stops (Fig 41).

The backpacks allow the cusp-fossa relationships to remain relatively level in that all occlusal stops can be kept almost on the same plane. At the same time, not only does this concept result in an esthetic and natural morphologic appearance, but it also facilitates fast and complete disclusion. A stable centric relation and the necessary clearance in the immediate occlusal vicinity are additional advantages that neither occlusal records nor articulators can represent. To this day, there is practically no way to record the true movements as they occur directly on the tooth. For this, one would have to resort to a stereographic record (functionally generated pathway)[20,21] with all its benefits but also with its disadvantages (Figs 42 and 43).

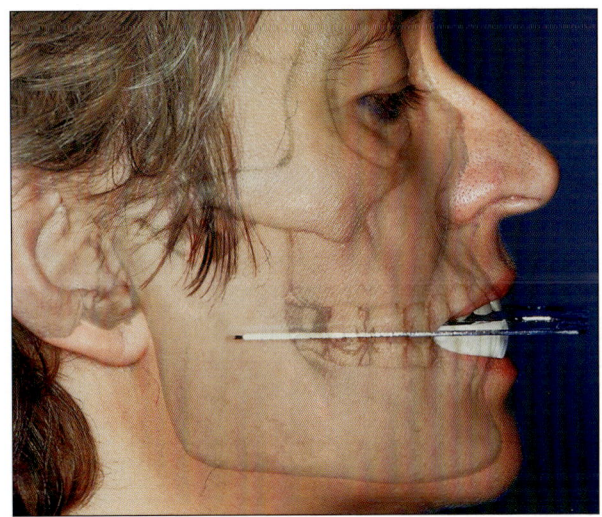

Fig 44 Bite fork is used to check the relationship between the occlusal planes and the cranium.

PLANES

Another aspect that is unfortunately frequently neglected is related to the various planes, of which the most important ones are defined as follows:

- *Occlusal plane:* A plane supported by the mandibular central incisors and the distobuccal cusps of the mandibular second molars.
- *Occlusal line:* The sagittal curvature of the dentition relative to the masticatory plane, ie, the anatomical curve formed by the teeth, called the curve of Spee (named after Ferdinand Spee, who described this curve in 1890). Behind the mandibular canine tip, this curve drops down slightly, turning to horizontal in the region of the first molars and ascending in the region of the second molars.[22,23]
- *Esthetic plane*[24] ("glass-plate plane"): If we visualize the occlusal plane as a glass plate on which we place the maxilla, ideally the teeth will be in contact as follows: central incisors, yes; lateral incisors, no (lateroprotrusion); canines, yes; first premolars, yes (buccally); second premolars, yes (buccally and palatally); first molars, yes (mesiopalatally); second molars, no.

The occlusal plane and the so-called occlusal line are important because they are responsible for correct disclusion and for the correct transfer of forces to the entire cranium and the body as a whole.[25]

How can we ensure that the occlusal plane can be checked immediately and integrated directly into our procedures? Probably the simplest method is the use of the Candulor bite fork (Candulor AG, Rielasingen/Worblingen, Germany). When fitted to the patient, as shown for the maxilla in Fig 44, it serves to check the so-called esthetic plane, which must be in harmony with the occlusal plane. The esthetic plane should run parallel to the bipupillary line. As Fig 44 clearly shows, this is not the case for the patient depicted. The issue is whether this is an anatomic problem or a challenge that needs to be resolved prosthodontically. Looking at the patient's smile, additional serious visual deficiencies become apparent. They are best resolved by using provisional therapeutic restorations, allowing the patient to become accustomed to her new appearance, phonetics, and function. The definitive restoration would then simply implement the result in ceramics and add the final touches (Figs 45 to 49).

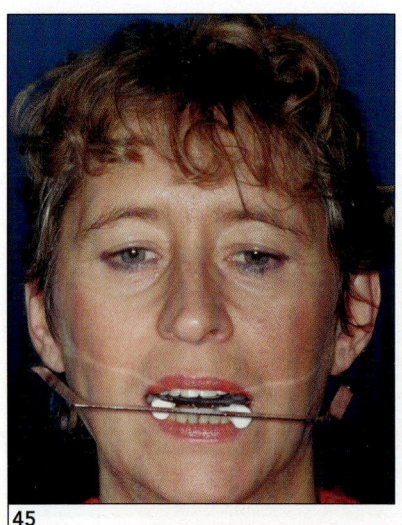

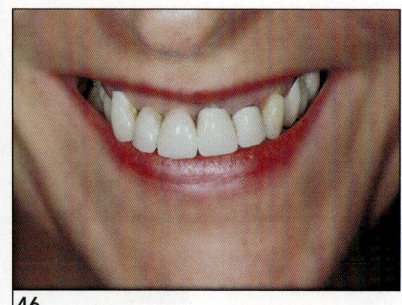

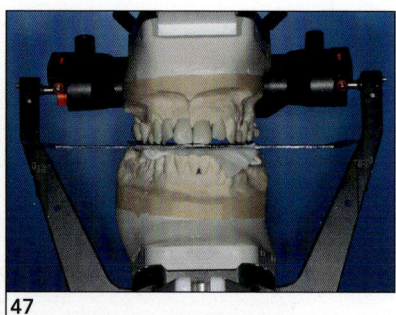

Figs 45 to 49 Planes are used for reference and can be finalized in temporal sequence, using therapeutic provisional restorations. Dentist: M. Schlee.

Figs 50 and 51 This unit is ideally suited for analyzing the various planes. These two photographs show the same patient before and after comprehensive prosthetic restoration of both jaws. Dentists: S. and B. Vanderborght.

45

46

47

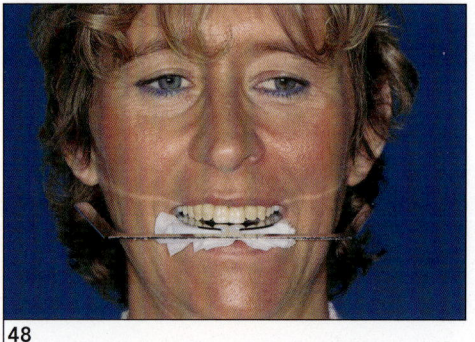

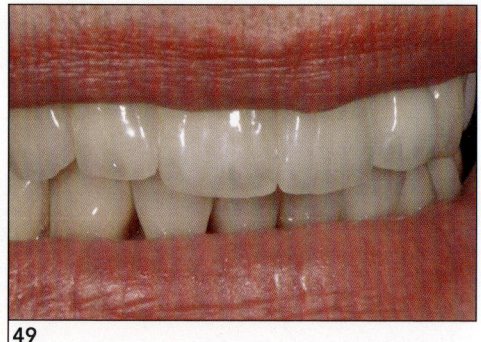

48

49

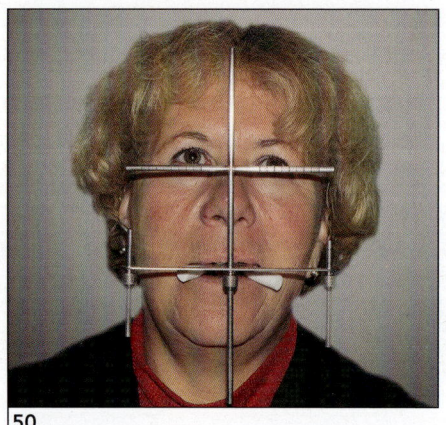

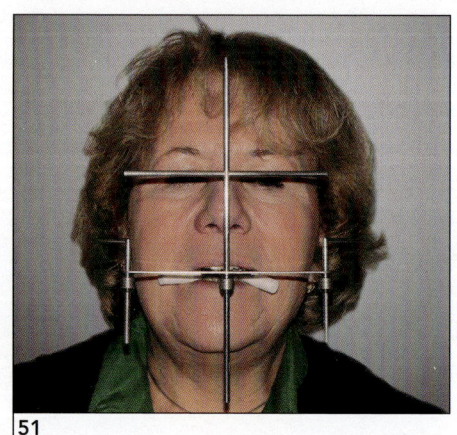

50

51

The HeadLines unit[26] (MediPlus, Unterleinleiter, Germany) may be used as an alternative to the Candulor bite fork. The underlying idea is the same as for the Candulor bite fork, but this unit additionally features a parallel indicator for the bipupillary line and two nanorough height-adjustable arms that, depending on the respective setting, can provide information about Camper's plane (Figs 50 and 51).

Correct arrangement of the planes can greatly enhance the patient's esthetic satisfaction.

CASE 1 (Figs 52 to 61)

Fig 52 Patient presents with implants in the maxillary right quadrant that are less than ideally placed.

Fig 53 Untrimmed cast with abutments in place.

Figs 54 and 55 Definitive restorations include veneers next to metal-ceramic crowns on implants and natural teeth.

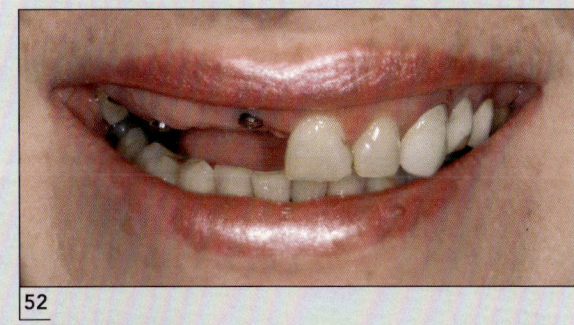
52

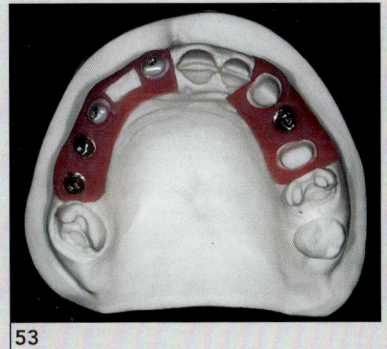
53

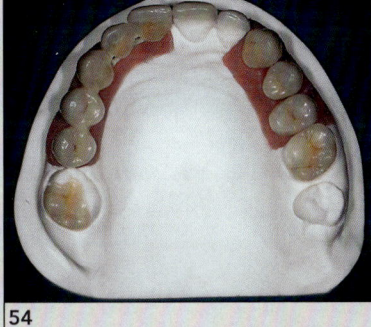
54

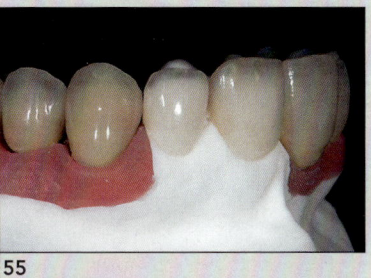
55

Fig 56 Maxillary arch immediately prior to definitive restoration.

Fig 57 Occlusal view of definitive restoraton.

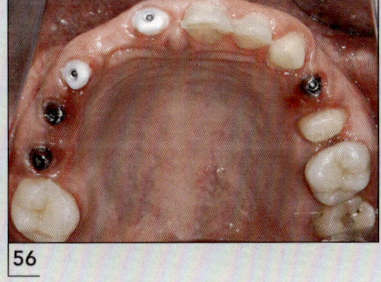
56

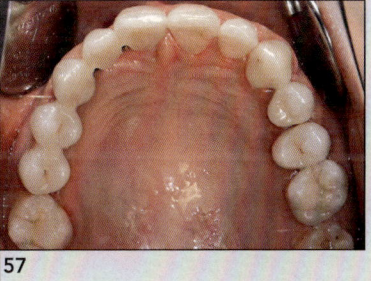
57

CASE 1

Complex cases require a broad arsenal of ideas and tools. The requirements are as diverse as the solutions to be provided, which must be found and provided individually for each patient.

Special difficulties arise if there are various problems in one patient that must be resolved with different types of restorations. This patient presented with implants in the right quadrant that had been provided elsewhere. Although they had been inserted according to the treatment plan, the plan itself was deficient. The problems were so complex that the patient required a complete oral rehabilitation. She had been promised that the prosthetic work would involve only her right quadrants; understandably, she was not very happy at the end of the first consultation. Treatment planning was adjusted to provide for the rehabilitation of the maxilla first, postponing the mandible for the time being and thus distributing the financial burden. The implant system used (right quadrant) did not leave much room for either an attractive emergence profile or for gingival grafts to achieve better soft tissue harmony. Ultimately, it was necessary to resort to a combination of an implant-supported fixed partial denture, veneers, metal-ceramic crowns supported by natural teeth and by implants, and ceramic onlays. For esthetic reasons, zirconia abutments were used on the two anterior implants (Figs 52 to 60).

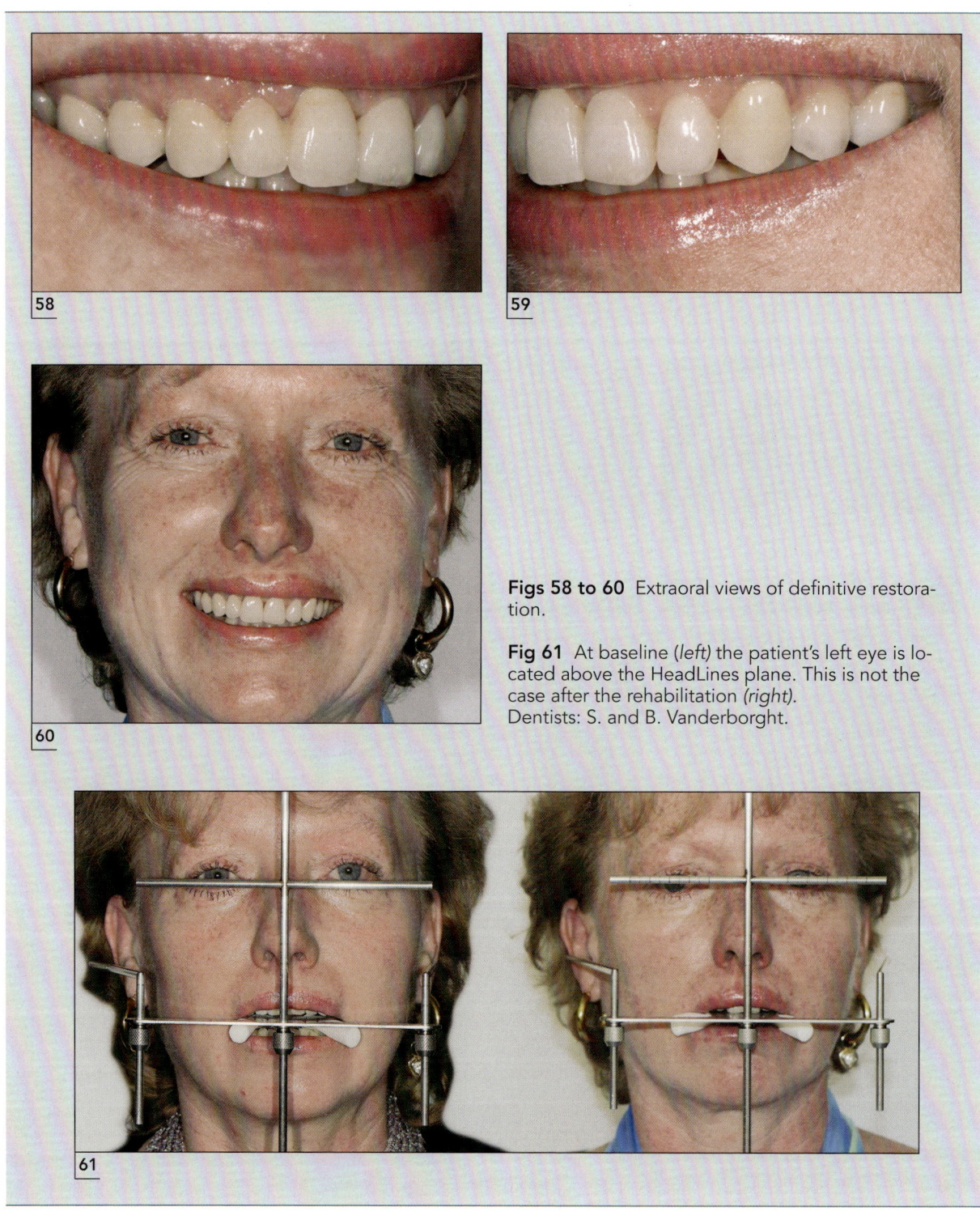

Figs 58 to 60 Extraoral views of definitive restoration.

Fig 61 At baseline (*left*) the patient's left eye is located above the HeadLines plane. This is not the case after the rehabilitation (*right*).
Dentists: S. and B. Vanderborght.

A comparison of the baseline planes with the planes after rehabilitation showed important differences in the details. At baseline, the patient's left eye was located above the HeadLines plane (Fig 61). The positions of the lateral arms were nearly perfect. This is an excellent way, and really the only way, to check the completed prosthesis on the articulator and, of course, directly on the patient.

CASE 2 (Figs 62 to 81)

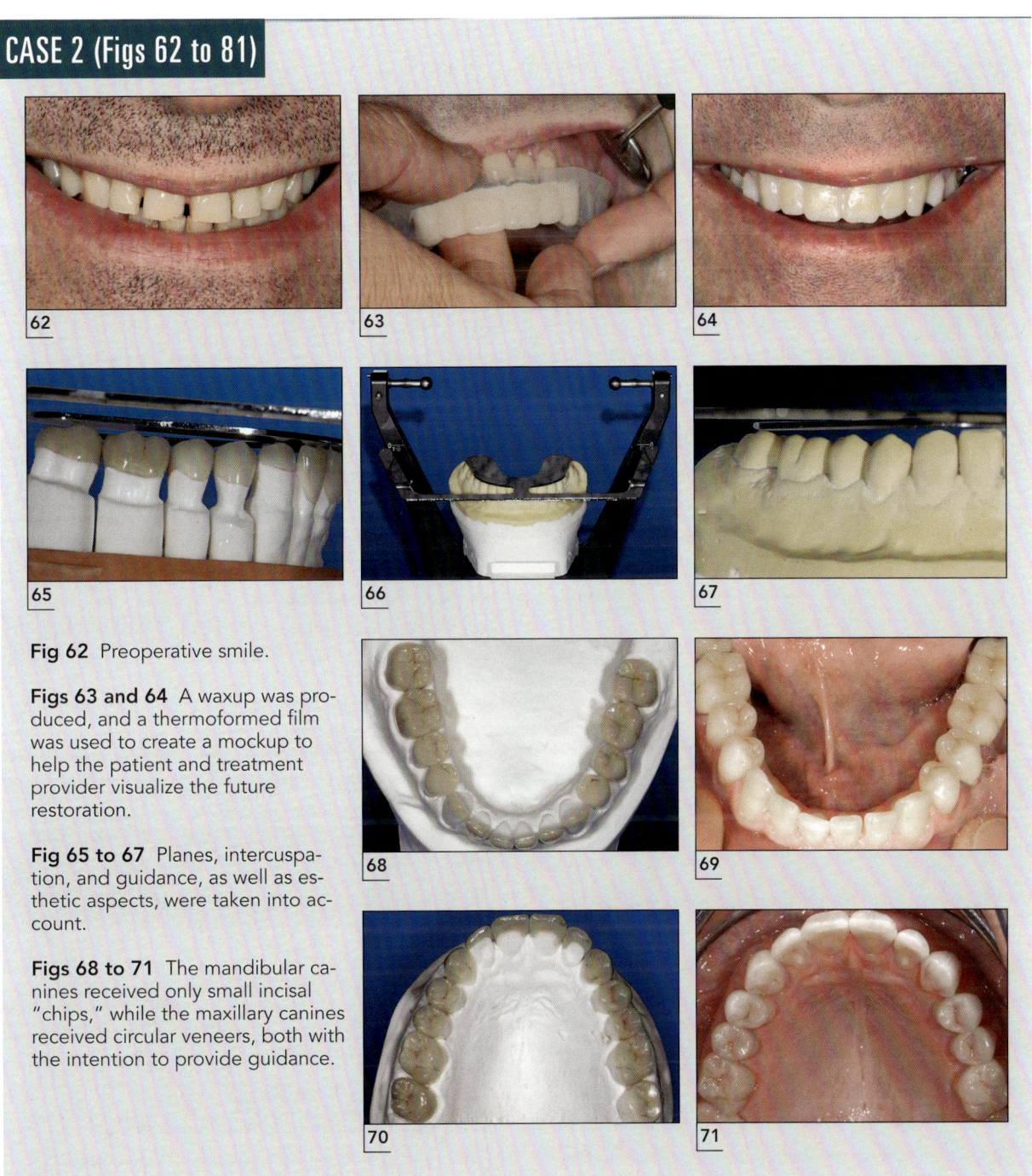

Fig 62 Preoperative smile.

Figs 63 and 64 A waxup was produced, and a thermoformed film was used to create a mockup to help the patient and treatment provider visualize the future restoration.

Fig 65 to 67 Planes, intercuspation, and guidance, as well as esthetic aspects, were taken into account.

Figs 68 to 71 The mandibular canines received only small incisal "chips," while the maxillary canines received circular veneers, both with the intention to provide guidance.

CASE 2

This patient also required a complex rehabilitation. A plastic mockup was created for the patient and the treatment provider to get a first overall impression. The treatment plan provided for a combination of veneers, ceramic onlays, and metal-ceramic crowns, supported in part by natural teeth and in part by implants. The mandible was restored first. Of course, the planes were continuously checked both during and after the placement of the restoration. The maxilla was essentially restored in the same manner. The completed restorations were inserted and cemented (Figs 62 to 75).

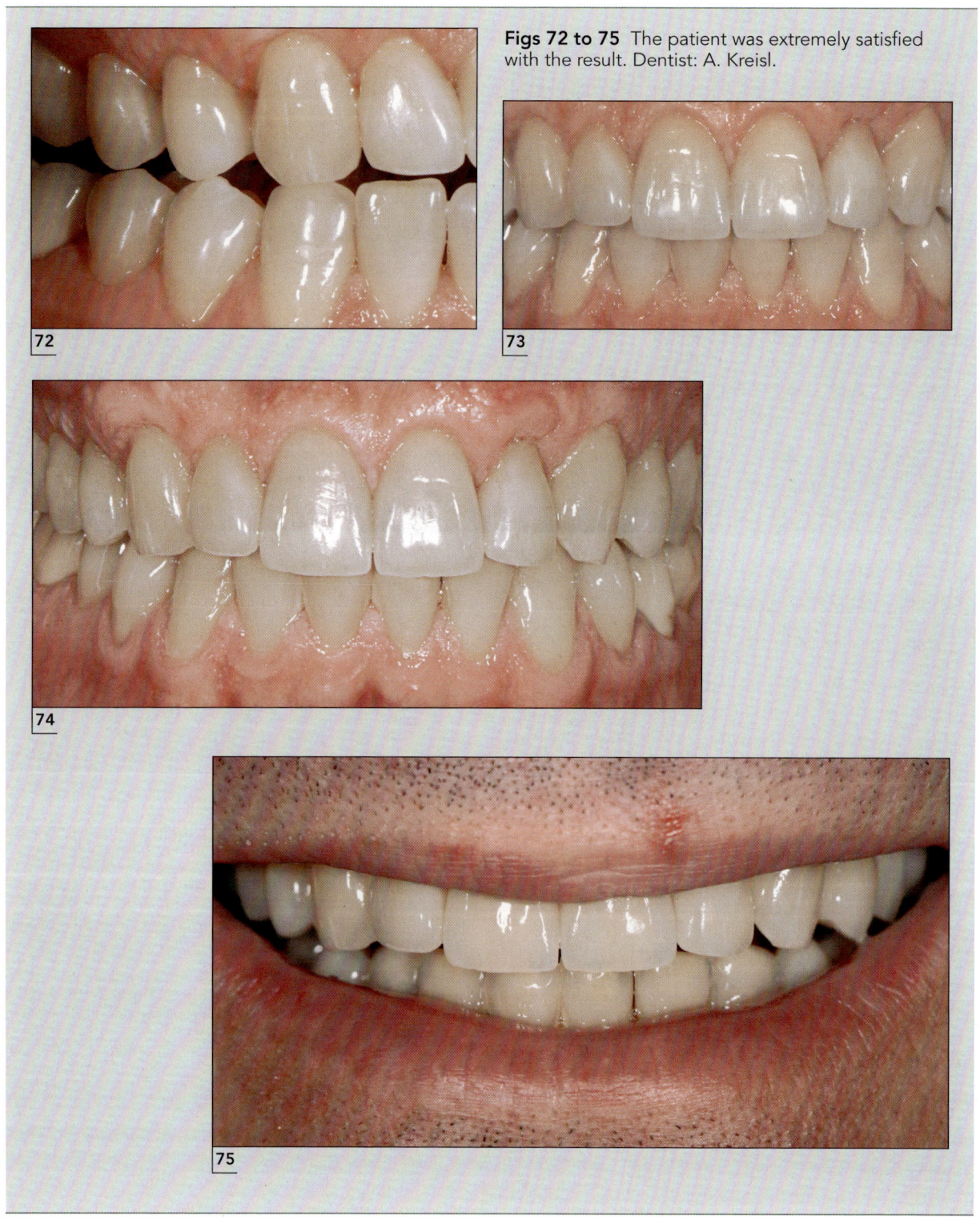

Figs 72 to 75 The patient was extremely satisfied with the result. Dentist: A. Kreisl.

For better functional control, new impressions were taken and new casts produced. These, too, were mounted arbitrarily in an articulator, so that the overall function including laterotrusions could be checked. As a segmented cast was also provided, it was possible to remove the teeth individ-

Figs 76 to 81 A more detailed functional check can be performed on the articulators using casts of the intraoral situation. Segmented teeth can be removed individually on the laterotrusive side, thus investigating the guidance offered by the next tooth in line, avoiding disturbances to the nonworking side. Dentist: A. Kreisl.

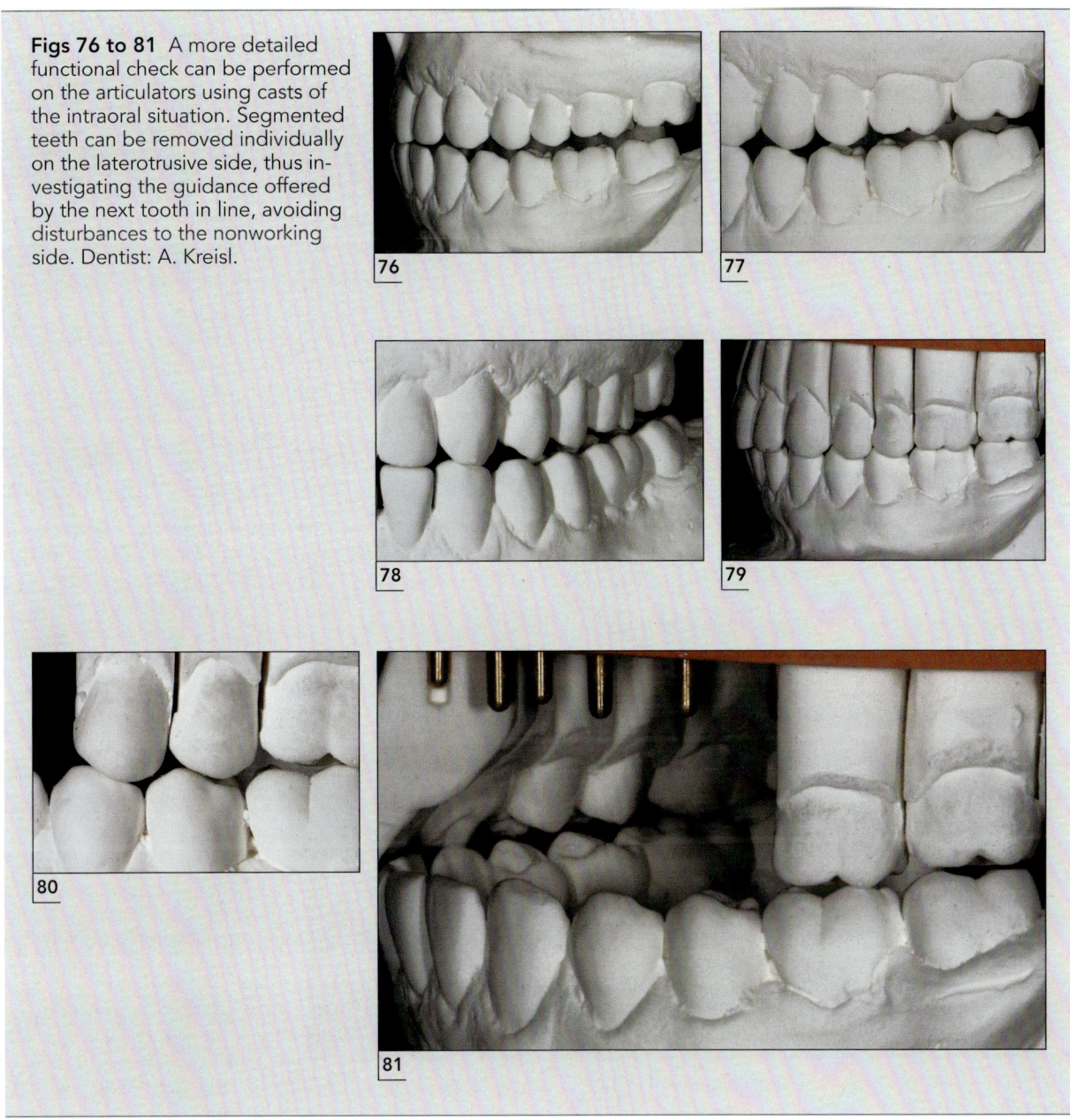

ually for even more control over functional details. The result illustrates the principle of sequential laterotrusion with canine dominance.[27–30.] Canine dominance means that removing the canine results in guidance by the maxillary first premolar and, possibly, the maxillary lateral incisor; if these are removed, guidance is provided by the maxillary second premolar; and if this, too, is removed, by the maxillary first molar. None of this may disturb the occlusal balance on the nonworking side. In a eugnathic natural dentition, this would mean that the maxillary canine is abraded first, then the first and second premolars, and, finally, the first molar. The principle of the distributed planes had already been taken into account by the dental technician when designing the restorations. Considering how difficult it is to adhesively cement veneers and ceramic onlays in a satisfactory manner, the challenge involved in inserting such restorations becomes obvious (Figs 76 to 81).

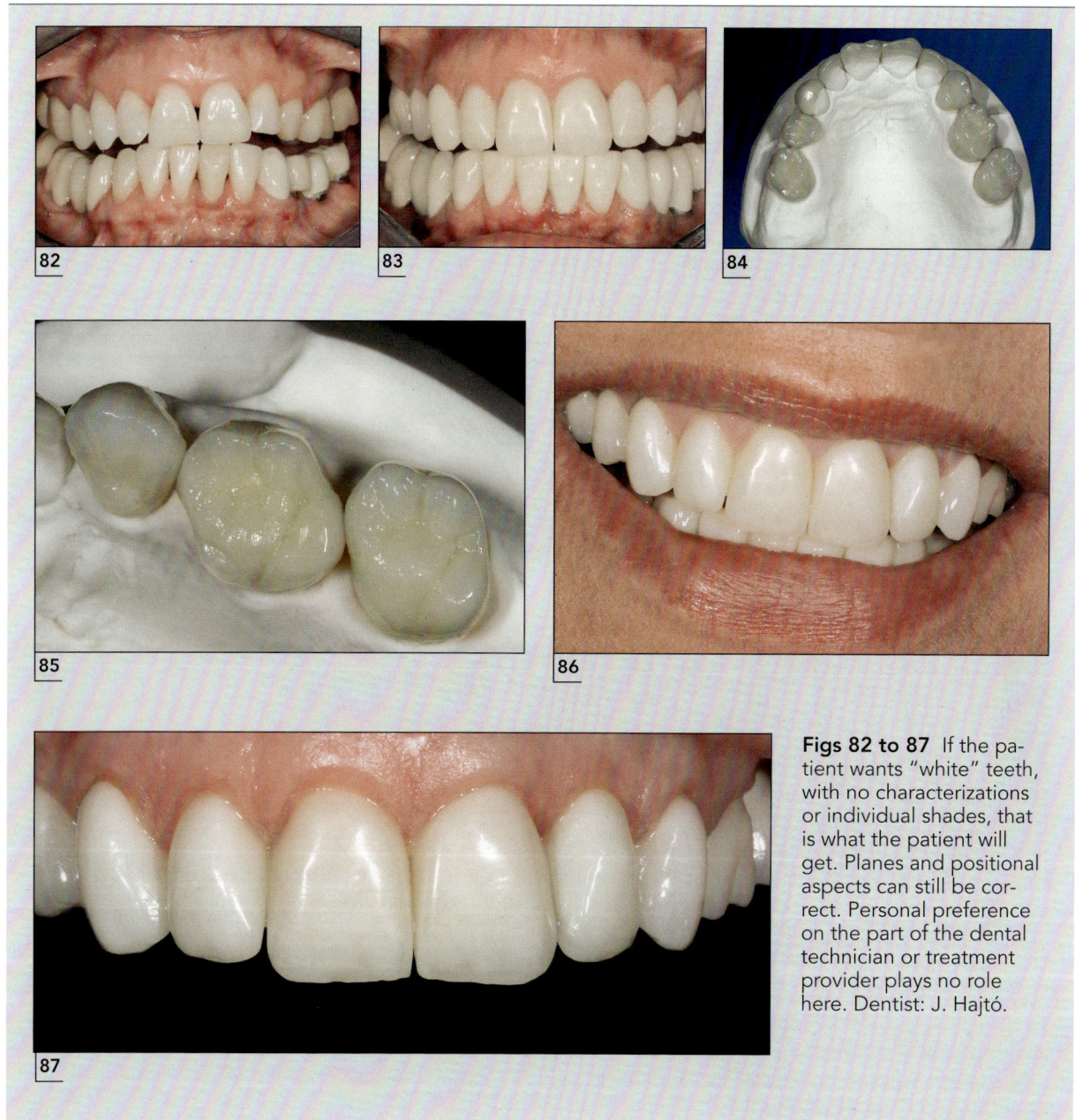

Figs 82 to 87 If the patient wants "white" teeth, with no characterizations or individual shades, that is what the patient will get. Planes and positional aspects can still be correct. Personal preference on the part of the dental technician or treatment provider plays no role here. Dentist: J. Hajtó.

FUNCTION AND BRIGHT TEETH

Function and esthetics must never be treated separately. The contribution of shade is secondary. If the patient desires white teeth and does not want to see individual characterizations or complex shades, we have to comply while still providing excellent function. Patient cases may be complex in structure, mixing all-ceramic crowns, veneers, and metal-ceramic crowns while ensuring that no or next to no visual discrepancy appears (Figs 82 to 87).

Restorations supported by implants pose a different kind of challenge. Again, patients frequently request bright teeth. The dental technician will comply, but will certainly appreciate being able to provide shaded areas, natural positional textures, or similar enhancements (Figs 88 to 93).

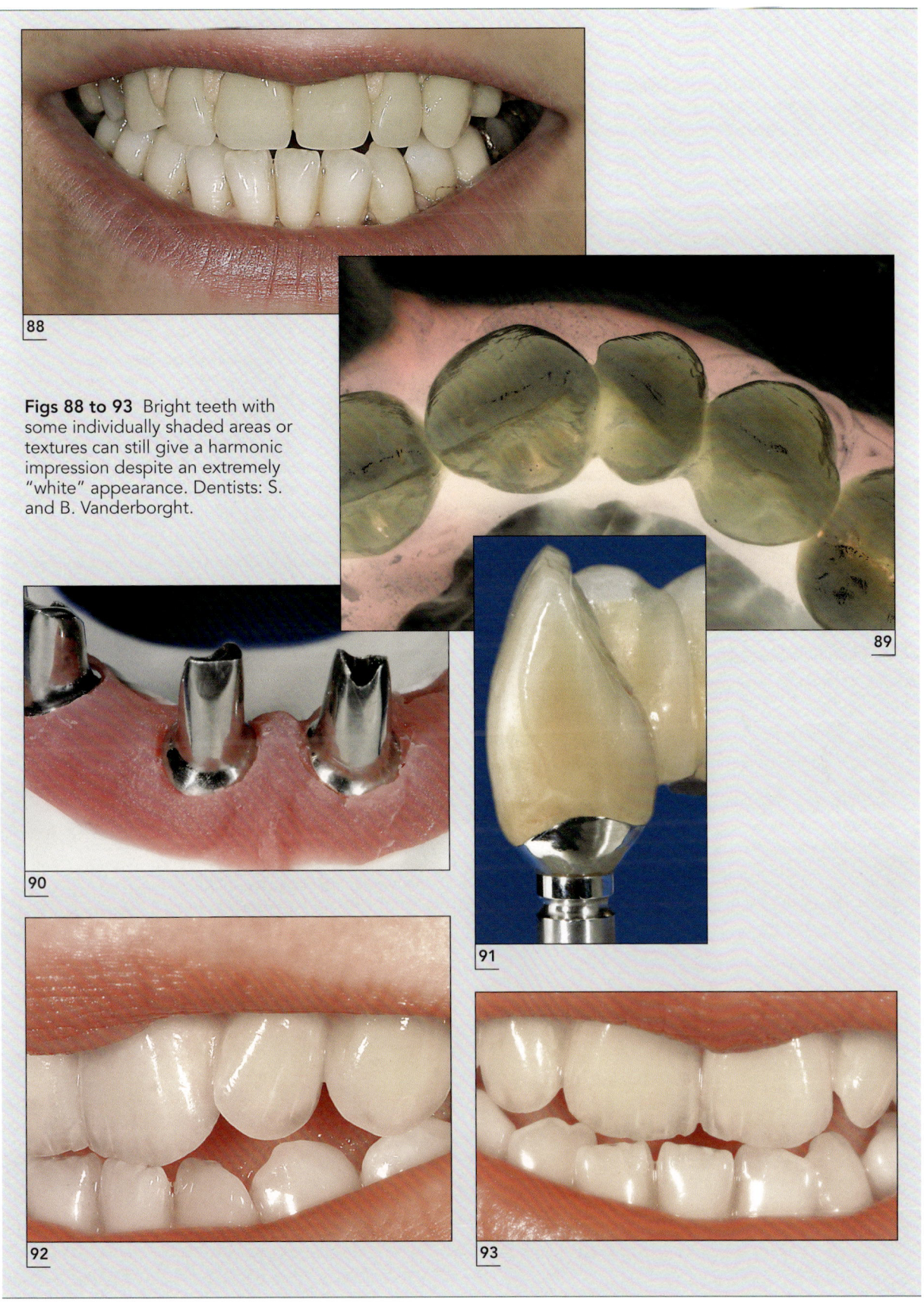

Figs 88 to 93 Bright teeth with some individually shaded areas or textures can still give a harmonic impression despite an extremely "white" appearance. Dentists: S. and B. Vanderborght.

REFERENCES

1. Schäffer H. Keramikinlays, Materialkundliche und klinische Aspekte—experimentelle Untersuchungen [Thesis]. Berlin: Quintessenz, 1993.

2. Hahn R. Vollkeramische Einzelzahnrestauration [Thesis]. Berlin: Quintessenz, 1997.

3. Hohmann W. Dentalkeramik auf der Basis hydrothermaler Gläser. Berlin: Quintessenz, 1993.

4. Bumann A, Lotzmann U. Funktionsdiagnostik und Therapieprinzipien. Stuttgart: Thieme, 2000.

5. Buth K. Zur funktionellen Gestaltung des Kauflächen-komplexes bei festsitzendem Zahnersatz mit hilfe der FGP—Technik und unter Anwendung von Kugelsegment-fertigteilen. Jahrestagung der Arbeitsgemeinschaft Dentale Technologie, May 1989.

6. End E. Die physiologische Okklusion des menschlichen Gebisses. München: Verlag Neuer Merkur, 2005.

7. Lundeen H, Gibbs C. Mandibular movement and ist clinical significance [in German]. Phillip J Restaur Zahnmed 1987;4(2):87–97.

8. Lundeen H, Gibbs Ch. The Function of Teeth. US: L and G Publishers, 2005.

9. Staehle H. Effect of the articulator joint on shaping the masticatory surface [in German]. Dtsch Zahnarztl Z 1984;39:356–359.

10. Lückerath W. Das transversale und vertikale Bewegungsspiel des Unterkiefers im Bereich der Kauflächen und der Kiefergelenke [Thesis], 1991.

11. McCollum BB, Stuart CE. A research report, published by Stuart, P.O. Box 1298, Ventura, CA 93001, 1955.

12. Stuart CE, Golden IB. Gnathological instruments. In: The History of Gnathology. Ventura, CA: Stuart CE, 1984.

13. Polz MH. Biomechanical basis of occlusal mastictory surface design [in German]. Zahntechnik (Zur) 1981(2); 39:126–134.

14. Polz MH. Die biomechanische Aufwachstechnik bei Inlay- und Onlay-Restaurationen. In: in Caesar HH. Inlay- und Onlay-Techniken. München: Verlag Neuer Merkur, 1987.

15. Polz MH. Die biomechanische Kaufläche und deren Anwendung in allen okkluslalen Beziehungen. Jahrestagung der Arbeitsgemeinschaft Dentale Technologie, May 1989.

16. Hugger A. Gelenknahe elektronissche Erfassung der Unterkieferfunktion und ihr Umsetzung in den Artikulator [Thesis]. Berlin: Quintessenz, 2000.

17. Lotzmann U. Studien zum Einfluss der okklusalen Prä-Therapie auf die zentrische Kieferrelation [Thesis]. Berlin: Quintessenz, 1999.

18. Koeck B. Experimentelle Untersuchungen zur Dynamik des Unterkiefers während des Nachtschlafes [Thesis]. Berlin: Quintessenz, 1982.

19. Schmierer A. Kiefergelenksfunktionen—die retrusive Surtrusion des Laterotrusionskondylus. Zahnarzt Magazin 1991;4:24–35.

20. Dawson P. Grundzüge der Okklusion. München: Verlag Zahnärztliches Schrifttum, 1978.

21. Lex Ch. FGP-Technik, praktischer Arbeitskurs bei BSI. Fürth, Germany, 1989.

22. Gysi A. Das Aufstellen der Zähne für Vollprothesen. Zürich: Schweizerische Zahntechniker Vereinigung, 1948.

23. Hajto J. Anteriors [in German]. Fuchstal, Germany: Teamwork Media, 2006:180.

24. Gysi A. The Gysi Method [in German]. DeTrey, 1932.

25. Rossaint A, Lechner J, van Assche S. Das Cranio-sacrale System. Heidelberg: Hüthig, 1996:59.

26. Schöttl R, Bertram U, Karg R, Losert-Bruggner B. Präzision der Modellposition im Artikulator bei der Übertragung mit mittelwertigen Gesichtsbögen. ICCMO Kompendium 2004. Erlangen: International College of Cranio-Mandibular Orthopedics, 2004:109–120.

27. Slavicek R. Die funktionellen Determinanten des Kauorgans [Thesis]. Wien, 1984.

28. Slavicek R, Mack H. Die funktionelle Morphologie der Okklusion. Dent Labor 1980;28:1307–1318.

29. Slavicek R. Das Kauorgan. Klosterneuburg: Gamma Med.-Wis, 2000.

30. Reusch D, Lenze PG, Fischer H. Rekonstruktion von Kauflächen undn Frontzähnen. Westerburg, Germany: Westerburger Kontakte, 1990.

FLAPLESS IMPLANT SURGERY IN CONJUNCTION WITH BONE AUGMENTATION AND SOFT TISSUE MANAGEMENT: A CASE REPORT

Franck Bonnet, DDS[1]

Minimally invasive surgery has revolutionized surgical practice by decreasing the duration of both the surgical and healing phases. The traditional access for bone grafting, soft tissue management, and implant placement is made using flap surgery. The original protocol is to leave the implants under a full-thickness flap for 4 to 6 months in order to eliminate bacterial contamination and avoid micromovements during osseointegration.[1,2] In recent decades, the second stage of implant flap surgery has been modified. Today, both implant placement and soft tissue management are performed at the same stage.[3]

The aim of minimally invasive surgery is to reduce periosteum delamination, preserve the soft tissue architecture, and improve the healing process. Various studies have shown that implant survival rates are similar with conventional or minimally invasive procedures.[4,5] However, it should be considered that minimally invasive procedures are more demanding and therefore require more learning. The use of computer-assisted surgical guides may reduce the effect of this learning curve.

This article will discuss the advantages and disadvantages of minimally invasive flapless surgery and present the proper surgical techniques, including soft tissue management and computer-guided implant placement.

FLAPLESS TECHNIQUE

Advantages

Minimally invasive surgery reduces pain, swelling, and the risk of hematomas. Postsurgical pain can have several origins: the technique, type of flap, and especially the trauma caused to the periosteum. While of course it is impossible to guarantee a pain-free recovery, it is clear that the flapless technique reduces the amount and duration of pain.[6] The bleeding risk both pre- and postoperatively can be reduced through proper implant positioning. Maintaining vascularization should limit bone resorption, and bone remodeling will occur only as the bone adapts functionally to the implant.[4,7] Esthetically, maintaining the soft tissue ar-

[1]Private practice, Cannes-Le Cannet, France.

Correspondence to: Dr Franck Bonnet, 28 Bd Gambetta, 06110 Cannes-Le Cannet, France. E-mail: ffbonnet@wanadoo.fr

chitecture, preserving the papilla, and avoiding vertical incisions close to the implant site will allow for smoother healing and better overall results.[8]

Disadvantages

The lack of visibility makes flapless surgery more difficult. When placing the implant, it is important to pay careful attention to the implant position to avoid damaging the oral situation and jeopardizing the final result. Due to the complexity of the procedure, inexperienced clinicians may be advised to use conventional techniques. Further, intraoperative findings may prompt the clinician to switch to an open flap approach. Again, such a decision calls for a skilled, experienced clinician.

Hard and Soft Tissue Analysis

In order to obtain reliable implant osseointegration and good esthetics, the clinician must analyze the quality and quantity of the hard and soft tissues before implant surgery.[9,10] When evaluating the bone level, it is important to assess the shape of the bone ridge, including its height, thickness, and concavity. Further, extensive knowledge of the oral anatomy is important to avoid damaging the vascular system and nerves of the mouth.[11] Clinical observations should be supplemented with three-dimensional scanning to better visualize the bony structures. Many authors have discussed the use of computer software to create a precise surgical template.[12–20]

When evaluating the soft tissues, clinicians should assess the thickness and height of fibrous keratinized tissue, the quality of the fibromucosal attachment, and the position of the mucogingival line. The relation of the soft tissues to the underlying bone, implant positions, and planned emergence profile must also be considered. In the esthetic zone, a minimum thickness of 1.5 to 2 mm of keratinized fibromucosa is desirable around the implants.[21,22] Therefore, a thick strip of mucosa should be preserved or created when using a flapless surgical procedure.

CASE REPORT

The patient was a 20-year-old female in good general health. She was a nonsmoker with good oral hygiene and a high level of motivation. Her maxillary right central incisor was missing and had been replaced with a long-term provisional bonded prosthesis (Figs 1a and 1b). The patient requested a more esthetically pleasing restoration.

The edentulous space was smaller than the contralateral central incisor (Figs 2a and 2b). The bone quantity was low, showing a width of 2 to 3 mm at the coronal aspect of the bone crest (Fig 3). Soft tissue analysis revealed sufficient papillae but reduced tissue volume due to bone resorption. The mucogingival junction was positioned 5 mm coronal to the adjacent teeth. The frenum presented a challenging situation.

Bone Augmentation

The goal was to augment the bone volume while preserving the soft tissue architecture. For this purpose, it was decided to use the tunnel technique (Figs 4a to 4r). The tunnel, created with a small vertical incision, preserves blood circulation and reduces the risk of flap necrosis.

One vertical incision was made, and the full-thickness mucosa was raised carefully (Figs 4a to 4d). The site was measured to prepare a collagen resorbable barrier membrane (Bio-Gide, Geistlich, Wolhusen, Switzerland), which was placed on the inner part of the periosteum (Figs 4e to 4i). Next, a xenograft was placed with a syringe between the bone and collagen membrane (Figs 4j to 4n). The goal was to create a space between the bone and membrane filled with bovine hydroxyapatite (Bio-Oss, Geistlich) (Figs 4o to 4r). Guided bone regeneration is well-documented in the literature and permits osseointegration after implant placement.[23] The use of the tunnel technique in association with guided bone regeneration offers superior soft tissue preservation and a reduced risk of surgical complications.

Five months later, a computer-guided surgical template (Procera, Nobel Biocare, Göteborg, Swe-

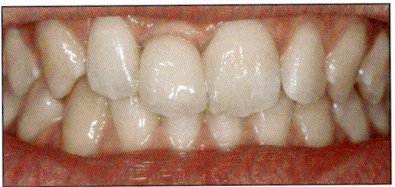 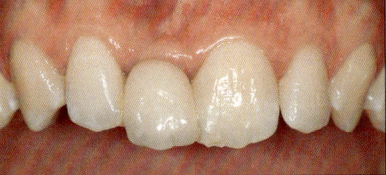

Figs 1a and 1b Initial situation. The existing restoration was esthetically unsatisfactory.

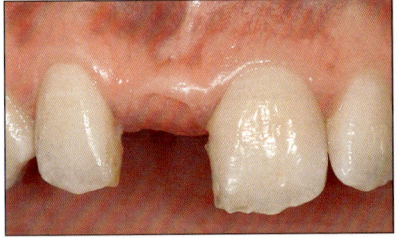 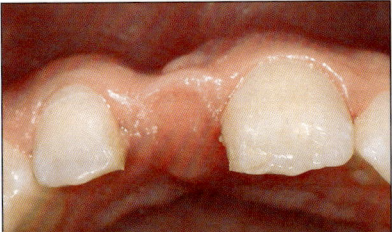

Figs 2a and 2b With the restoration removed, the edentulous space is smaller than the contralateral incisor.

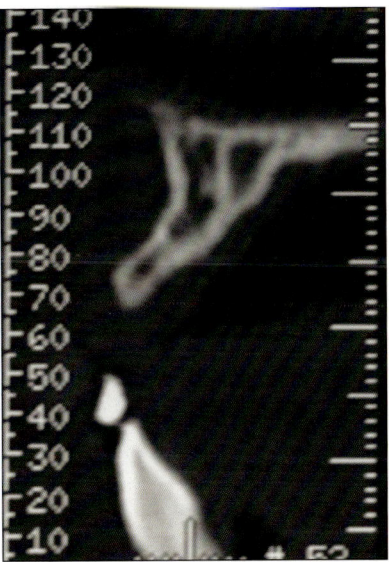

Fig 3 Initial radiographs revealed inadequate bone quantity.

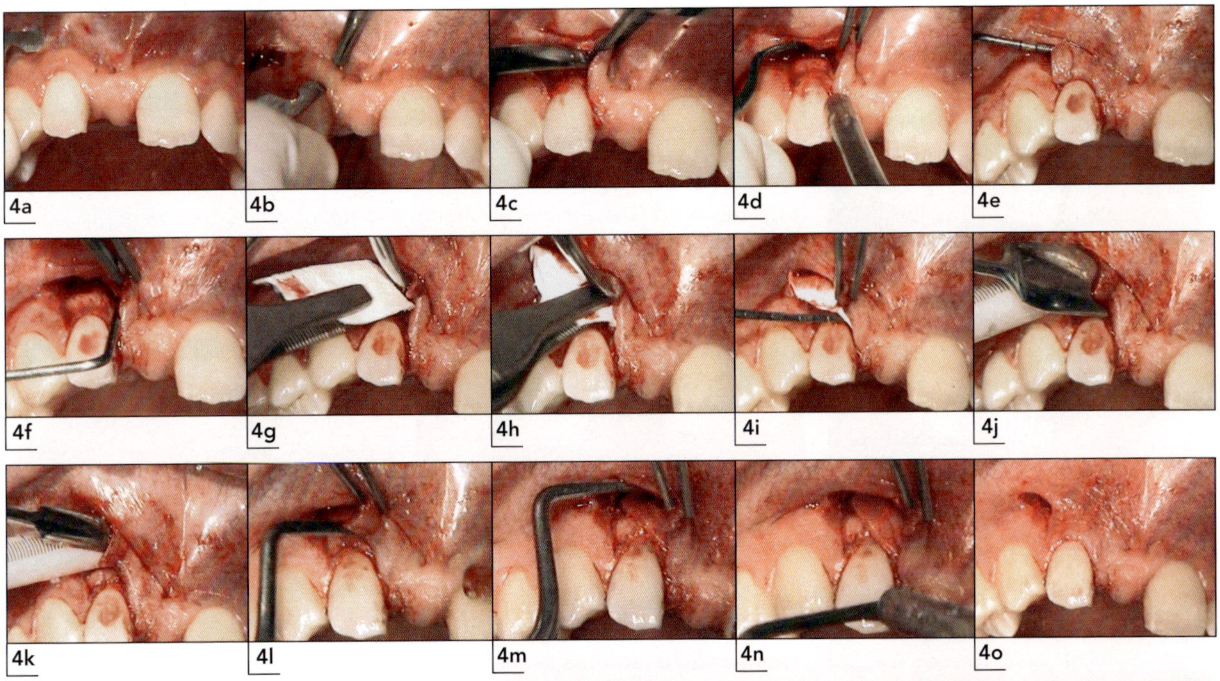

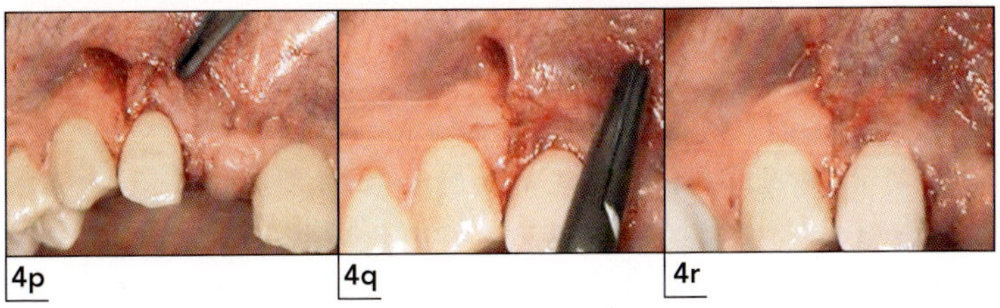

Figs 4a to 4r Bone augmentation using the tunnel technique.

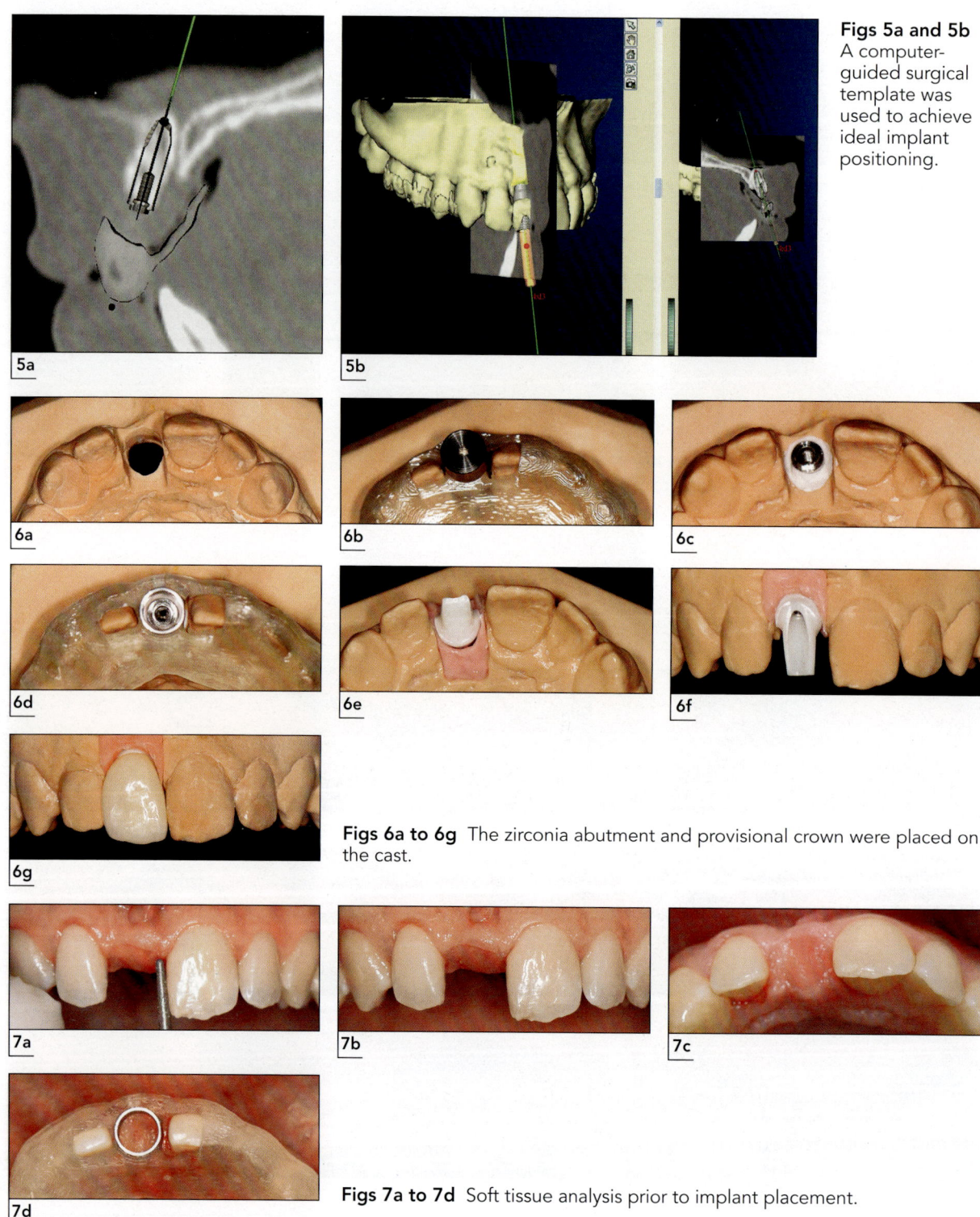

Figs 5a and 5b A computer-guided surgical template was used to achieve ideal implant positioning.

Figs 6a to 6g The zirconia abutment and provisional crown were placed on the cast.

Figs 7a to 7d Soft tissue analysis prior to implant placement.

den) was used for ideal implant positioning at the central incisor site (Figs 5a and 5b). A cast was then fabricated with an esthetic zirconia abutment and provisional crown (Figs 6a to 6g). The soft tissue position was also planned on the cast. Following anesthesia on the day of surgery, the surgical guide was placed to analyze the soft tissue modifications prior to implant placement (Figs 7a to 7d).

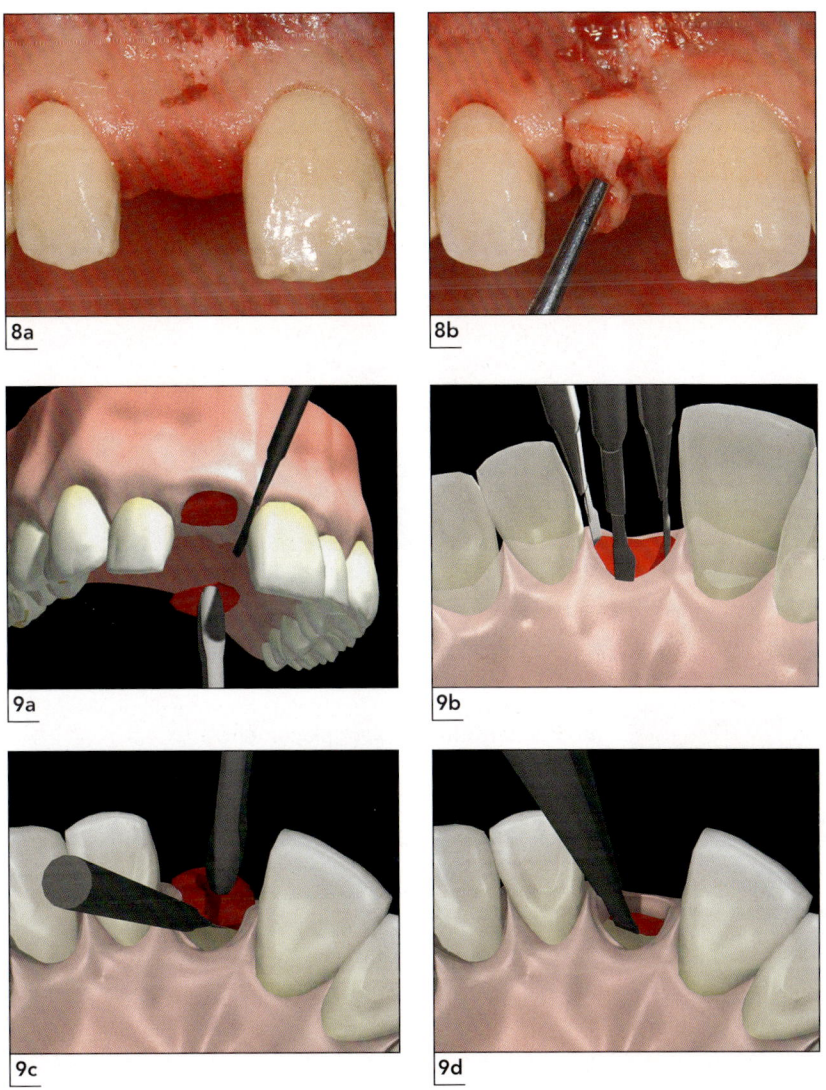

Figs 8a and 8b The frenum was displaced to begin the soft tissue augmentation procedure.

Figs 9a to 9d Computer model showing the modified roll flap technique.

Soft Tissue Augmentation

At the same time as implant placement, the frenum was displaced and a modified roll flap technique was used to access to the bone crest to improve the quality and quantity of the fibromucosa without buccal incisions (Figs 8a and 8b). This technique is appropriate if there is inadequate buccal soft tissue width in conjunction with intact papillae.

After deepithelization (Fig 9a), mesial, distal, and palatal incisions (Fig 9b) were made to raise the palatal and crestal connective tissue, which was positioned in a bucally created envelope (Figs 9c and 9d). The incisions should be more or less extended palatally, depending on the buccal volume that needs to be filled in. Tissue reconstructed in this way has shown good medium-term (4-year) stability.[24]

10a

10b

10c

11a

11b

11c

11d

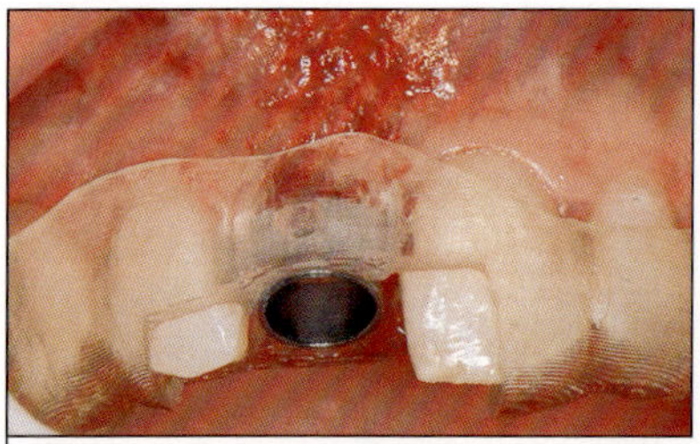

Figs 10a to 10c Implant placement using the surgical guide.

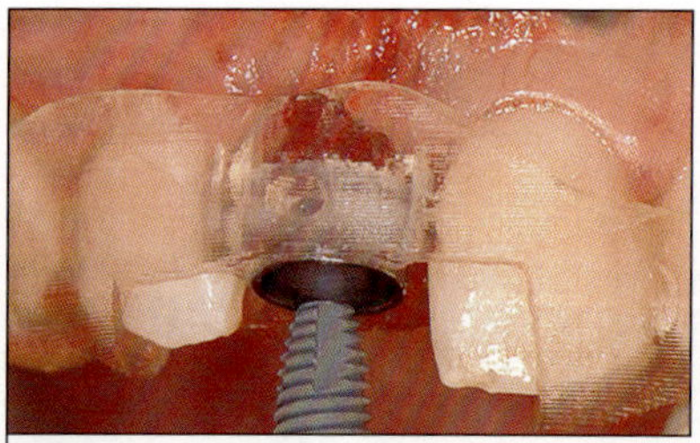

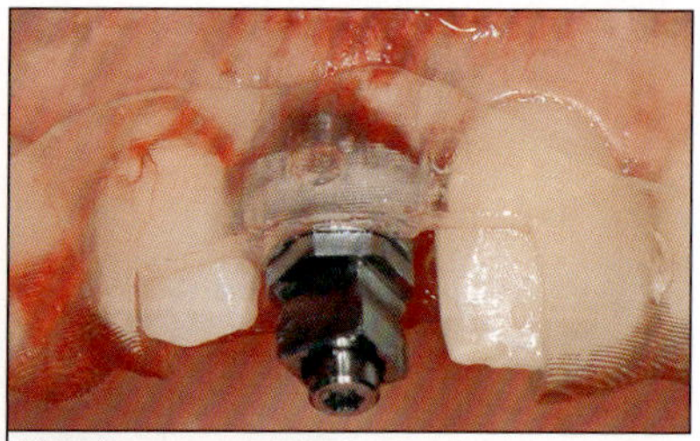

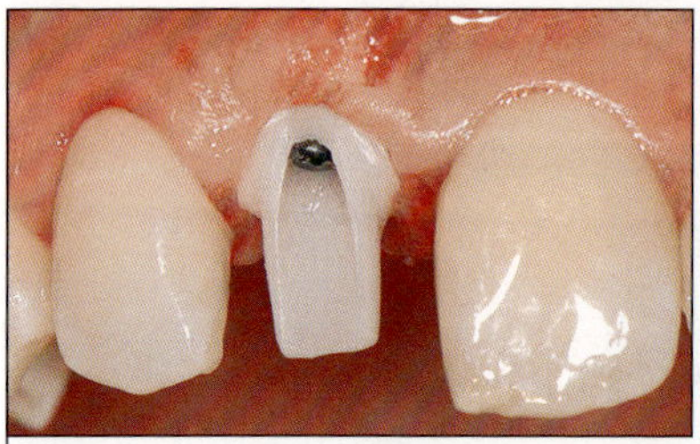

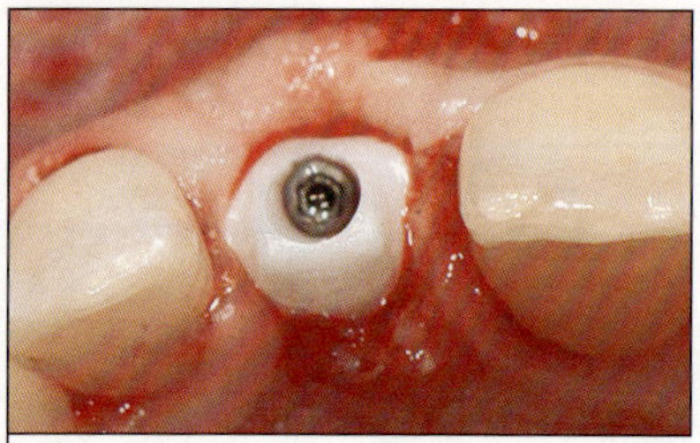

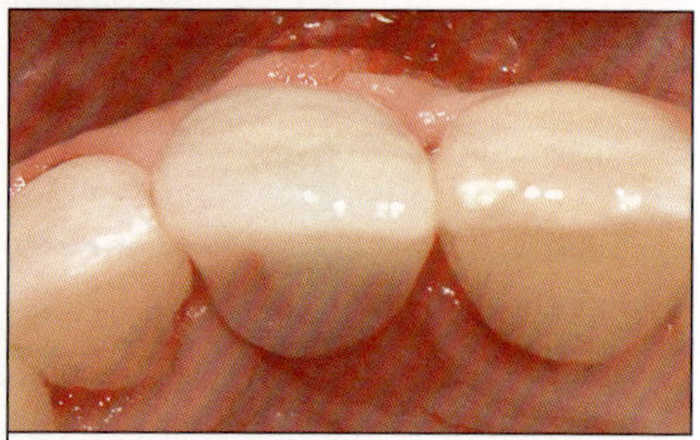

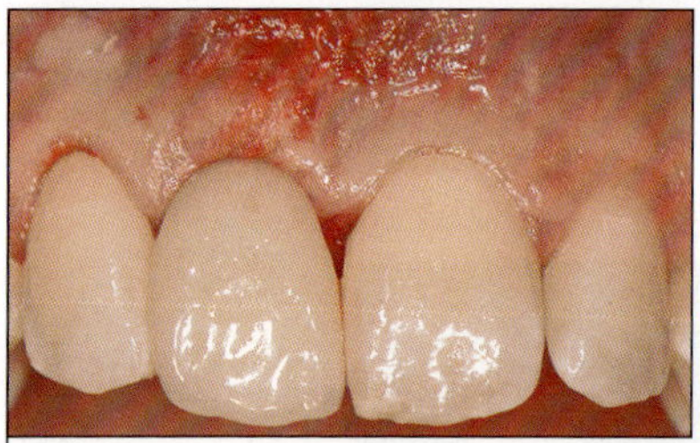

Figs 11a to 11d The zirconia abutment and provisional crown were placed immediately after implant placement.

Fig 12 Healing phase after 2 weeks.

Fig 13 Healing phase after 4 weeks.

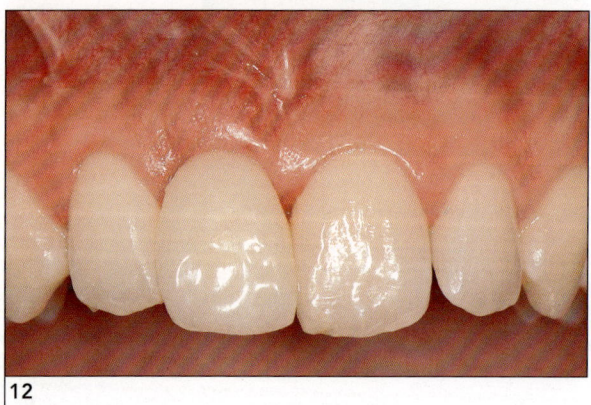

12

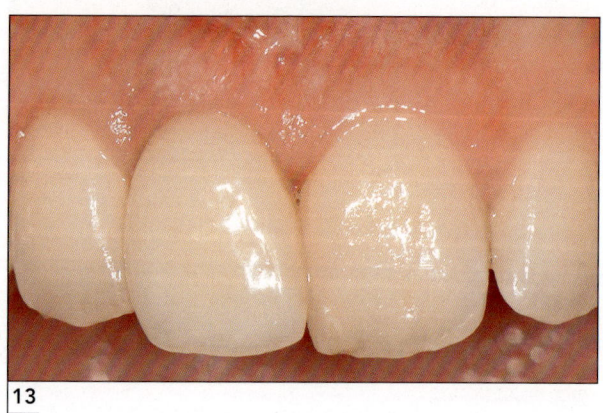

13

Implant Placement

At the same appointment, the implant was placed with a flapless procedure. To reduce the difficulty of this blind surgery, a surgical guide was used (Figs 10a to 10c). Immediately after implant placement, the prefabricated zirconia abutment and provisional crown were placed (Figs 11a to 11d). The goal at this stage is to create good soft tissue adhesion to the final abutment and to design the emergence profile. Figures 12 and 13 show the healing process at 2 and 4 weeks, respectively.

Four months later, an impression was made and a Procera zirconia crown (Nobel Biocare) was placed. Good communication between the clinician and technician was necessary to achieve esthetic integration of the definitive prosthesis with the patient's smile (Figs 14a to 14h).

Figs 14a to 14h After 4 months of healing, the definitive crown was placed.

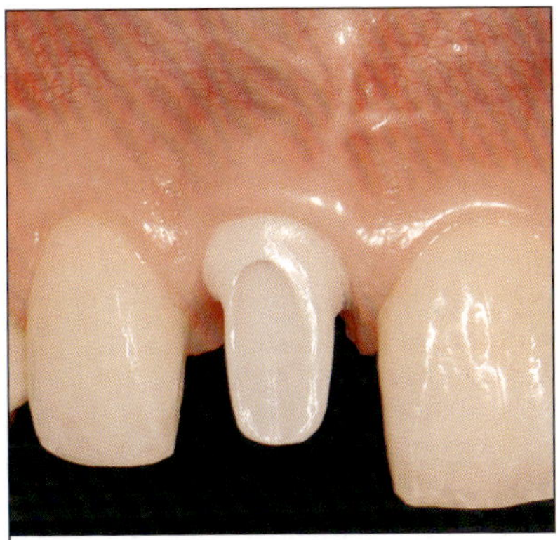

14a

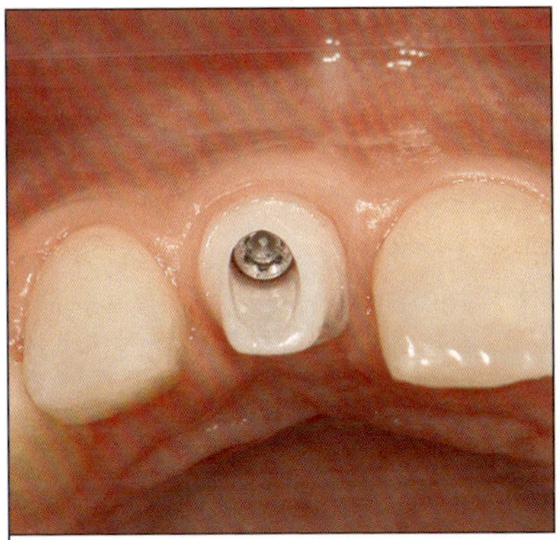

14b

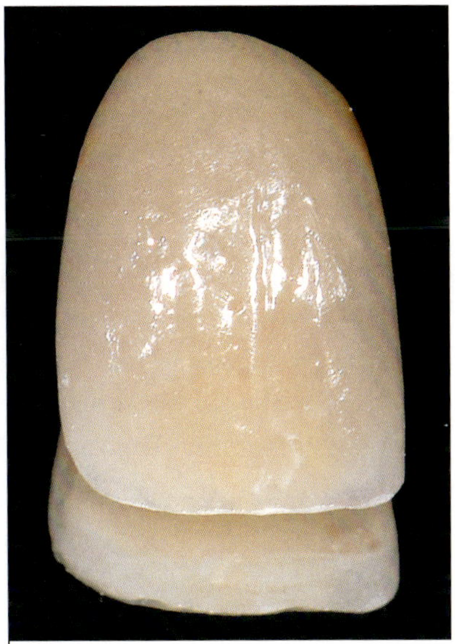

14c

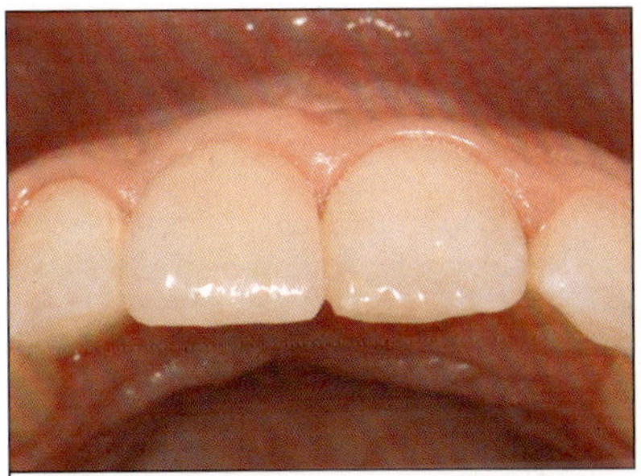

14d

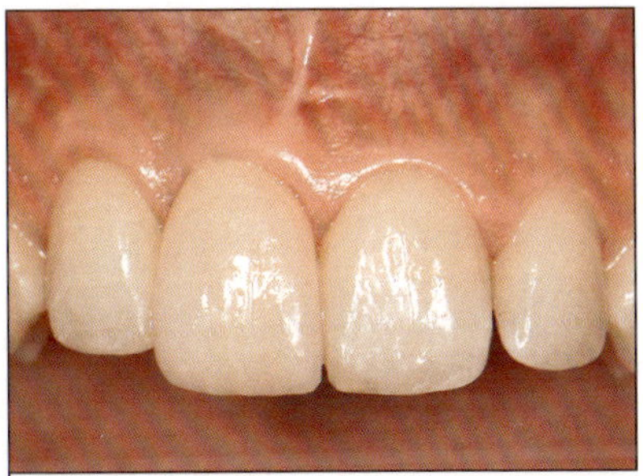

14e

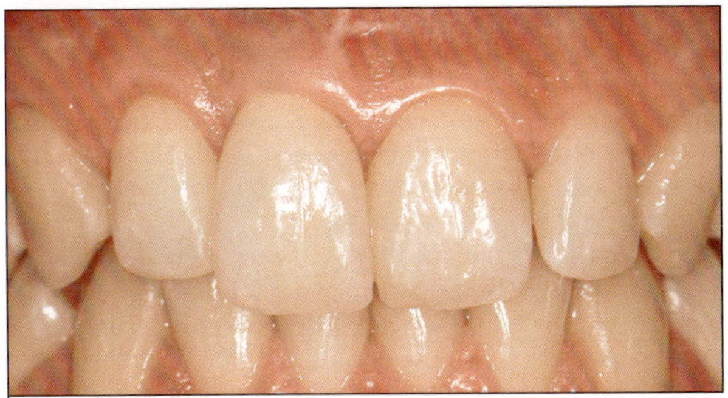

14f

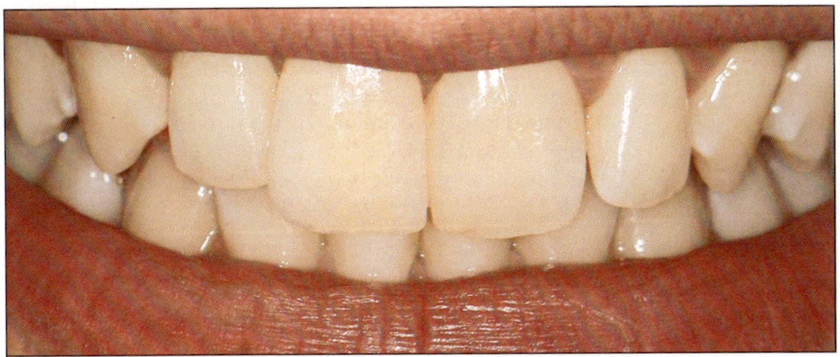

14g

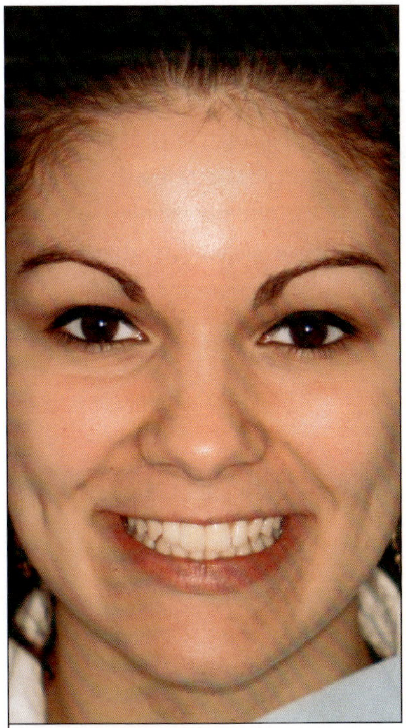

14h

DISCUSSION

The benefits of the flapless technique were discussed previously. In some cases, however, a flapless approach may be contraindicated. Adequate bone levels are necessary to maintain the graft material and promote osteoconduction. Insufficient bone levels may encourage the use of conventional surgical techniques. Further, the soft tissue architecture should be carefully assessed prior to treatment planning. The quality and quantity of soft tissues in relation to the size and position of the implant should be sufficient to indicate a flapless approach.

CONCLUSIONS

Flapless surgery preserves the hard and soft tissues, reduces the length of the surgical and healing phases, and improves patient comfort. The limitations of these surgical procedures depend on the quantity and quality of the soft and hard tissues. The lack of visualization requires greater surgical skill than conventional procedures. Further, because intraoperative findings may require raising a flap, only experienced clinicians with knowledge of conventional surgical techniques should attempt flapless procedures. Computer-based surgical guides should be used to promote ideal implant positioning. When used carefully in the proper situations, this surgical protocol allows patients to benefit from improved implant treatment.

ACKNOWLEDGMENTS

Special thanks to Dr Pascale Montagné, Dr Guillaume Becker, and Mr Jean-Pierre Casu.

REFERENCES

1. Brånemark PI, Hansson BO, Adell R, et al. Osseointegrated implants in the treatment of the edentulous jaw. Experience from a 10-year period. Scand J Plast Reconstr Surg Suppl 1977;16:1–132.

2. Adell R, Lekholm U, Brånemark PI. A 15-year study of osseointegrated implants in the treatment of the edentulous jaw. Int J Oral Surg 1985;10:387–418.

3. Becker W, Becker BE. Flap designs for minimization of recession adjacent to maxillary anterior implant sites: A clinical study. Int J Oral Maxillofac Implants 1996;11:46–54.

4. Rocci A, Martignoni M, Gottlow J. Immediate loading in the maxilla using flapless surgery, implants placed in predetermined positions, and prefabricated provisional restorations: A retrospective 3-year clinical study. Clin Implant Dent Relat Res 2003;5 Suppl 1:29–36.

5. Berdougo ML, Fortin T, Blanchet E, Isidori M, Bosson JL. Flapless implant surgery using an image-guided system. A 1- to 4 year comparative multicenter retrospective clinical study in Lyon. Int J Oral and Maxillofac Implant 2007, abstract 22(4).

6. Fortin TH, Bosson JL, Isidori M, Blanchet E. Effect of flapless surgery on pain experienced in implant placement using an image guided system. Int J Oral Maxillofac Implants 2006;21:298–304.

7. Becker W, Goldstein M, Becker BE, Sennerby L. Minimally invasive flapless implant surgery: A prospective multicenter study. Clin Implant Dent Relat Res 2005;7 Suppl 1:S21–S27.

8. Wöhrle P. Single tooth replacement in the aesthetic zone with immediate provisionalization: Fourteen consecutive case reports. Pract Periodontics Aesthet Dent 1998;9:1107–1114.

9. Wennstrom J, Bengazi F, Lekholm U. The influence of the masticatory mucosa on the peri-implant soft tissue condition. Clin Oral Implants Res 1994;5:1–8.

10. Warrer K, Buser D, Lang NP, Karring T. Plaque induced peri-implantitis in the presence of absence of keratinized mucosa. An experimental study on monkeys. Clin Oral Implants Res 1995;6:131–138.

11. Renouard F, Tulasne JF. Risque anatomique en chirurgie implantaire. Réalités Cliniques 1992;3:311–325.

12. Fortin TH, Coudert JL, Champleboux G, Sautot P, Lavallee S. Computer-assisted dental implant surgery using computed tomography. J Image Guid Surg 1995;1:53–58.

13. Verstreken K, Van Cleynenbreugel J, Marchal G, Naert I, Suetens P, Van Steenberghe D. Computer-assisted planning of oral implant surgery: A three-dimensional approach. Int J Oral Maxillofac Implants 1996;11:806–810.

14. Fortin TH, Champleboux G, Lormee I, Coudert JL. Very precise dental implant placement on bone using surgical guides in conjunction with medical imaging techniques. J Oral Implantol 2000;26:300–303.

15. Tardieu P, Vrielinck I, Escolano E. Computer-assisted implant placement. A case report: Treatment of the mandible. Int J Oral Maxillofac Implants 2003;18: 599–604.

16. Van Steenberghe D, Malevez C, Van Cleynenbreugel J, et al. Accuracy of drilling guides for transfer from three-dimensional CT-based planning to place of zygoma implants in human cadavers. Clin Oral Implants Res 2003;14:131–136.

17. Fortin TH, Bosson JL, Coudert JL, Isidori M. Reliability of preoperative planning of an image-guided system for oral implant placement based on 3-dimensional images: An in vivo study. Int J Oral Maxillofac Implants 2003;18: 886–893.

18. Fortin TH, Isidori M, Blanchet E, Perriat M, Bouchet H, Coudert JL. An image-guided system drilled surgical template and trephine guide pin to make treatment of completely edentulous patients easier: A clinical report on immediate loading. Clin Implant Dent Relat Res 2004;6: 111–119.

19. Gillot L, Cannas B. Mise en charge immédiate avec une prothèse élaborée avant la phase chirurgicale. L'information Dentaire 2005;31:1871–1876.

20. Vaida C, Mattout P, Lascu L. Le concept Nobelguide, la planification implantaire en 3D sur ordinateur. J Parodontologie d'Implantologie Orale 2006;25:263–280.

21. Müller HP, Eger T. Gingival phenotypes in young male adults. J Clin Periodontol 1997;24:65–71.

22. Goasling GD, Robertson PB, Maham CJ, Morrison WW, Olson JV. Thickness of facial gingiva. J Periodontol 1977; 48:768–771.

23. Khoury F, Antoun H, Missika P. Bone augmentation in Oral Implantology. Chicago: Quintessence, 2007.

24. Bonnet F. Minimally invasive surgery of the healed ridges: Classification and surgical techniques. J Parodontologie d'Implantologie Orale. Vol 26(4).

ZIRCONIA IMPLANT FIXED PARTIAL DENTURE REPLACING MULTIPLE MISSING TEETH IN THE ESTHETIC ZONE: A CASE REPORT AND TECHNICAL ASPECTS

Davide Riva, ODT[1]
Luca Pizzoni, DDS, MS[2]

Patients' esthetic and functional demands are increasing every year. To satisfy these often challenging requests, new devices and techniques for implant and prosthetic treatments have been developed. The aim of this article is to describe the technical and clinical procedures necessary to achieve optimal functional and esthetic results using one such promising prosthetic option—the zirconia implant fixed partial denture (FPD)—via the presentation of a challenging clinical case.

In recent years, zirconia has been presented as a suitable material for implant-supported restorations, particularly when high esthetic demands are present. The development of computer-aided design/computer-assisted manufacture (CAD/CAM) technology allows for a high level of precision, as well as the chance to work with a reliable, industrialized product. However, research in both the dental

material and clinical fields is still ongoing. For computer numeric controlled–milled titanium frameworks, the precision of fit has been tested in vitro,[1–3] and the clinical performance has been followed in the long term.[4–6] On the other hand, although the fracture resistance of zirconia frameworks has been tested in vitro,[7] clinical data on the long-term success of these restorations are still limited.[8]

CASE REPORT

The patient was a 71.1-year-old woman in a good general medical condition. Her chief complaints were pain and swelling of the palatal mucosa in the area of the maxillary right canine and first premolar, which had occurred 3 days prior to presentation, and the poor esthetics of her smile, which had worsened over the previous year.

Her oral examination revealed palatal swelling and inflammation in the areas mentioned above. A one-piece gold resin FPD in the maxilla spanning from first molar to first molar was present and appeared separated (as a result of decay) from the

[1]Milan, Italy.
[2]Lecturer, Department of Odontology, Instituto Ortopedico Galeazzi, University of Milan, Italy.

Correspondence to: Mr Davide Riva, Via Vela 3, 20133 Milan, Italy. Fax: 3902 2952 3411. E-mail: driva@fastwebnet.it

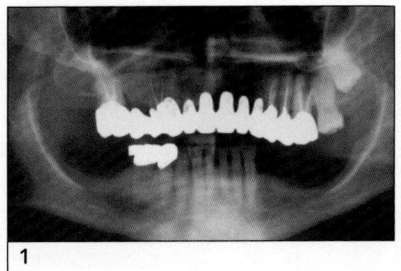 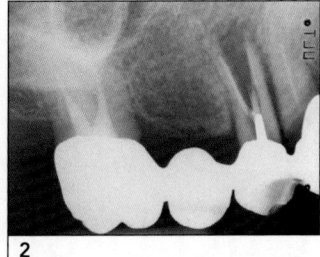

Fig 1 Pretreatment panoramic radiograph.

Fig 2 Pretreatment intraoral radiograph.

root of the right canine, which was palatally dislocated. Without any tooth support in the anterior region, the FPD had gradually changed inclination, while the anterior pontic elements moved up in the buccal mucosa. The patient had healthy but worn mandibular incisors and canines. The mandibular right and second premolars had been treated with gold resin crowns. A mandibular removable prosthesis was present in the remaining lateral segments.

The periodontal examination showed sufficient oral hygiene, with no probing pocket depths except for a 6-mm pocket on the mesial aspect of the maxillary left first molar and a 12-mm pocket palatal and buccal to the maxillary right first premolar with pus. The panoramic (Fig 1) and intraoral (Fig 2) radiographs revealed decay at the maxillary right canine and a vertical root fracture at the maxillary right first premolar. Both teeth had received previous endodontic treatment but showed radiolucent apical lesions. The maxillary right first molar and left premolars and first molar had also received endodontic treatment. The left second molar was healthy, while the third molar was impacted. All remaining teeth in the maxilla were missing. The patient showed generalized moderate horizontal bone resorption and a vertical defect mesial to the right first molar. Severe vertical and horizontal bone resorption was present in the mandibular lateral edentulous segments.

The patient showed no tooth exposure at rest or when smiling. A decreased lower face height was evident, and the patient's profile had a mild Class III tendency, with chin prominence and minimal upper lip support.

Technical Aspects

The solution, planned with the clinician, was to obtain a one-piece zirconia restoration that would be screwed directly at the implant level. This solution makes it possible to finalize the prosthesis in one CAD/CAM step; in contrast, an FPD over abutments would require more steps, leading to possible drawbacks in terms of precision, cost, and time. Further, the method selected is an optimal solution for cases in which the screw access holes are positioned in the occlusal and palatal/lingual areas. Another advantage is that the prosthesis can be removed if needed.

Treatment Plan

The treatment plan was as follows:

1. Systemic antibiotic therapy (1g amoxicillin every 12 hours for 6 days)
2. Scaling, root planing, and oral hygiene instruction
3. Extraction of the maxillary right canine and first premolar
4. Placement of provisional removable partial prostheses in the maxilla and mandible to reestablish the vertical dimension of occlusion
5. Composite resin restoration of the mandibular anterior teeth
6. Placement of osseointegrated implants at the maxillary right second premolar and canine and left central incisor and canine sites with the aid of a surgical guide from the waxup
7. Placement of a zirconia implant FPD

Figs 3 and 4 Intraoral views prior to implant placement.

Fig 5 Intraoral evaluation of the resin framework.

Fig 6 Extraoral evaluation of the resin framework. Note the upper lip support.

Fig 7 Intraoral view after implant placement.

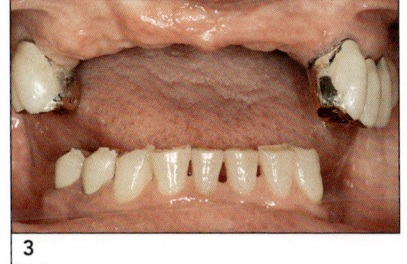

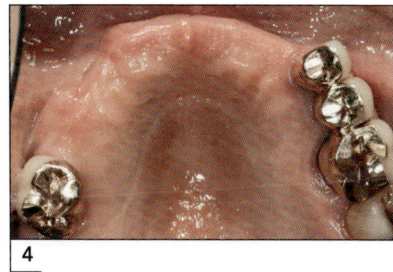

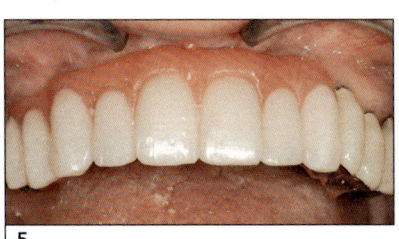

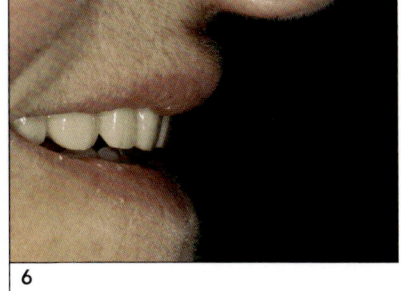

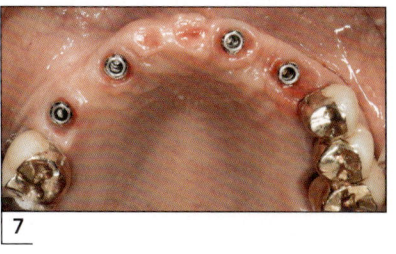

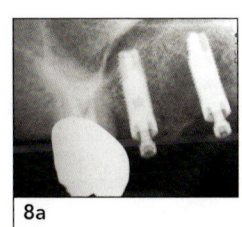

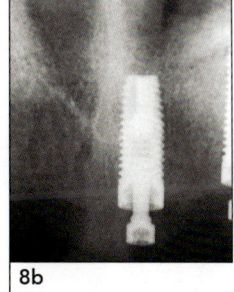

Figs 8a to 8c Intraoral radiographs after implant placement.

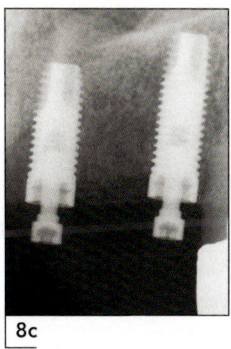

Since placing implants in the mandibular lateral segments would require bone augmentation, the patient preferred to continue use of a removable partial denture in that area. For financial reasons, she also chose to keep the gold resin crowns on the remaining maxillary teeth.

Treatment

After the extraction of the maxillary right canine and first premolar (Figs 3 and 4), the patient used a provisional removable partial denture in both arches, and a composite resin restoration of the mandibular anterior teeth was fabricated. Esthetics and function were evaluated in the provisional phase. Implant placement was carried out 5 months after extraction. Since the levels of keratinized gingiva and bone were sufficient, a flapless technique was used to minimize patient discomfort. All implants had a rough surface and dimensions of 4×13 mm, except for the implant at the maxillary left central incisor, which measured 4×11 mm. The bone quality was type 3, according to Lekholm and Zarb,[9] and the implant primary stability was good (32 Ncm). The implants were restored with a provisional resin FPD. The bone quality and implant stability, together with the fact that the patient was accustomed to wearing a removable prosthesis, suggested that immediate loading of the implants should not be used in this particular case. The manufacturing phase of the zirconia implant FPD began 6 months after placement of the provisional restorations (Figs 5 to 8).

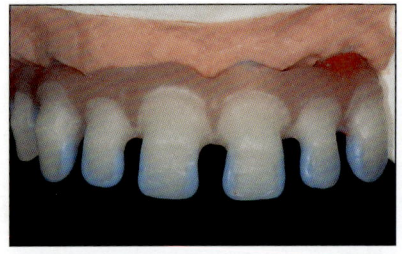 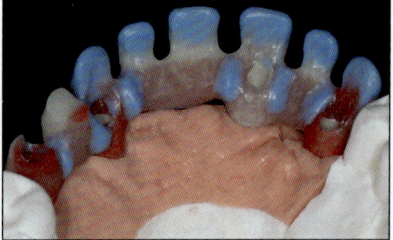

Figs 9a and 9b Frontal (a) and palatal (b) views of the resin framework.

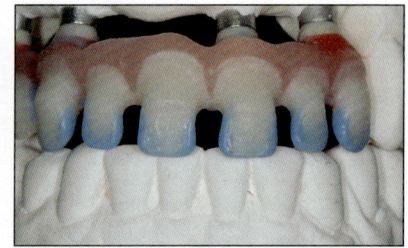

Fig 10 Resin framework on the master cast for the scanning procedure.

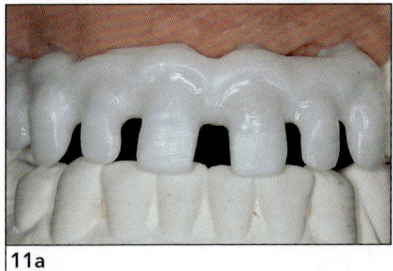 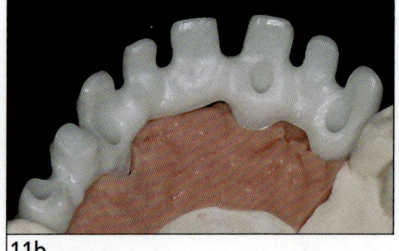 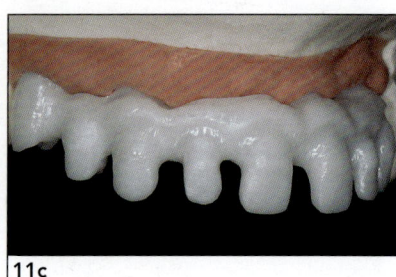

11a 11b 11c

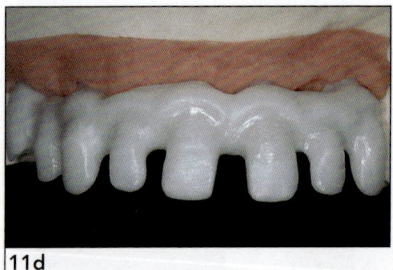 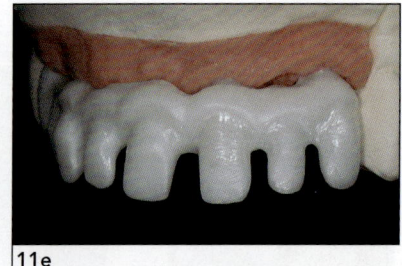

11d 11e

Figs 11a to 11e Zirconia framework on the master cast.

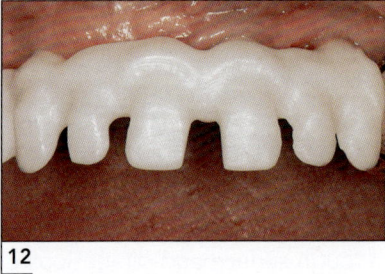 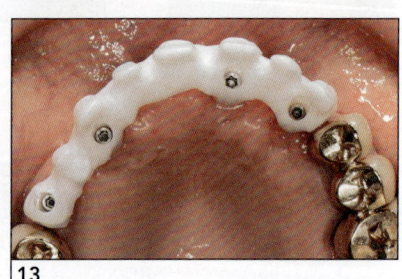

12 13

Figs 12 and 13 Intraoral views of the zirconia framework.

Technical Procedure

The master cast must replicate the correct position of each implant using a transfer impression. This should be accurately checked using a stone control key connecting all impression copings on each replica.

A resin framework was fabricated for the scanning procedure (Figs 9 and 10). Thanks to advanced scanning and CAD procedures, it is possible to obtain a product with the following beneficial properties:

1. Framework design offering correct support to the veneering ceramics. The design should incorporate all information obtained from the diagnostic waxup and provisional phase. Moreover, it is important to respect the dimensions of the framework, particularly in the connection areas (Figs 11 to 13).
2. High-density sinterized material (industrial machined zirconium oxide) that ensures good resistance and stability during the baking procedures.[7]
3. Optimal marginal connection thanks to the latest CAD/CAM technology.[8]

Fig 14 Liner application on the zirconia framework.

Fig 15 Zirconia framework after baking of the liner.

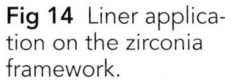

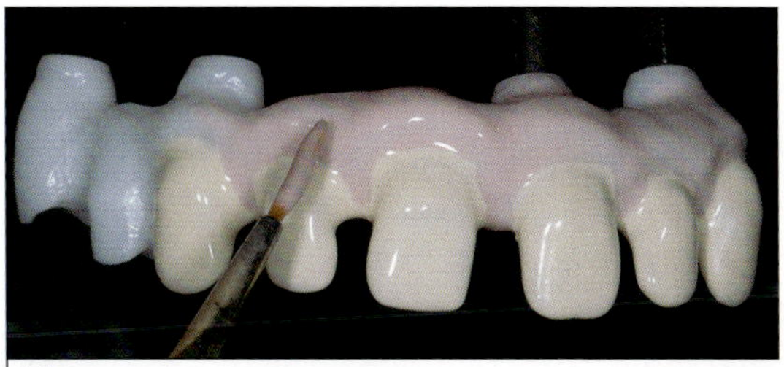

Figs 16a to 16d First layering stage. *(a)* Buildup of the dentin core. *(b)* Application of incisal effects. *(c)* Application of enamel and transparent layers. *(d)* Layering of the gingival area.

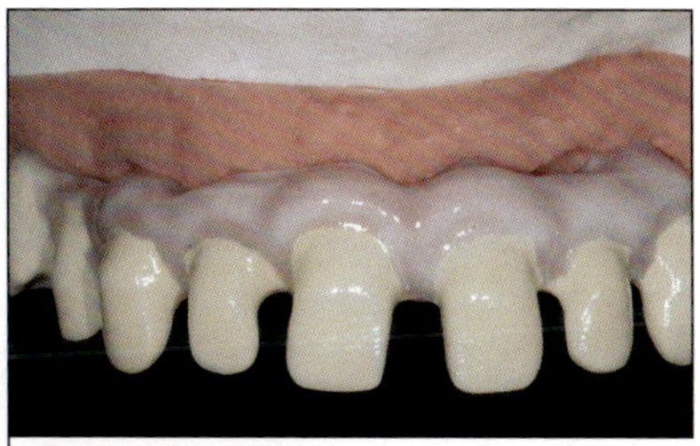

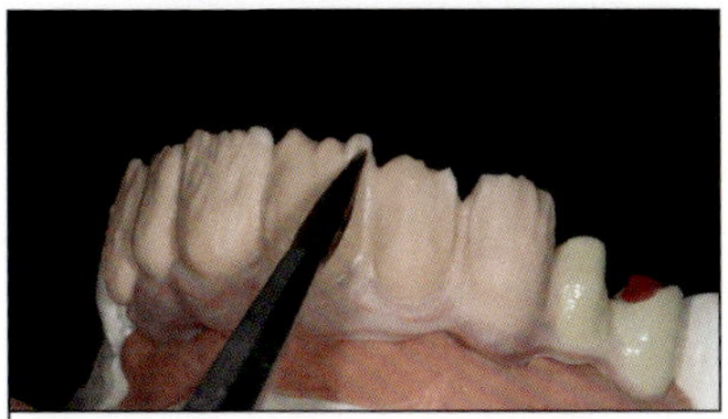

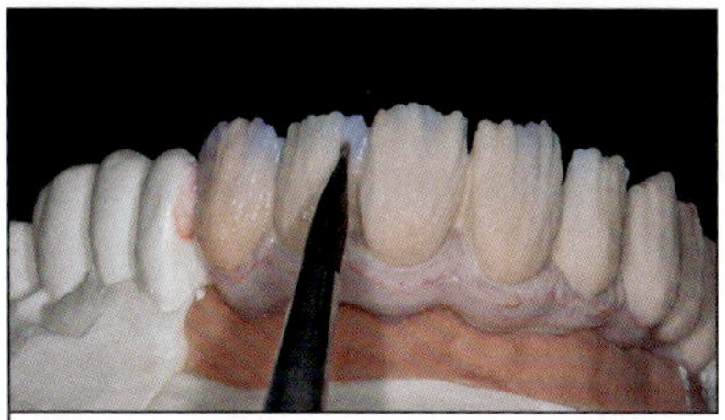

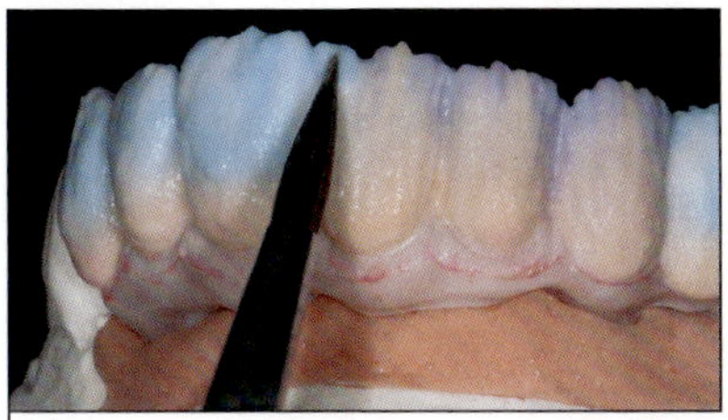

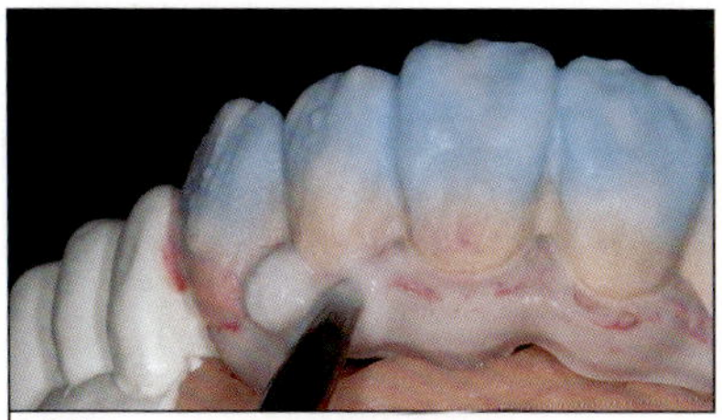

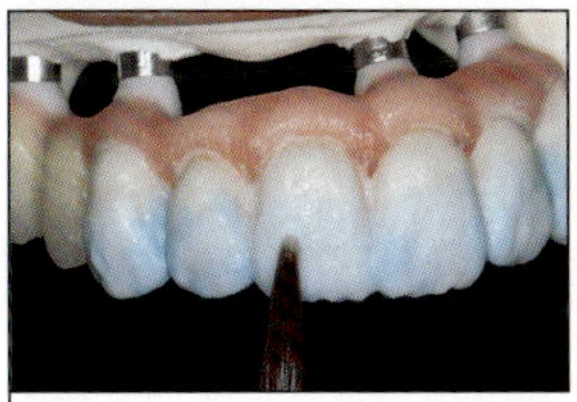

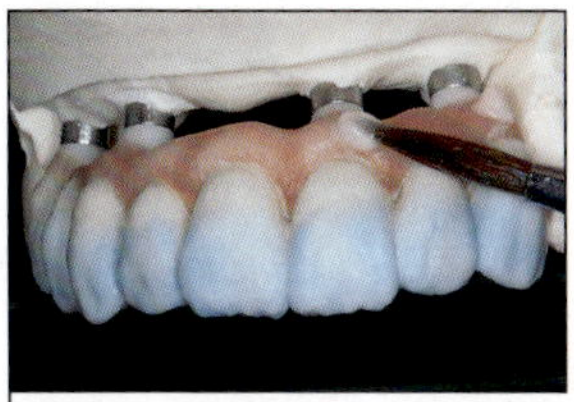

Figs 17 and 18 Second layering stage using transparents and pink ceramic.

Layering Procedure

Ceramic layering begins with liners. In tooth areas, a liner is used to achieve a warm substrate for the chosen color. In gingival areas, a pink liner is applied (Figs 14 and 15).

In long-span FPDs, as in this case, it is better to simplify the layering process by using only a few masses; this way, the technician can focus on finding the right combination between the dentin core design and enamel layer to obtain natural light dynamics (Fig 16a). Incisal effects can be used to emphasize this aspect, but it is important to maintain good control of their position; in other words, too little is better than too much (Fig 16b). At this stage, the shape can be completed using enamel and transparent layers (Fig 16c). Regarding the gingival areas, a couple of pink masses can be combined (Fig 16d).

The second layering is a critical phase, because it is of primary importance to maintain humidity during all stages of application (Figs 17 and 18). In

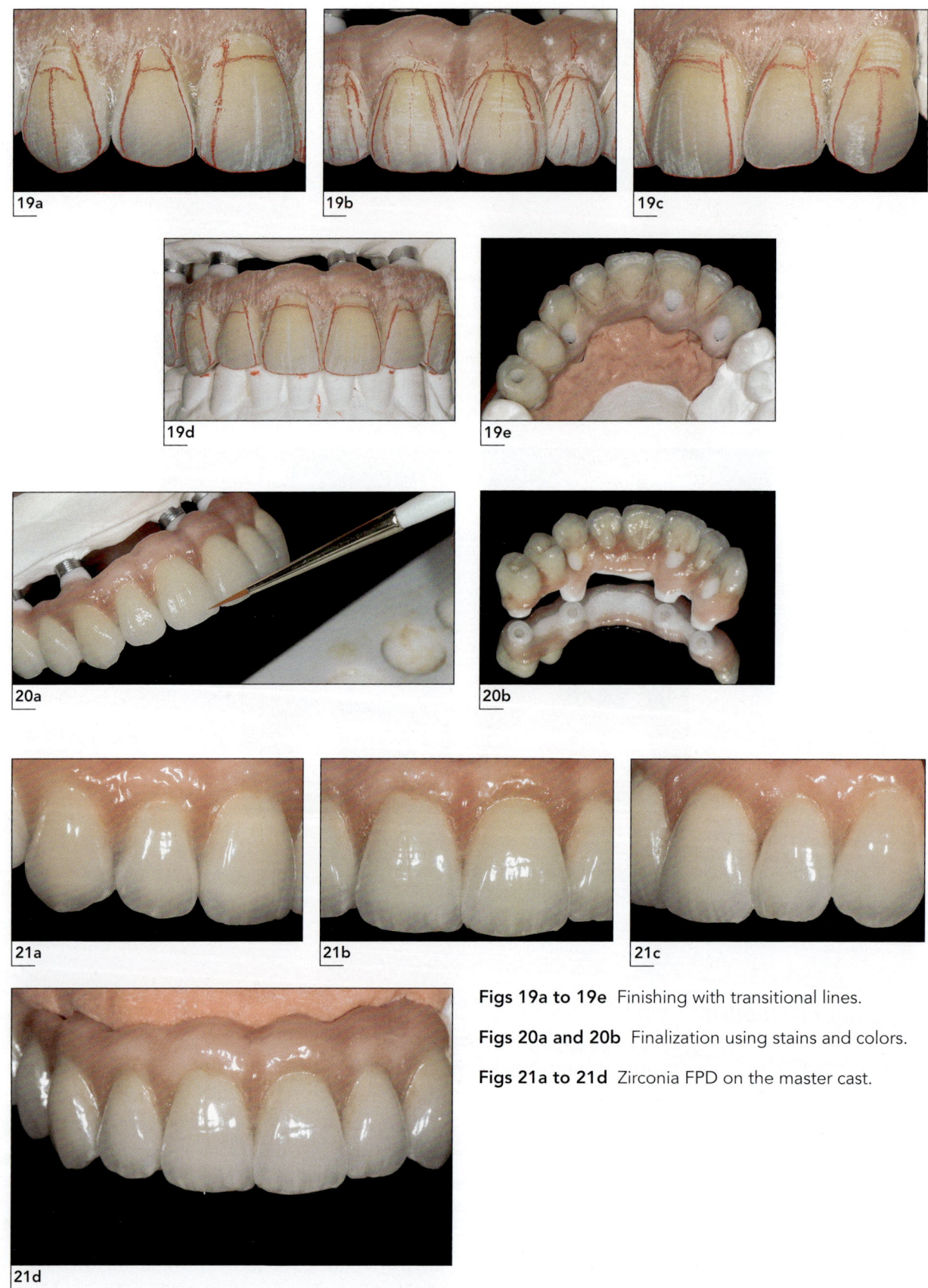

19a

19b

19c

19d

19e

20a

20b

21a

21b

21c

21d

Figs 19a to 19e Finishing with transitional lines.

Figs 20a and 20b Finalization using stains and colors.

Figs 21a to 21d Zirconia FPD on the master cast.

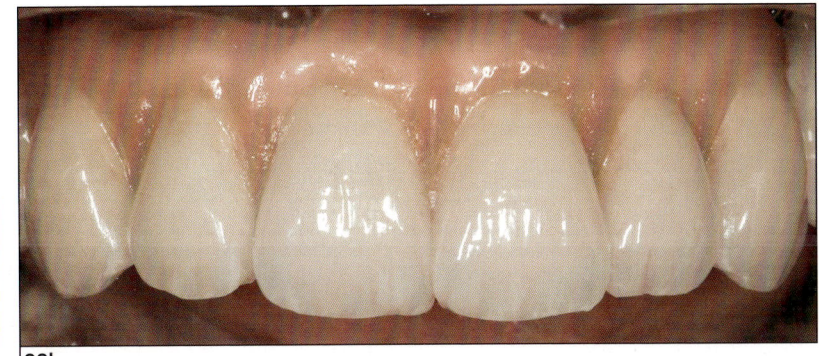

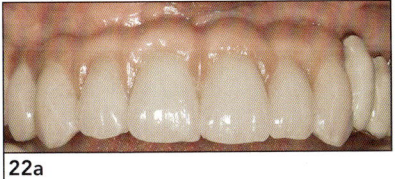

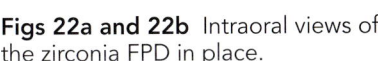

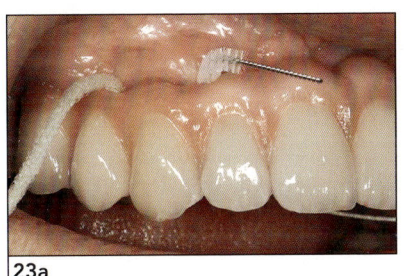

Figs 22a and 22b Intraoral views of the zirconia FPD in place.

Figs 23a and 23b It is important to leave space between the framework and gingiva for oral hygiene devices.

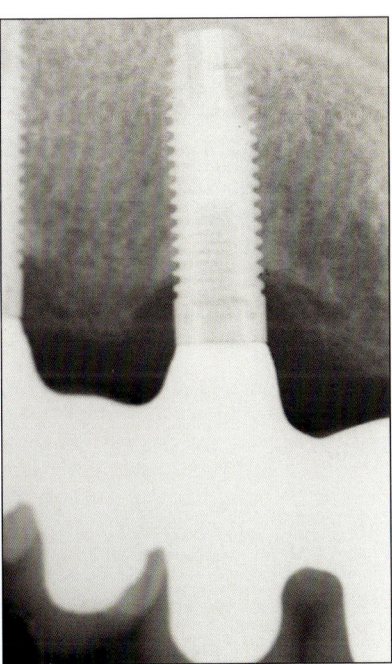

Figs 24a to 24c Intraoral radiographs of the implants with the zirconia FPD attached only at the maxillary right second premolar in order to check the passive fit.

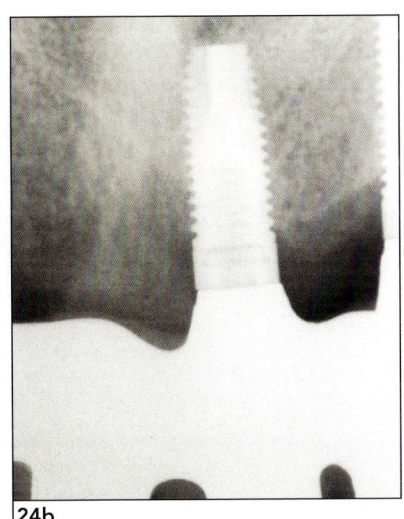

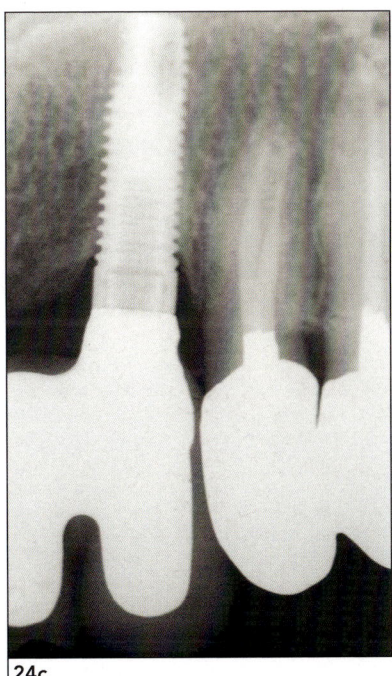

this regard, it helps to add a drop of stain liquid to the masses. Ceramic layering is an important part of achieving a natural appearance; however, the esthetic result also depends on a variety of other considerations, most importantly, the dynamic of light on the surfaces. This depends primarily on the positions of the transitional lines (Fig 19). In this case, the interaction between the teeth and ceramic gingiva produced a natural esthetic result (Figs 20 to 24).

CONCLUSIONS

New technological achievements combining CAD/CAM procedures and industrial framework production allow clinicians and technicians to satisfy patients' functional and esthetic demands. Further, these techniques offer prosthetic devices with high resistance and precision that can be produced with less complex and time-consuming procedures. Nevertheless, the diagnostic and treatment planning phases maintain their utmost importance, together with the clinical and technical skills of all members of the treatment team. In particular, the technician should focus on the design and esthetic components of the restoration.

ACKNOWLEDGMENTS

Mr Riva thanks his collaborator, Roberto Dulevio, for the excellent effort that always characterizes his work, as well as his assistant, Michaela Riva, for her help assembling this article.

REFERENCES

1. Al-Fadda SA, Zarb GA, Finer Y. A comparison of the accuracy of fit of 2 methods for fabricating implant-prosthodontic frameworks. Int J Prosthodont 2007;20:125–131.

2. Takahashi T, Gunne J. Fit of implant frameworks: An in vitro comparison between two fabrication techniques. J Prosthet Dent 2003;89:256–260.

3. Ortorp A, Jemt T, Bäck T, Jälevik T. Comparisons of precision of fit between cast and CNC-milled titanium implant frameworks for the edentulous mandible. Int J Prosthodont 2003;16:194–200.

4. Ortorp A, Jemt T. Clinical experiences of CNC-milled titanium frameworks supported by implants in the edentulous jaw: 1-year prospective study. Clin Implant Dent Relat Res 2000;2:2–9.

5. Ortorp A, Jemt T. Clinical experience of CNC-milled titanium frameworks supported by implants in the edentulous jaw: A 3-year interim report. Clin Implant Dent Relat Res 2002;4:104–109.

6. Ortorp A, Jemt T. Clinical experiences of computer numeric control–milled titanium frameworks supported by implants in the edentulous jaw: A 5-year prospective study. Clin Implant Dent Relat Res 2004;6:199–209.

7. Vult von Steyern P. All-ceramic fixed partial dentures. Studies on aluminum oxide– and zirconium dioxide–based ceramic systems. Swed Dent J Suppl 2005;(173):1–69.

8. Raigrodski AJ. Contemporary materials and technologies for all-ceramic fixed partial dentures: A review of the literature. J Prosthet Dent 2004;92:557–562.

9. Lekholm U, Zarb, GA. Patient selection and preparation. In: Branemark PI, Zarb GA, Albrektsson T (eds). Tissue-Integrated Prostheses: Osseointegration in Clinical Dentistry. Chicago: Quintessence, 1985.

THE USE OF SIX ANTERIOR METALLOCERAMIC TEETH IN A MAXILLARY COMPLETE OVERDENTURE

Bruno R. Chrcanovic, DDS[1]
Rolf Ankli, DPT[2]

An overdenture is a removable complete or partial prosthesis with a denture base covering one or more natural teeth or implants. The overdenture concept for removable partial denture treatment is well-established. One of the first published reports in the dental literature was by Ledger in 1856,[1] which encouraged clinicians to leave root stumps under artificial teeth.

The reasoning for the overdenture concept is based on the conservative management of remaining dentition. The remaining teeth in partially edentulous arches may be spaced in such a way that the arrangement of replacement teeth is severely restricted. In these cases, the situation can be greatly improved if the offending teeth are endodontically treated, coronally amputated, and used as overdenture abutments.[2] This increases

[1]Private practice, Belo Horizonte, Brazil.
[2]Belo Horizonte, Brazil.

Correspondence to: Dr Bruno R. Chrcanovic, Av. Raja Gabaglia 1000 sala 1209, Gutierrez, Belo Horizonte, Minas Gerais, CEP 30380-090, Brazil. E-mail: brunochrcanovic@hotmail.com

tooth support of the overlying base, encourages bone retention, and improves stability.

As an alternative method to improve the overall esthetics of prosthetic treatment, this article describes a clinical case of overdenture construction with six anterior metalloceramic teeth built in a conventional acrylic resin base. This method may also be used for conventional complete dentures.

CASE REPORT

The middle-aged female patient was in the middle of treatment with another dental clinician and technician. The pretreatment panoramic radiograph showed the presence of 19 teeth (Fig 1). When she presented at the author's dental office, only the six anterior teeth with a partial removable prosthesis remained in the maxilla, along with a provisional removable prosthesis over four implants in the mandible (Figs 2 to 4). The other dental clinician had planned to remove all remaining maxillary teeth and place a maxillary overdenture over implants; however, the patient was unsatisfied with

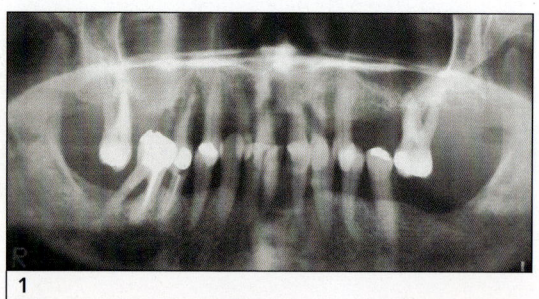

Fig 1 Pretreatment panoramic radiograph.

Figs 2 and 3 Patient's smile at the initial presentation.

Fig 4 Radiographic status after initial treatment by another clinician.

Figs 5 and 6 Periapical radiographs of the maxillary anterior teeth.

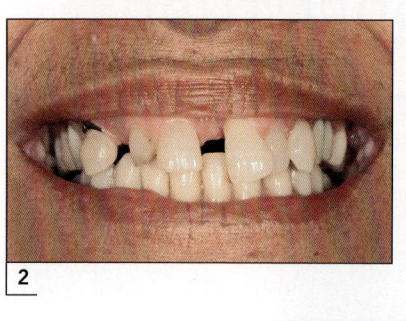

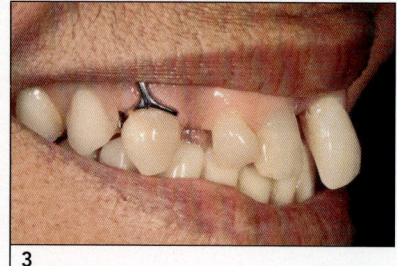

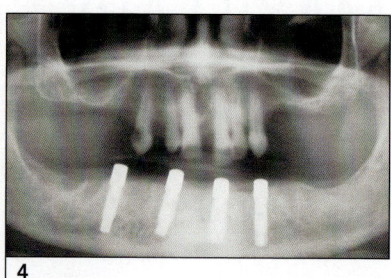

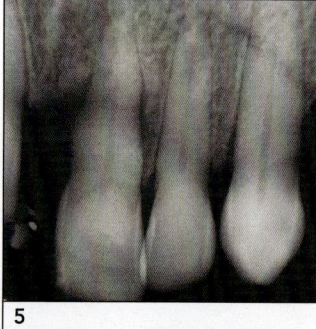

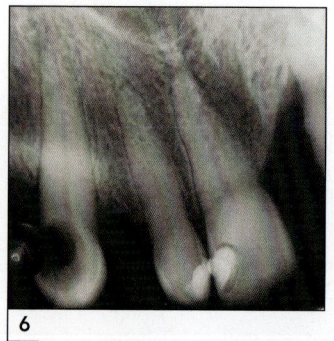

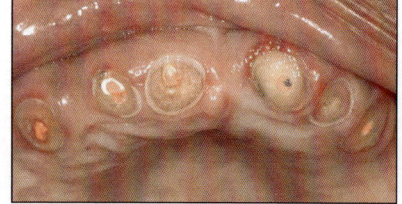

Fig 7 Tooth roots reduced to the gingival level after endodontic treatment.

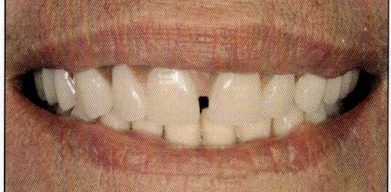

Fig 8 Maxillary provisional prosthesis in place.

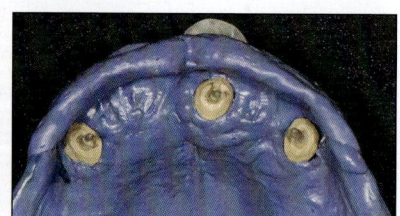

Fig 9 Cast gold pins transferred in an individual tray.

this clinician and wanted to conclude the definitive maxillary work with another treatment team. After taking new periapical radiographs of the maxillary anterior teeth (Figs 5 and 6), it was decided to place an overdenture over the natural roots.

All remaining teeth were periodontally and endodontically treated and then reduced to the level of the gingiva (Fig 7). A provisional prosthesis was then placed (Fig 8). Three teeth—the right first premolar,

right central incisor, and left canine—were chosen to support attachments. The three other teeth—the right canine, left central incisor, and left lateral incisor—were restored with photopolymerized acrylic resin. The three pulp canals were prepared, and an impression was made. Three cast pins with caps were inserted into the pulp canal and then transferred in an individual tray (Fig 9). A working cast with the pins (Fig 10) was then fabricated and used

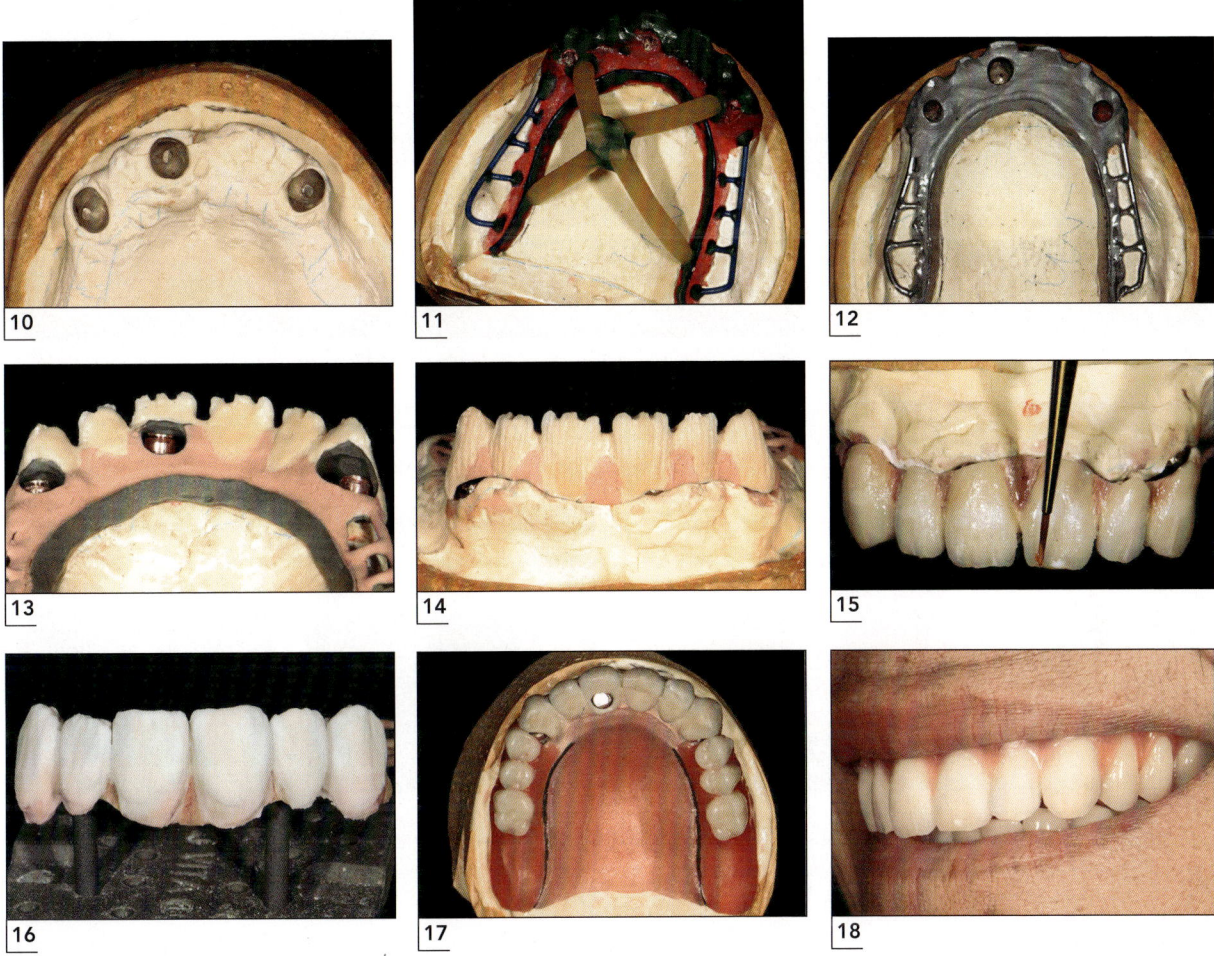

Fig 10 Working cast with the transferred cast gold pins.

Fig 11 Fabrication of the metal structure prior to casting.

Fig 12 Metal structure after casting.

Fig 13 Holes were made in the structure to retain the attachment's female part.

Fig 14 Metal structure after wash-opaque, opaque, and effect liners.

Fig 15 Characterizations after the first porcelain firing.

Fig 16 Replacement teeth just before the second porcelain firing.

Fig 17 Posterior acrylic resin teeth mounted and covered palatally with wax for the try-in.

Fig 18 Try-in of the maxillary overdenture.

to place Dalla Bona attachments (Dalbo attachments, Cendres & Métaux, Biel-Bienne, Switzerland). These attachments were soldered to the pins, and the metal infrastructure was fabricated (Figs 11 and 12). Holes were made in the structure to promote acrylic retention of the attachment's female part during the acrylization process (Fig 13). Pink opaque resin was used to mask the dark color of the metal. Opaque and effect liners were applied (Fig 14). The VITA VM13 ceramic system (VITA Zahnfabrik, Bad Säckingen, Germany) was used. Some characterizations were made after the first porcelain firing (Fig 15), which was followed by a second firing (Fig 16). Next, the unfinished structure was mounted with the posterior acrylic resin teeth (Vivadent, Schaan, Liechtenstein) (Fig 17) for try-in before final glazing (Fig 18).

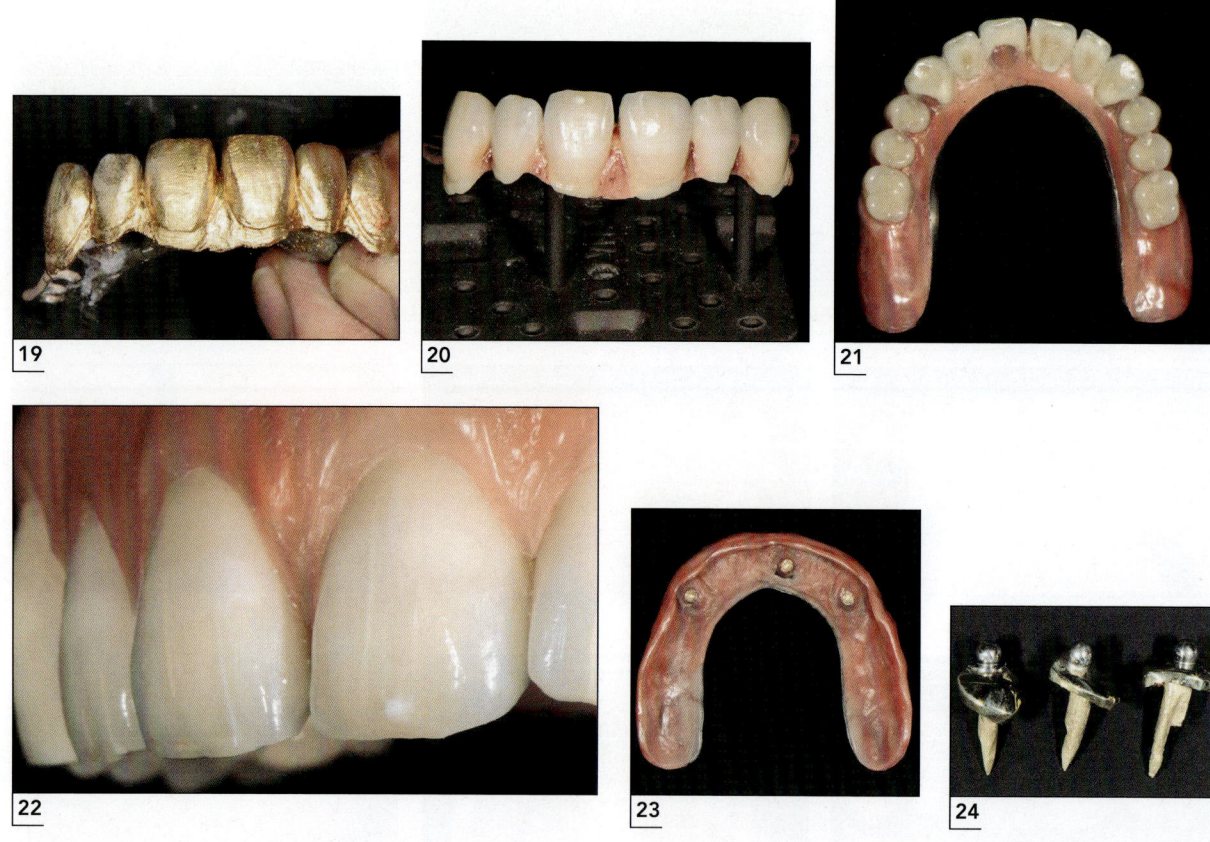

19

20

21

22

23

24

Fig 19 Gold powder used to visualize the porcelain texture.

Fig 20 Replacement teeth after glazing.

Fig 21 Prosthesis after acrylization.

Fig 22 Close-up view of the acrylic gingiva.

Fig 23 The attachment's female part located on the inner side of the prosthesis.

Fig 24 The attachment's male part welded to the cast gold pins.

After patient, clinician, and technician approval, the porcelain texture was elaborated (Fig 19), and porcelain finishing was completed with the glazing process (Fig 20). Acrylization was then carried out (Fig 21). The appearance of the acrylic gingiva was excellent (Fig 22). The inner side of the prosthesis contained the female part of the attachment (Fig 23), while the pins contained the male part (Fig 24). The pins were then cemented onto the selected roots (Figs 25 and 26). Figures 27 to 30 show the final result. The patient requested a small diastema between the central incisors.

DISCUSSION

In partially edentulous arches, one or more remaining teeth may be unsuitable for inclusion as abutments for direct retainers. The teeth may be severely compromised by decay, show irreparable fracture of the coronal structure, have shortened roots, or be displaced to such a degree that they cannot reasonably be considered for use as conventional abutments. If bone retention in the area of such a tooth is a pertinent factor in the treatment plan, the root structure should be retained to permit its use as an overdenture abutment. When

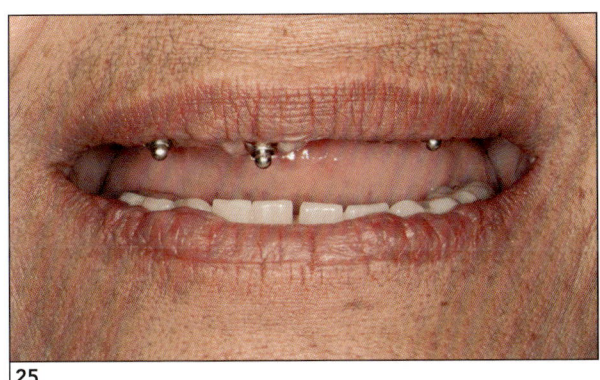

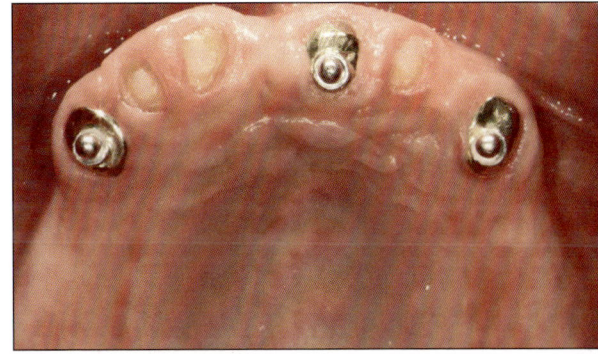

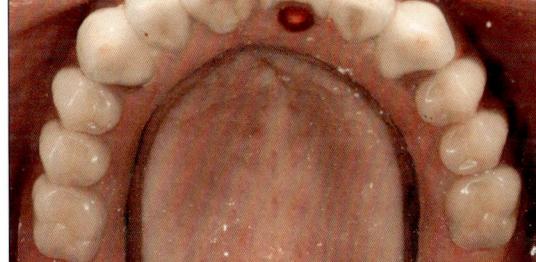

Figs 25 and 26 Cast gold pins cemented to the roots.

Figs 27 to 30 Final result.

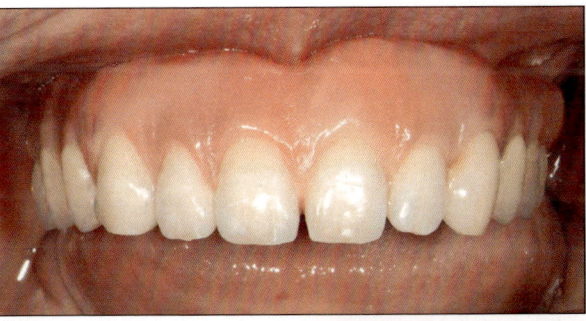

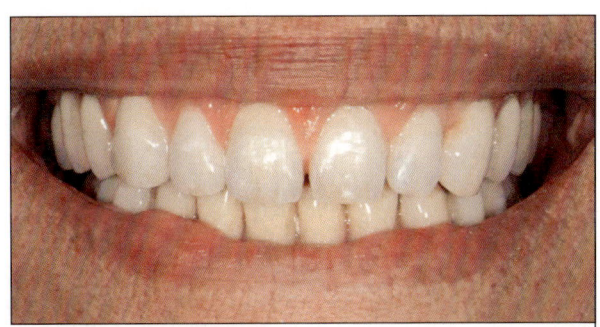

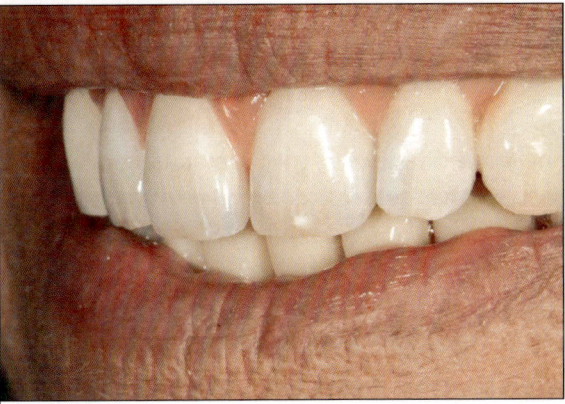

the remaining tooth structure is severely compromised, a coronal prosthesis can be prepared to accept a variety of attachments, including magnets, clips, snaps, and O-rings. All of these attachments provide positive retention while engaging minimal vertical space.

Atwood[3] and Tallgren[4] demonstrated that extracting a patient's remaining dentition with or without long-term complete or partial denture restoration significantly reduces the quantity and quality of the residual ridges. Miller[5] and Crum and Rooney[6] reported less reduction of the residual ridges when using a mandibular overdenture supported by canine roots as opposed to a conventional mandibular complete denture.

In this case, preserving the maxillary anterior residual ridge was necessary to prevent the sequellae of anterior hyperfunction syndrome, or *combination syndrome*, a term coined originally by Kelley in 1972.[7] The clinical signs and symptoms of combination syndrome consist of loss of osseous tissue in the anterior maxilla, formation of hyperplastic tissue, overgrowth of the maxillary tuberosities, increased pneumatization of maxillary sinuses, papillary hyperplasia, denture stomatitis of the palatal mucosa underlying the maxillary complete denture, disorientation of the plane of occlusion, and extrusion and periodontal pathology around remaining mandibular anterior teeth, causing loss of osseous tissue in the anterior maxilla.[8] By retaining one or more roots in the maxillary anterior region under an overdenture, this cycle of destructive changes may be prevented.

The mechanism of alveolar ridge maintenance through root retention occurs because of the root's ability to convert the compressive force of denture bearing into tensile force to the bone via the periodontal ligament. Occlusal forces generated during mastication are directed through the denture teeth and acrylic resin base to both the abutment roots and the mucosa overlying the supporting residual ridge. This stimulatory effect is transmitted through all fibers of the periodontal ligament and, as long as the forces are not excessive, promotes maintenance of the crestal bone and roots. Because clinical crowns are not present, forces are directed down the long axes of the abutments without torque or tipping.[8]

Because of the maintenance of periodontal ligament proprioceptors, patients treated with overdentures can more effectively regulate the range and type of chewing cycle in masticatory reflex and discriminate loads greater than 2,000 g better than complete-denture wearers.[9] Further, these patients demonstrate increased masticatory muscle efficiency[10] and 79% chewing efficiency compared with 59% in patients treated with complete dentures.[11]

For the partially edentulous patient, preserving the remaining teeth provides great psychologic comfort. In general, patient acceptance of overdentures is superior to conventional dentures, especially in the mandibular arch. This is because patients generally prefer to retain some of their natural dentition, even in an altered form.

Improper maintenance of periodontal health and dental caries is the leading cause of overdenture abutment loss. However, maintaining periodontal health with overdentures can actually be easier than maintaining periodontal health with the natural dentition, as long as the patient is given proper oral hygiene instructions. Crown removal provides physical access that makes it easier to maintain proper oral hygiene on isolated overdenture abutments.

Treating patients with overdentures is more costly than with conventional prostheses. This is due to the additional expense of endodontics and periodontal therapy or implant surgery when the roots of the natural teeth are missing. Further, there is the added cost of restoring the root stumps with attachments, although the resulting restoration will be substantially less costly than a fixed prosthesis.

This case was even more expensive than a usual overdenture with prefabricated teeth; however, the use of metalloceramic replacement teeth improved the overall esthetics. It should also be noted that the patient must be careful when removing the prosthesis to avoid breakage of the fragile porcelain anterior teeth.

CONCLUSION

Good preliminary results of a provisional prosthesis are essential to the final esthetic outcome. Conservative treatment planning should always be carried out when possible. Even with the rise of implant restorations, the use of viable dental roots with overdenture rehabilitation remains a valid treatment that may be attractive to patients who are opposed to more invasive oral surgeries.

REFERENCES

1. Ledger E. On preparing the mouth for the reception of a full set of artificial teeth. Br J Dent Sci 1856;1:90–96.
2. Castleberry DJ. Philosophies and principles of removable partial overdentures. Dent Clin North Am 1990;34:589–592.
3. Atwood DA. Reduction of the residual ridges. A major oral disease entity. J Prosthet Dent 1971;26:266–279.
4. Tallgren A. The continuing reduction of the alveolar ridges in complete denture wearers: A mixed longitudinal study covering 25 years. J Prosthet Dent 1972;27:120–132.
5. Miller PA. Complete dentures supported by natural teeth. J Prosthet Dent 1958;8:924–928.
6. Crum RJ, Rooney GE Jr. Alveolar bone loss in overdentures—A 5 year study. J Prosthet Dent 1978;40:610–613.
7. Kelley E. Changes caused by a mandibular removable partial denture opposing a maxillary complete denture. 1972. J Prosthet Dent 2003;90:213–219.
8. Renner RP. The overdenture concept. Dent Clin North Am 1990;34:593–606.
9. Pacer FJ, Bowman DC. Occlusal force discrimination by denture patients. J Prosthet Dent 1975;33:602–609.
10. Nagasawa T, Okane H, Tsuru H. The role of the periodontal ligament in overdenture treatment. J Prosthet Dent 1979;42:12–16.
11. Rissin L, House JE, Manly RS, et al. Clinical comparison of mastigatory performance and electromyographic activity of patients with complete dentures, overdentures, and natural teeth. J Prosthet Dent 1978;39:508–511.

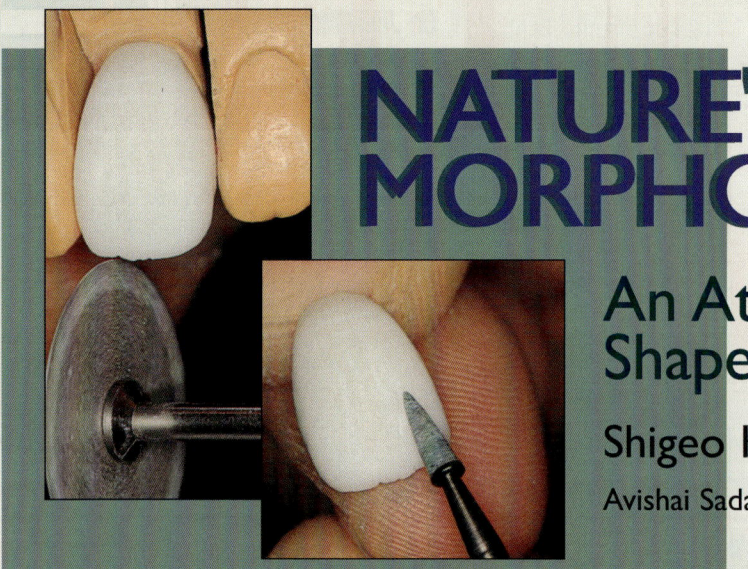
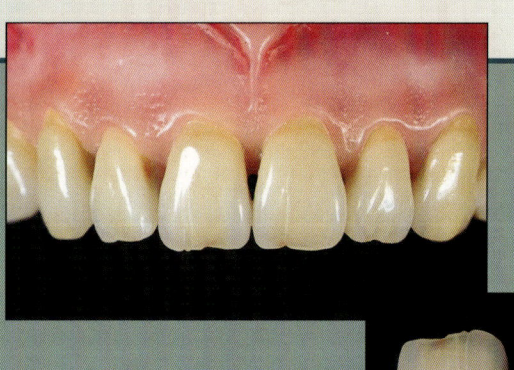
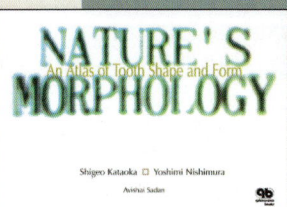
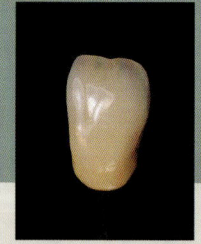
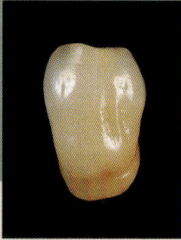
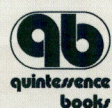

MICRODENTISTRY:
A PATH TO EXCELLENCE

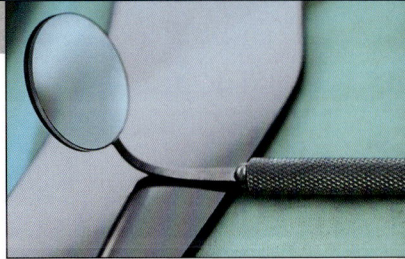

Claudia Cia Worschech, DDS, MS, PhD[1]

U ntil recently, the only magnification used in the dental profession came in the form of eyeglass-mounted oculars with or without illumination accessories.[1] In the nineteenth century, operative dentistry was considered an entirely mechanical practice with almost no relation to technique or the physical or biological properties of dental materials[2] and little equipment was necessary. As the science of dentistry progressed, however, new materials were developed and with them came more complex restorative techniques that required optimal visibility.

Depending on the course of action, restorative procedures require different degrees of magnification. One of the many advantages of using microscopes over loupes or operating telescopes is the ability to change magnification easily and quickly without interrupting the procedure. A properly configured microscope for restorative dentistry should have a magnification range of 2.5× to 15×.[3]

There are several positions from which to execute work. Many clinicians prefer the 9 o'clock (Fig 1) or 12 o'clock (Fig 2) positions. The entire team works better because instruments and materials are within easy reach and movements are ergonomic. Observing through binoculars is common, and these positions are very important in achieving perfect ergonomics and precision in details (traditional way). Likewise, a dentist and auxiliary team can observe all steps of the treatment looking at an LCD, as is often done in the office of the author (Fig 3); this makes it possible to visualize in detail each step of the procedure (alternative way).

[1]Private practice, São Paulo, Brazil.

Correspondence to: Dr Claudia Cia Worschech, Rua Florindo Cibin, 313 Americana, São Paulo, CEP 13465-000, Brazil. E-mail: claudiacw@terra.com.br

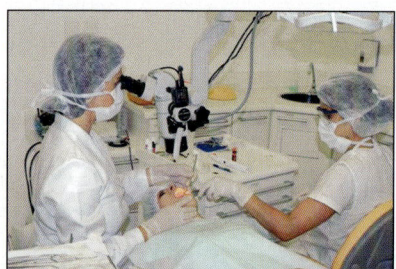

Fig 1 A dentist working in a 9 o'clock position.

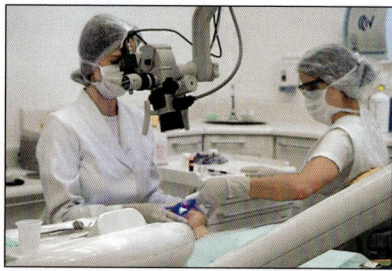

Fig 2 A dentist working in a 12 o'clock position.

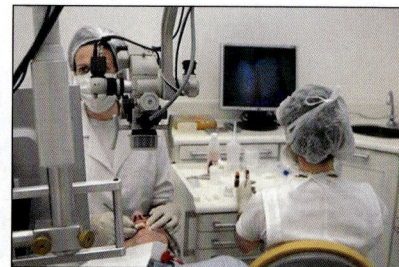

Fig 3 An alternative position in which the dentist and assistant simultaneously view an LCD to execute procedures.

Fig 4 Under 6× magnification, it is possible to note the transition between the tooth and resin restoration.

Fig 5 Under 10× magnification, restorative composite shows superficial roughness, which can decrease the restoration's longevity.

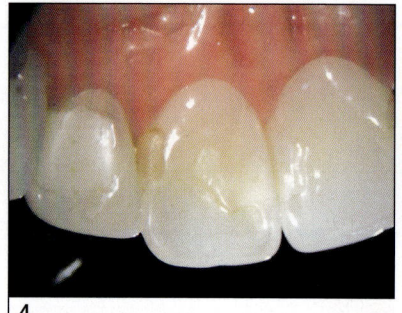

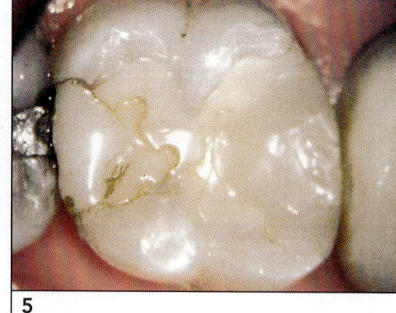

Operating microscopes provide clarity and detail so vivid and revealing because coaxial illumination is controlled for a shadow-free visual field. Dental professionals have recognized that the quality of the light in the working field is just as important as magnification and recognize the potential for improved precision in both diagnostic and treatment procedures.[4] Operating microscopes help clinicians provide exact diagnostics of carious lesions, cervical adaptations, gaps, cracks, polishing, shape, and texture. Further, they allow clinicians to make precise impressions and provide prophylaxis. All of these benefits hinge on the clinician's willingness to learn new skills.

One critical factor of esthetics, periodontal health, and longevity of restorations is the precision of margins at the periodontal-restorative interface. Improper margins can cause overhangs and overcontouring that may ultimately result in caries, periodontal inflammation and breakdown, and compromised esthetics. To prevent pathology at the restorative tooth interface, each phase of an esthetic treatment must be performed with precision and care.[5] Micropathology is usually invisible or not compelling at less than 12× magnification.

This includes signs of occlusal wear, microleakage, early recurrent decay, and isolated periodontal inflammation surrounding crude dentistry that violates the parameters of marginal integrity.[6]

Every time we replace restorations (esthetic or nonesthetic) because of recurrent caries lesions or superficial or intrinsic discolorations of resin that damage the esthetic restoration's quality, some healthy tissue needs to be removed. Identifying the transition between teeth and restorations and seeing these structures with magnification and high-quality light translates to less wear, less removal of healthy dental tissue, and greater preservation of teeth (Figs 4 and 5).[7] Forgie et al investigated differences in cavity preparation size using normal vision and surgical magnification (2.6×); they concluded that experienced clinicians performed larger preparations with unaided vision compared to those performed with magnification.[8]

The replacement of amalgam restorations or esthetic treatment often leads to ever larger restorations that have shorter life spans than their predecessors, and the replacement procedures themselves may cause damage to adjacent healthy teeth.[9]

Fig 6 Initial caries can be diagnosed with a microscope.

Fig 7 Under 16× magnification, details become extremely vivid.

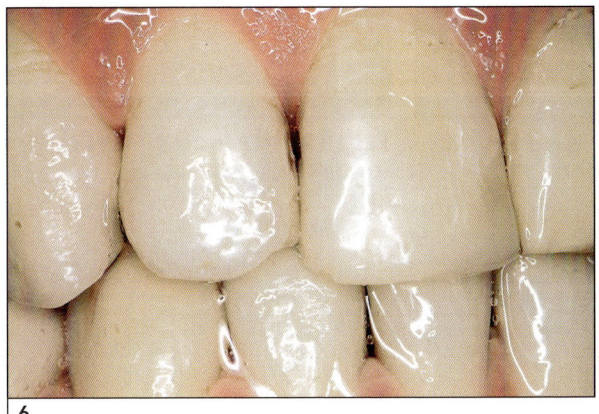

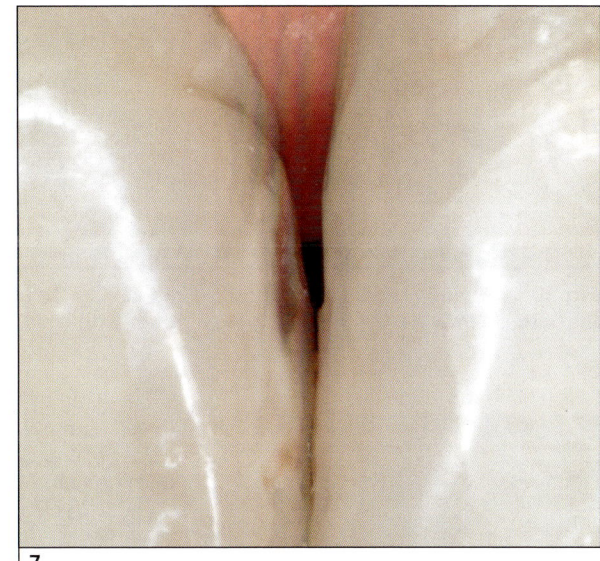

Figs 8 and 9 Gary Carr mirrors provide nitid, clear images. Their flexibility provides more confortable movements inside the mouth and during procedures.

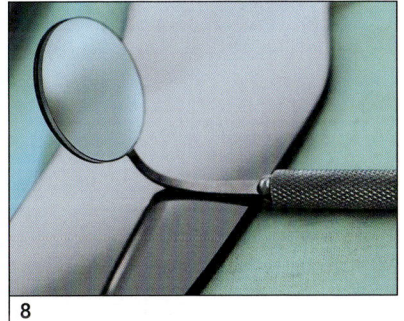

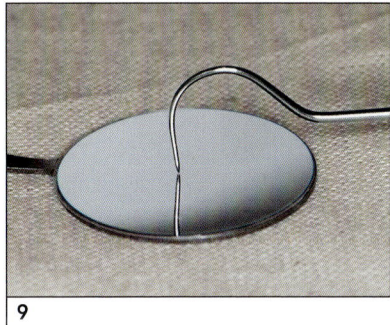

Improved lighting coupled with magnification provide a clear distinction between surfaces that may look similar in color or texture under traditional working conditions. Decay, dentin, enamel, composite, and porcelain are easily distinguishable from one another and can be seen with unprecedented detail under the scrutiny of the microscope.[4]

MAGNIFICATION IN DIAGNOSIS

Caries lesions

Although magnification represents great progress for the dental profession, as well as the general population, the trend toward fewer and smaller cavities has brought with it new questions as to how to diagnose smaller lesions,[9] especially because early diagnosis can mean minimally invasive dental procedures and the best possible treatment and results (Figs 6 and 7). For correct examination and accurate observation, special instruments and materials, such as small, flexible mirrors, microburs, and modified materials, need to be introduced in the clinical armamentarium to take full advantage of this treatment modality (Figs 8 and 9). However, even if an extra-small access cavity is achieved with the aid of a microscope and microburs, there are no restorative material delivery systems capable of taking advantage of such small openings.[10]

Cracks

Clinicians have used magnification to observe cracks (Figs 10 to 12) for nearly a decade. Pat-

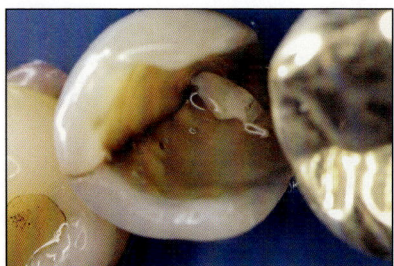

Fig 10 Note the cracks and gaps that can be treated.

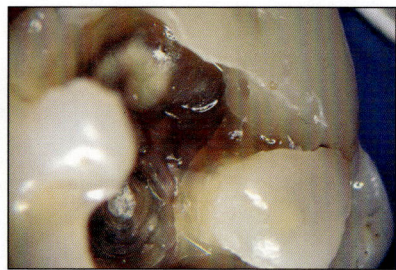

Fig 11 Cracks and gaps can be noted with more facility.

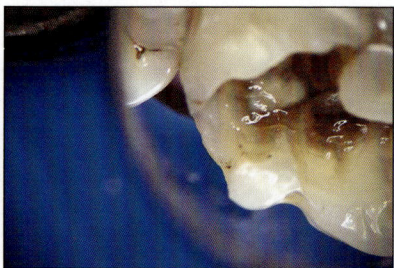

Fig 12 Cracks that cause pain and discomfort in patients must be identified early to avoid dire consequences.

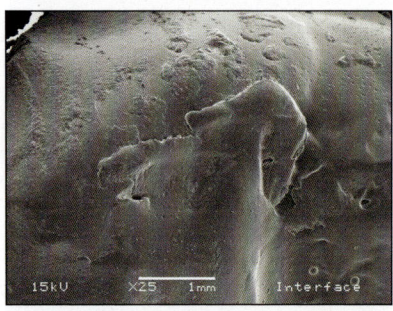

Fig 13 *(Left)* A scanning electron microscope easily identifies how polishing can modify a restoration's behavior. In clinical procedures, margins must be smooth.

Fig 14 *(Right)* Clinical photograph showing the margin between tooth and resin in a posterior tooth.

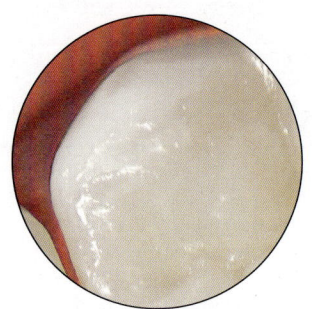

terns have become clear that can lead to appropriate treatment prior to development of symptoms or destruction of tooth structure. Conversely, many cracks are not structural and can lead to misdiagnosis and overtreatment. Methodic microscopic examination, an understanding of crack progression, and an appreciation of the types of cracks will guide a clinician in making appropriate decisions. Teeth can have structural cracks in various stages. To date, diagnosis and treatment often occur at final stages of crack development.[11]

Without the information provided by high-powered microscopic inspection, many teeth with structurally significant cracks would have otherwise been treated only when they became symptomatic. This can result in more complicated, involved treatment or even a catastrophic event that leads to tooth loss[12]: Most of these superficial fractures are relatively undetectable with normal vision, but when viewed under high power, hairline cracks appear as crevasses.[13]

MAGNIFICATION IN ADHESIVE RESTORATION

Adhesive restoration eliminates the need for more extensive and retentive preparations. Enamel-like composites offer long-lasting tooth structure replacement with minimum requirements for restorative bulk; little or no healthy tooth material needs to be removed to allow for an adequate thickness of restorative material.[9] However, esthetic and cosmetic procedures calling for invisible margins and tooth-restoration interface transitions are far easier and less stressful when magnification is available. If the margins are undetectable under magnification, they will certainly not be visible to the naked eye (Figs 13 and 14). Fine internal and external colorations and characterizations are virtually impossible to achieve without appropriate magnification.

Bonded restoration presents unique and difficult finishing requirements and therefore demands great care and precision to create a margin that is smooth and nonirritating to the gingival tissues. As

CASE 1 (Figs 15 to 20)

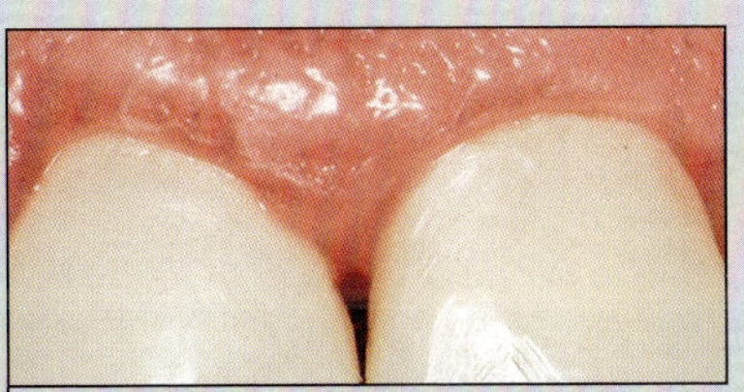

Fig 15 The right maxillary central incisor restored under 12× magnification, and the left maxillary central incisor restored without magnification.

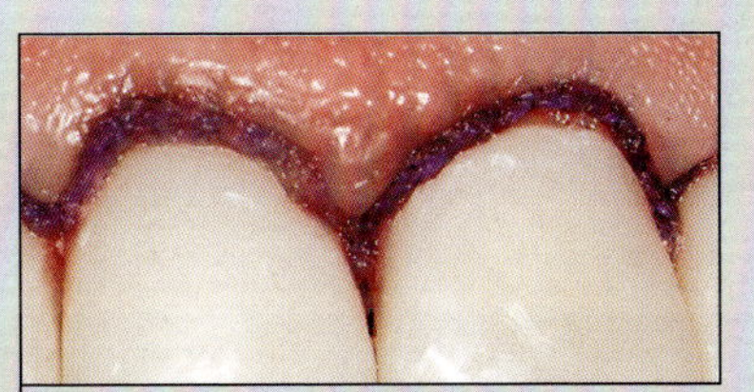

Fig 16 Gingival retractors in place.

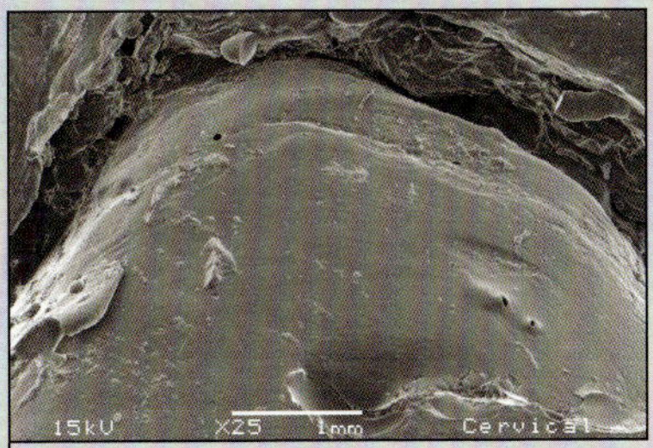

Fig 17 Under a scanning eletron microscope, the correct adaptation between the tooth and direct restoration is apparent. Note the cervical region.

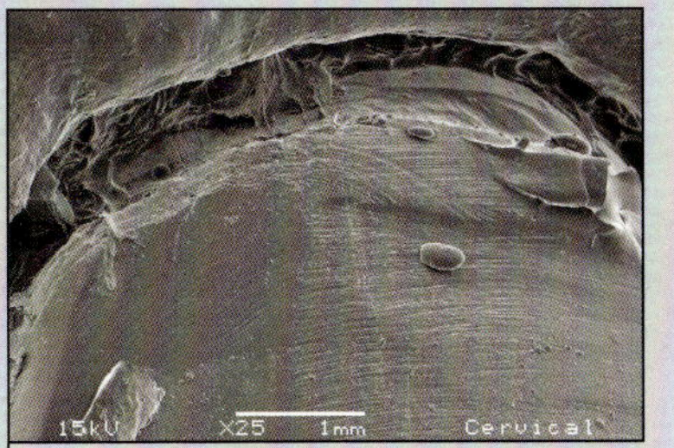

Fig 18 Under a scanning eletron microscope, the incorrect adaptation between the tooth and direct restoration is visible.

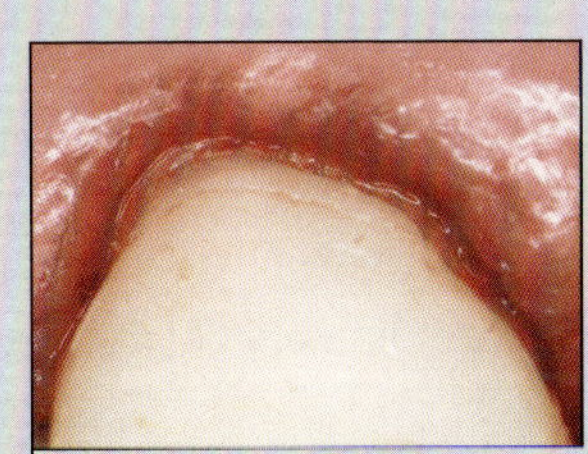

Fig 19 Clinical detail of the right central incisor.

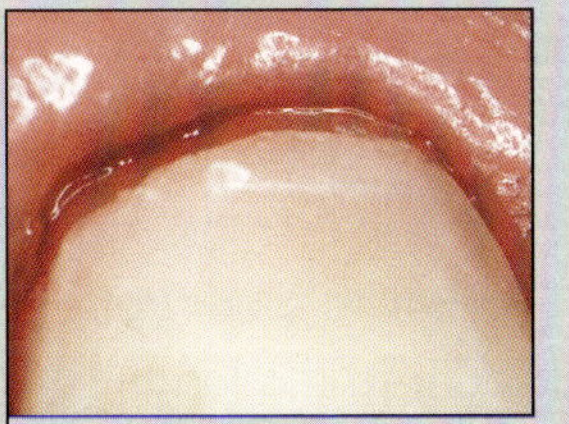

Fig 20 Clinical detail of the left central incisor. Note the inexact interface.

one progresses through the regimen of finer and finer burs and finishing disks, it becomes more difficult to evaluate the surface texture of the finished crestal edge. Only when this junction is fine-tuned under magnification can one be assured that the gingival tissues will not inflame, bleed, recede, or expose the critical tooth-restoration interface.[13]

CLINICAL EXAMPLES

Case 1

Figures 15 and 16 show the great difference between direct restoration (4 Seasons, Ivoclar Vivadent, Schaan, Liechtenstein) performed under magnification and that executed with the naked eye. The maxillary right central incisor was restored under microscope view, while the left central incisor was restored without magnification. Both were finished and polished. A retractor (Ultradent Products, South Jordan, Utah, USA) was then applied for several minutes; after the retractor was removed, impressions were made using a silicone material (Virtual, Ivoclar Vivadent). Specimens were prepared for analysis with an electron microscope (SEM), and photos revealed impressive details about the clinical procedure.

Figure 17 shows the cervical region of the maxillary right central incisor where the interface between composite resin and the tooth is smooth and displays evidence of correct polishing of margins. In Fig 18 (left central incisor), we can see that the composite resin and tooth structure are not level. The same clinician executed both esthetic restorations, although for the right central incisor (Fig 19), 12× magnification was used. In the case of the left central incisor (Fig 20), the clinician's naked eye could not as accurately set or finish the composite resin.

CASE 2 (Figs 21 to 23)

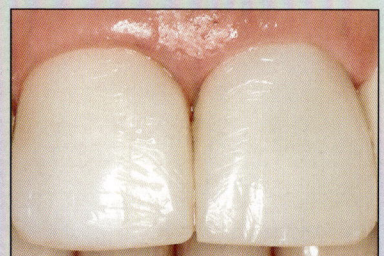
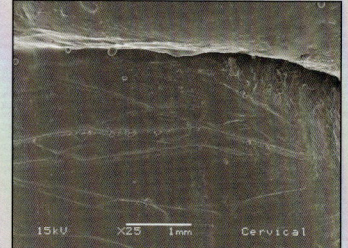
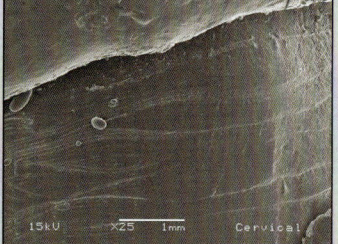

Fig 21 Correct finishing and polishing of restoration margins.

Figs 22 and 23 SEM photos indicate that there is a superficial smoothness and a correct match between the tooth and restorative material.

This suggests that magnification helps provide smooth margins and correct adaptations because is possible to see the limits. If it is possible to see well, it is possible to work better, and the clinical results contribute to the longevity of direct and indirect restorations.

Case 2

Another clinical case demonstrates this point well. In Fig 21, both teeth (maxillary right and left central incisors) were restored under microscope. Precise finishing of margins of the direct facets is evident (4 Seasons, Ivoclar Vivadent, and Renamel Microfill, Cosmedent, Chicago, Illinois, USA). There is no gap or bubble inside the resin. You can see texture, but it is also possible to see a smooth superficial margin. This clinical situation is certainly very favorable, and the longevity of the restoration should be good.

In Figs 22 and 23, under SEM, perfect superficial margins are shown. The risks undertaken to provide microtexture are clear, although there is a continual and intimate transition between tooth and composite resin in both teeth. Note the gingival margins. Both teeth received direct facets.

Case 3

Residual materials left around restorations can cause gingival irritation and marginal inflammation. This can be avoided with simple procedures and accurate visibility on the part of the dentist. When adhesive accumulates near gingival tissue, inflammation often results; pain and discomfort could indicate replacement of the entire restoration (Fig 24). Dentists could not observe this minute detail around the composite restoration without some form of magnification (Figs 25 and 26).

Case 4

Esthetic restorations with imperfect margins can cause damage. The margins sometimes retain pigment and leave an unattractive appearance. Often these restorations are replaced in an effort to improve appearance and eliminate wear on healthy tissue. Figures 27 and 28 demonstrate through high magnification how the interface between natural dentition and resin can be rough as a result of imperfect polishing or adhesive technique. After the restoration is replaced (Renamel Microfill, Cosmedent), the superficial smoothness is apparent (Figs 29 and 30).

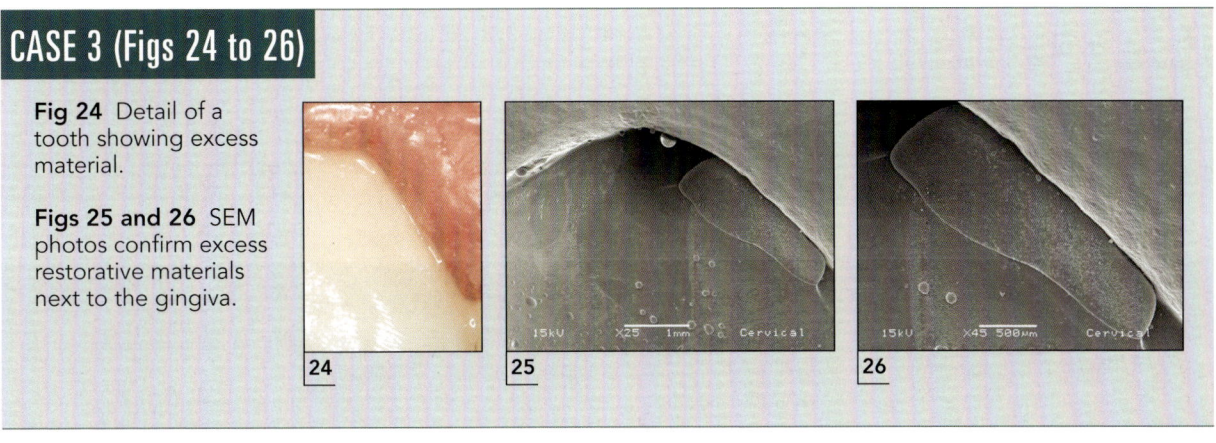

CASE 3 (Figs 24 to 26)

Fig 24 Detail of a tooth showing excess material.

Figs 25 and 26 SEM photos confirm excess restorative materials next to the gingiva.

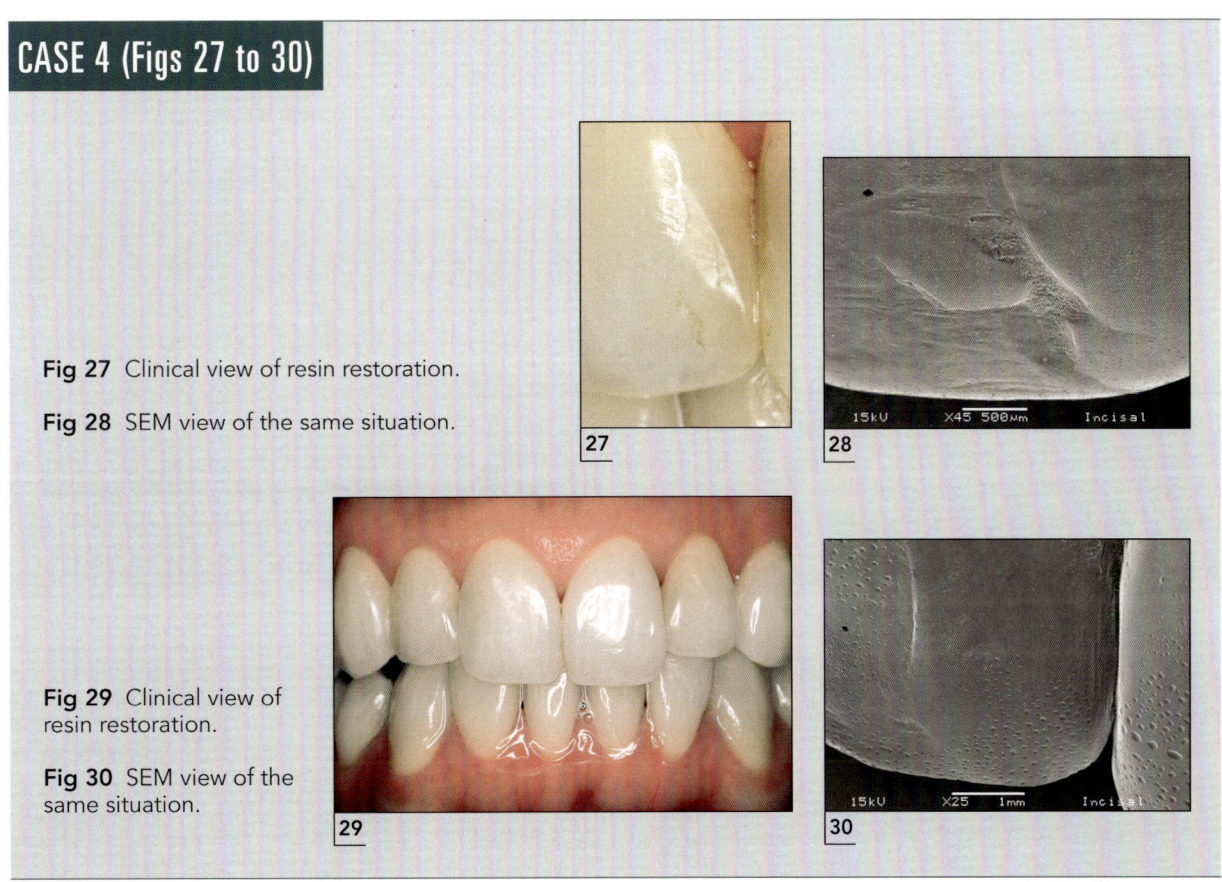

CASE 4 (Figs 27 to 30)

Fig 27 Clinical view of resin restoration.

Fig 28 SEM view of the same situation.

Fig 29 Clinical view of resin restoration.

Fig 30 SEM view of the same situation.

Case 5

If direct restoration cannot sufficiently repair a tooth, indirect restorations may be an option. In this case, impressions are very important. Under magnification, gingival retractors are positioned with precision, and it is not as difficult to get detailed impressions, as shown in Figs 31 and 32 (Elite H-D, Ivoclar Vivadent).

CASE 5 (Figs 31 to 32)

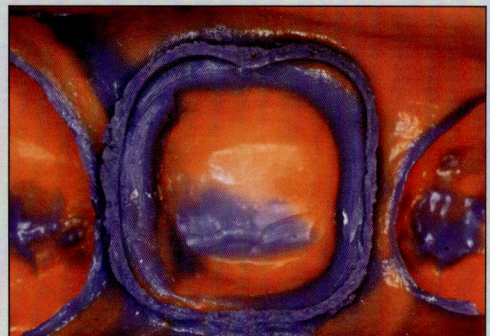

Fig 31 Detailed impression.

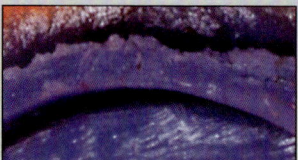

Fig 32 Note the thickness of the impression material.

CASE 6 (Figs 33 to 36)

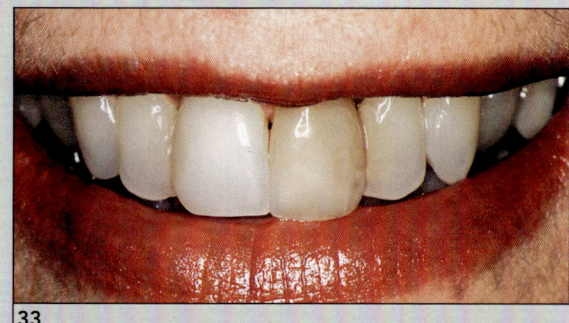

33

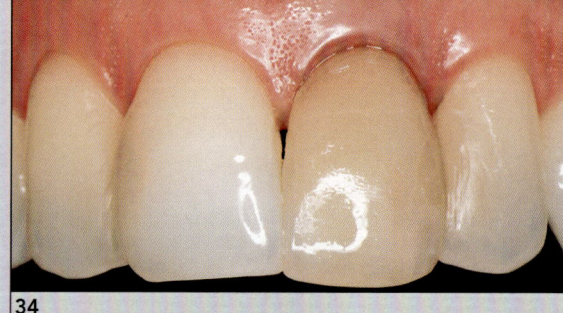

34

Figs 33 and 34 Porcelain laminate on the maxillary left central incisor shows dark color.

Figs 35 and 36 The maxillary left central incisor with laminate in position. Note the precise integration between gingival tissue and porcelain restoration.

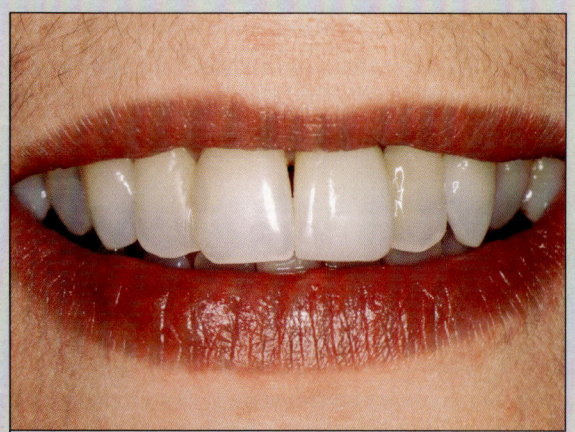

35

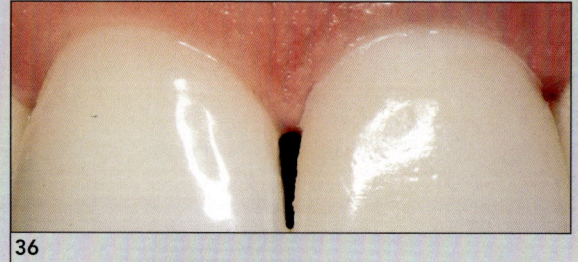

36

Case 6

Perfect adaptation of all-ceramic restorations is becoming achievable with magnification. Note in Figs 33 to 36 how a single ceramic laminate in the maxillary left central incisor is integrated with gingival tissue and remains in sync with adjacent teeth and gingival tissue.

CONCLUSIONS

Clinicians need to be able to accept new ways to work and new philosophies. Microscopes must be incorporated into dental routines, and this can be a challenge for many professionals who imagine retaining old concepts of ergonomic movements or positions after purchasing a microscope.[14] Continual refinement is necessary after clinicians learn new techniques.

The path to excellence in dentistry consists of perceiving tiny details, taking special care in manipulating materials, and precisely viewing the structures to be treated. The learning curve with the microscope can be long or short, depending on the person and how much time he or she invests. Good training is essential.

ACKNOWLEDGMENTS

The author would like to acknowledge State University of Campinas, Piracicaba Campus, São Paulo, Brazil, as well as give special thanks to Dr Mario De Góes for his permission and orientation of SEM utilization. Special thanks also to technician Marcos Celestrino and Alliança Laboratory, São Paulo, Brazil, for the laminate ceramic execution.

REFERENCES

1. Sheets CG, Paquette JM, Hatate K. The clinical microscope in an aesthetic restorative practice. J Esthet Restor Dent 2001;13:187–200.
2. Worschech CC, Moura, JR, Fonseca, DM. Micro-operative dentistry: Why do it? Quintessence Dent Technol 2007; 31:199–205.
3. Carr GB. Microscope photography for the restorative dentist. J Esthet Restor Dent 2003;15:417–425.
4. Friedman M, Mora A, Schmidt R. Microscope-assisted precision dentistry. Compend Contin Educ Dent 1999;20: 723–735.
5. Sheets CG. The periodontal-restorative interface: Enhancement through magnification. Pract Periodont Aesthet Dent 1999;11:925–931.
6. Clark D. Maximizing the return on investment of an operating microscope. Dent Econ 2004;94(5).
7. Worschech CC. Replacement of esthetic restorations: Can we see the limits? R. Dental Press Estet, Maringá 2006;3(4) 77–90.
8. Forgie AH, Pine CM, Pitts NB. Restoration removal with and without the aid of magnification. J Oral Rehabil 2001; 28:309–313.
9. Freedman G, Goldstep F, Seif T. Ultraconservative resin restorations: "Watch and wait" is not acceptable treatment. Dent Today 2000;19:66–71.
10. Friedman MJ, Landesman HM. Microscope-assisted precision (MAP) dentistry. A challenge for new knowledge. J Calif Dent Assoc 1998;26:900–905.
11. Clark DJ, Sheets CG, Paquette JM. Definitive diagnosis of early enamel and dentin cracks based on microscopic evaluation. J Esthet Restor Dent 2003;15:391–401.
12. Garcia A. Dental magnification: A clear view of the present and close-up view of the future. Compendium 2005;26:459–463.
13. Arens DE. Introduction to magnification in endodontics. J Esthet Restor Dent 2003;15:426–439.
14. Gondim E Jr, Murgel CAF, Sousa Filho FJ. Microscópio cirurgico: la nueva frontera de la Odontología clínica Del siglo. Fola/Oral 1997;3:147–152.

PLAN NOW TO ATTEND

Addressing your need for knowledge about the newest procedures and techniques, Quintessence Publishing is offering seminars by leading dental researchers and clinicians at our suburban Chicago headquarters. Each seminar will give you the opportunity to learn about the newest advances in your field, acquire hands-on experience with top-of-the-line equipment, and meet industry leaders. Seminars are limited to 40 attendees to provide you with a first-rate educational experience. On-site breakfast, lunch, and coffee breaks, included in your registration fee, will maximize your educational and professional contact with the speaker and your colleagues.

SPRING 2008 SCHEDULE

UELI GRUNDER   MARCH 2 (SUNDAY)

Esthetics in Implant Therapy: Surgical and Restorative Integration
Full-Day Lecture Course

ALAN ROSENFELD AND GEORGE A. MANDELARIS
MARCH 28 (FRIDAY HALF DAY) / MARCH 29 (SATURDAY FULL DAY)

Principles of Computer-Guided Implantology—Level I*
Lecture and Hands-on Course
*Level II course planned for Fall 2008

TOMASO VERCELLOTTI   APRIL 12 (SATURDAY)

New Ultrasonic Implant Site Preparation Technique to Improve Implant Surgery
Lecture and Hands-on Course

DOMENICO MASSIRONI   APRIL 26 (SATURDAY)

Precision Tooth Preparation for Esthetic Restorations
Full-Day Lecture Course

NAOKI AIBA   MAY 17 (SATURDAY)

DENTSCAPE: Dental Photography for Functional Esthetics
Lecture and Hands-on Course

DALE A. MILES   MAY 30 (FRIDAY)

The CAT's out of the Bag: Cone-Beam CT for Dentistry
Full-Day Lecture Course

Seminar Location
Quintessence Publishing Office, Hanover Park, Illinois

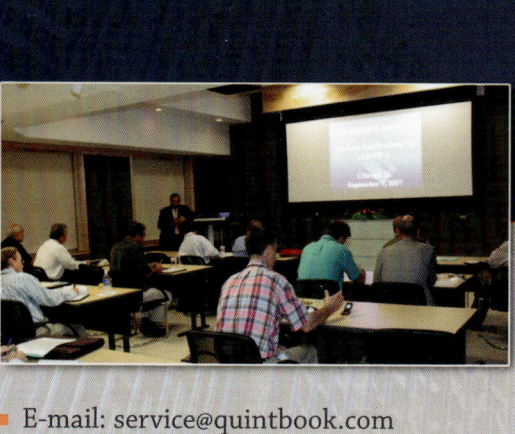

For details and registration visit www.quintpub.com

Quintessence Publishing Co, Inc
4350 Chandler Drive, Hanover Park, IL 60133
Phone (630) 736-3600 ▪ Fax (630) 736-3633 ▪ E-mail: service@quintbook.com
Website: www.quintpub.com

« QuintessenceSeminars »

IMPROVING OCCLUSION IN REMOVABLE PARTIAL DENTURES: MODIFIED FLASKING PROCEDURES

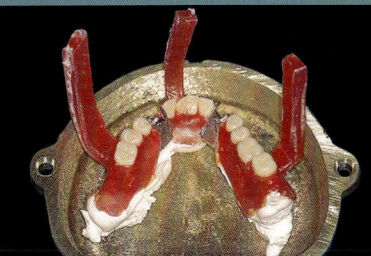

Michelle Roberta Vieira Silva, DDS[1]

Leonardo Marchini, DDS, MSD, PhD[2,3]

Vicente de Paula Prisco da Cunha, DDS, MSc, PhD[2,3]

Jarbas Francisco Fernandes dos Santos, DDS, MSD, PhD[2,3]

Occlusion is an exhaustively studied factor that should contribute to better performance in removable prosthodontics and a good functional relation with the stomatognathic components (muscles and temporomandibular joints). Achieving adequate occlusion is important for improving the patient's comfort and satisfaction with the dentures.[1,2]

Adequate occlusion is normally achieved in the artificial teeth waxup step. However, during the normal technical procedures for acrylic resin polymerization, polymerization shrinkage usually results in movement of the artificial teeth. This movement often leads to increased vertical dimensions, premature contacts, and anterior "open bite" of dentures.[3–6] Flasking and deflasking procedures also contribute to occlusal alterations[6,7] by modifying the position of artificial teeth in relation to the complete denture base or the metal framework of removable partial dentures.

For technical procedures involving removable partial dentures, alterations of teeth position in relation to the metal framework are allowed by placing the metal framework and artificial teeth on opposite sides of the flask. This article presents a technique to minimize the occlusal alterations this can cause by use of a plaster wall to fix the relative position of the metal framework and teeth.

DESCRIPTION OF THE TECHNIQUE

The patient used herein to describe the technique already had a removable partial denture (RPD) in the maxillary arch. This RPD was well-adapted, and the patient reported it felt comfortable. The two canines were the only teeth remaining in the mandibular arch.

[1]Private practice, São José dos Campos, SP, Brazil

[2]School of Health Sciences, University of Vale do Paraíba, São José dos Campos, SP, Brazil.

[3]Department of Dentistry, University of Taubaté, Taubaté, SP, Brazil.

Correspondence to: Dr Leonardo Marchini, Av Adhemar de Barros, 1136 Ap 153, 12245-010 São José dos Campos, SP, Brazil. E-mail: leomarchini@directnet.com.br

Teeth waxup and functional impression of edentulous ridge

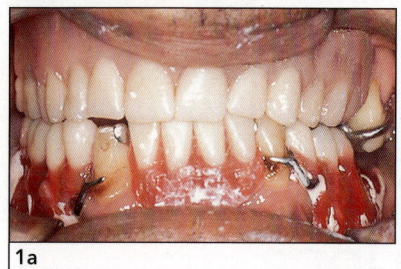

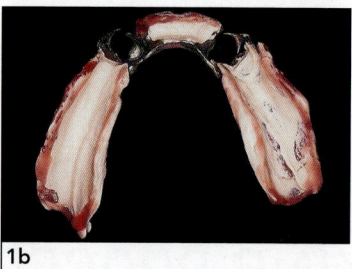

Fig 1a Waxup is tried in the mouth and occlusion is found acceptable.

Fig 1b Final functional impression of the edentulous ridge. Wax is used for border molding.

Fixing of RPD on false base and preparation of plaster wall

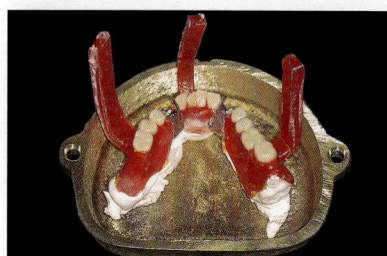

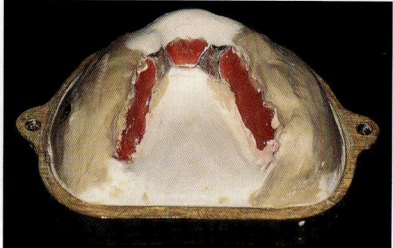

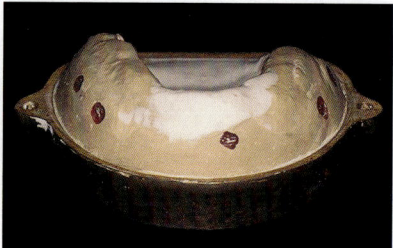

Fig 2a The RPD is placed in the flask base, which is filled with type II plaster. Note that wax is fixed over the buccal surfaces. This serves as a channel for the acrylic resin flow in a subsequent step.

Fig 2b A wall made of type III plaster is built over the buccal surfaces of the RPD and covers the artificial teeth completely. The lingual surfaces are not covered.

Fig 2c Buccal aspect of the plaster wall. Note the channels made of wax, with excess removed.

After a preliminary impression was made with irreversible hydrocolloid, and then delineating and RPD framework planning, fabrication, and set-up, the intermaxillary record was made and the mandibular RPD mounted in a semiadjustable articulator for artificial teeth waxup. The RPD base was not reinforced with resin, since that would have hindered processing the permanent base later.

The teeth waxup was tried in the mouth, and the occlusion achieved approved by the patient and dentist (Fig 1a). The functional impression of the edentulous ridge was made using zinc-eugenol paste and wax for border molding (Figs 1a and 1b). The impressions were filled with type III plaster.

The RPD was then placed in the base of the flask, after fixing sprues in the buccal areas for the acrylic resin flow (Fig 2a). A wall of plaster (type III)

was made over the buccal areas, covering the artificial teeth completely. The lingual areas were not covered with plaster (Figs 2b and 2c). All exposed plaster surfaces had to be expulsive. They were then isolated, and the middle part of the flask was placed and filled with type II plaster. After the plaster hardened, the flask was heated by immersion in boiling water. The flask was then opened, and all the wax was removed with boiling water (Figs 3a and 3b). Note, in Fig 3b, that the teeth and metal framework remained in the same relative position in the same part of the flask.

Heat-activated acrylic resin was placed on the plaster wall, over the RPD framework and onto the artificial teeth, and allowed to flow through the buccal sprues (Fig 3c). The flask was then closed, pressed under 1.5 tons of force (Fig 3d), and left in a water bath at 72°C for 12 hours to polymerize the acrylic resin.

Flasking, resin pressing, and polymerization

Fig 3a Flask opened after wax removal.

Fig 3b Lingual and internal aspects of the RPD in the plaster wall. Note that the artificial teeth and metal framework remain in the same part of the flask.

Fig 3c Pink heat-activated acrylic resin is placed on the plaster wall and flows down through the buccal sprues.

Fig 3d The flask is closed and pressed under 1.5 tons of force.

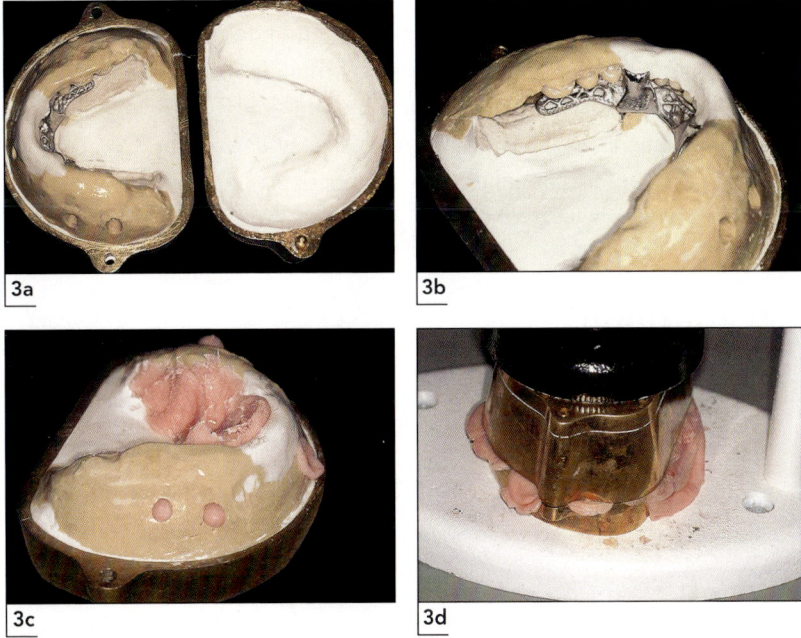

Deflasking and finishing

Fig 4a After removal of the flask base, the plaster that filled the functional impressions of the alveolar ridge is left behind and must be removed carefully to preserve the denture base.

Fig 4b Denture base after molding.

Fig 4c RPD after finishing and polishing procedures.

Fig 4d Final RPD in the patient's mouth. No major occlusal adjustments were necessary.

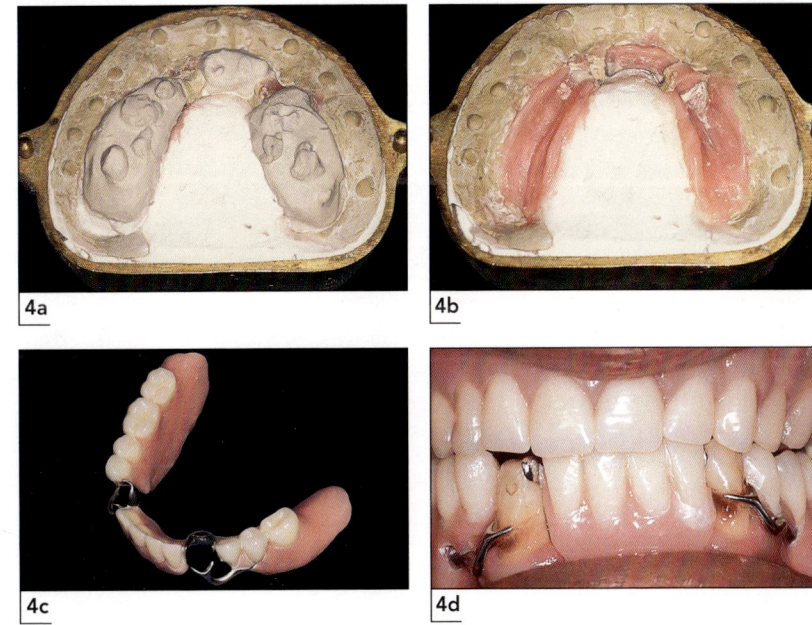

The deflasking procedures (Figs 4a and 4b) were carried out carefully, making sure the RPD base was adequate (Fig 4b). The wax flow channels in the buccal area had now turned into acrylic resin and were removed during the finishing procedures (Fig 4c).

The occlusal scheme obtained during the artificial teeth waxup was now visible in the acrylic dentures (Fig 4d), and no major occlusal adjustments were required.

CONCLUSION

The technique reported here produces optimal occlusion in removable partial dentures by maintaining the relative position between the metal framework and artificial teeth. This technique is easy and does not require additional equipment or costs.

REFERENCES

1. Dubojska AM, White GE, Pasiek S. The importance of occlusal balance in the control of complete dentures. Quintessence Int 1998;29:389–394.

2. Ruffino AR. Improved occlusal equilibration of complete dentures by augmenting occlusal anatomy of acrylic resin denture teeth. J Prosthet Dent 1984;52:300–302.

3. Abuzar MA, Jamani K, Abuzar M. Tooth movement during processing of complete dentures and its relation to palatal form. J Prosthet Dent 1995;73:445–449.

4. Kawara M, Komiyama O, Kimoto S, Kobayashi K, Nemoto K. Distortion behavior of heat-activated acrylic denture base resin in conventional and long, low temperature processing methods. J Dent Res 1998;77:1446–1453.

5. Sadamori S, Ishii T, Hamada T. Influence of thickness on the linear dimensional chang, warpage and water uptake of a denture base resin. Int J Prosthodont 1997;10:35–43.

6. Wesley RC, Henderson D, Frazier QZ, et al. Processing changes in complete dentures: Posterior tooth contacts and pin opening. J Prosthet Dent 1973;29:46–54.

7. Kobayashi N, Komiyama O, Kimoto S, Kawara M. Reduction of shrinkage on heat-activated acrylic denture base resin obtaining gradual cooling after processing. J Oral Rehabil 2004;31:710–716.